W9-CES-200

Cardiology Drug Update

Guest Editor

JOANNE M. FOODY, MD

CARDIOLOGY CLINICS

www.cardiology.theclinics.com

Consulting Editor

MICHAEL H. CRAWFORD, MD

November 2008 • Volume 26 • Number 4

SAUNDERS an imprint of ELSEVIER, Inc.

W.B. SAUNDERS COMPANY
A Division of Elsevier Inc.

Elsevier, Inc. ● 1600 John F. Kennedy Blvd. ● Suite 1800 ● Philadelphia, Pennsylvania 19103-2899

http://www.theclinics.com

CARDIOLOGY CLINICS Volume 26, Number 4
November 2008 ISSN 0733-8651, ISBN-13: 978-1-4160-6276-9, ISBN-10: 1-4160-6276-9

Editor: Barbara Cohen-Kligerman

Cardiology Clinics (ISSN 0733-8651) is published quarterly by Elsevier Inc., 360 Park Avenue South, New York, NY 10010-1710. Months of issue are February, May, August, and November. Business and editorial Offices: 1600 John F. Kennedy Blvd., Suite 1800, Philadelphia, PA 19103-2899. Customer Service Office: 6277 Sea Harbor Drive, Orlando, FL 32887-4800. Periodicals postage paid at New York, NY, and additional mailing offices. Subscription prices are $244.00 per year for US individuals, $378.00 per year for US institutions, $122.00 per year for US students and residents, $298.00 per year for Canadian individuals, $470.00 per year for Canadian institutions, $346.00 per year for international individuals, $470.00 per year for international institutions and $173.00 per year for Canadian and foreign students/residents. To receive student/resident rate, orders must be accompanied by name of affiliated institution, data of term, and the *signature* of program/residency coordinator on institution letterhead. Orders will be billed at individual rate until proof of status is received. Foreign air speed delivery is included in all *Clinics* subscription prices. All prices are subject to change without notice. **POSTMASTER:** Send address changes to *Cardiology Clinics*, Elsevier Periodicals Customer Service, 6277 Sea Harbor Drive, Orlando, FL 32887-4800. **Customer Service: 1-800-654-2452 (US). From outside of the US, call 1-407-563-6020. Fax: 1-407-363-9661. E-mail: Journals CustomerService-usa@elsevier.com**.

Reprints. For copies of 100 or more, of articles in this publication, please contact the Commercial Reprints Department, Elsevier Inc., 360 Park Avenue South, New York, NY 10010-1710. Tel.: 212-633-3812; Fax: 212-462-1935; Email: reprints@elsevier.com.

Cardiology Clinics is also published in Spanish by McGraw-Hill Interamericana Editores S. A., P.O. Box 5-237, 06500, Mexico D. F., Mexico; in Portuguese by Reichmann and Alfonso Editores Rio de Janeiro, Brazil; and in Greek by Dimitrios P. Lagos, 8 Pondon Street, GR115-28 Ilissia, Greece.

Cardiology Clinics is covered in *MEDLINE/PubMed (Index Medicus)*, *Excerpta Medica*, *The Cumulative Index to Nursing and Allied Health Literature* (CINAHL).

Printed in the United States of America.

Contributors

CONSULTING EDITOR

MICHAEL H. CRAWFORD, MD
Professor of Medicine, University of California
San Francisco; Lucie Stern Chair in Cardiology,
and Interim Chief of Cardiology, University of
California San Francisco Medical Center,
San Francisco, California

GUEST EDITOR

JOANNE M. FOODY, MD
Associate Professor, Harvard Medical School,
Brigham and Women's/Faulkner Hospitals,
Boston, Massachusetts

AUTHORS

CHRISTIE M. BALLANTYNE, MD
Baylor College of Medicine and Methodist
DeBakey Heart and Vascular Center, Houston,
Texas

HAROLD E. BAYS, MD
Louisville Metabolic and Atherosclerosis
Research Center, Louisville, Kentucky

MICHAEL DAVIDSON, MD
Chicago Center for Clinical Research, Chicago,
Illinois

**PRAKASH C. DEEDWANIA, MD, FACC,
FACP, FCCP, FAHA**
Professor of Medicine, University of California
School of Medicine; Chief, Division of
Cardiology; Director, Cardiovascular
Research, VA Central California Health Care
System, University of California, San Francisco
Program at Fresno, Fresno, California; and
Clinical Professor of Medicine, Stanford
University, Palo Alto, California

VIVIAN A. FONSECA, MD
Professor of Medicine, Tullis-Tulane Alumni
Chair in Diabetes; and Section Chief of
Endocrinology, Tulane University Health
Sciences Center, New Orleans, Louisiana

GARY S. FRANCIS, MD
Professor of Medicine, Department of
Cardiovascular Medicine; and Head,
Department of Clinical Cardiology, Cleveland
Clinic Lerner College of Medicine, Cleveland
Clinic, Cleveland, Ohio

USMAN JAVED, MD
Cardiology Fellow, Division of Cardiology, VA
Central California Health Care System,
University of California, San Francisco Program
at Fresno, Fresno, California

JENNIFER JOHN-KALARICKAL, MD
Assistant Professor, Tulane University Health
Sciences Center; and Director of Diabetes,
Medical Center of Louisiana, New Orleans,
Louisiana

OLGA KUZNETSOVA, PhD
Merck & Co., Inc., Rahway, New Jersey

ESENG LAI, MD, PhD
Merck & Co., Inc., Rahway, New Jersey

L. VERONICA LEE, MD
Assistant Professor of Medicine, Division
of Cardiology, Yale University School of
Medicine, New Haven, Connecticut

DARBIE MACCUBBIN, PhD
Merck & Co., Inc., Rahway, New Jersey

YALE B. MITCHEL, MD
Merck & Co., Inc., Rahway, New Jersey

HEMANTH NEELI, MD
Section of Hospital Medicine, Temple
University Hospital, Philadelphia, Pennsylvania

JOSEPHINE M. NORQUIST, MS
Merck & Co., Inc. North Wales, Pennyslvania

SUZANNE OPARIL, MD
Professor of Medicine, Vascular Biology and
Hypertension Program, University of Alabama
at Birmingham, Birmingham, Alabama

JOHN F. PAOLINI, MD, PhD
Merck & Co., Inc., Rahway, New Jersey

RICHARD PASTERNAK, MD
Merck & Co., Inc., Rahway, New Jersey

EDUARDO PIMENTA, MD
Faculty, Department of Hypertension and
Nephrology, Dante Pazzanese Institute of
Cardiology, Sao Paulo, Brazil

DANIEL J. RADER, MD
Institute for Translational Medicine and
Therapeutics, University of Pennsylvania
School of Medicine, Philadelphia,
Pennsylvania

CHRISTINE McCRARY SISK, BS
Merck & Co., Inc., Rahway, New Jersey

SCOTT D. SOLOMON, MD
Director, Non-Invasive Cardiology, Brigham
and Women's Hospital, Boston; and Associate
Professor, Harvard Medical School, Boston,
Massachusetts

PETER H. STONE, MD
Cardiovascular Division, Brigham and
Women's Hospital, Boston; Co-Director,
Samuel A. Levine Cardiac Unit; Director,
Clinical Trials Center, Associate Professor of
Medicine, Harvard Medical School, Boston,
Massachusetts

SAMUEL UNZEK, MD
Clinical Fellow, Department of Cardiovascular
Medicine, Cleveland Clinic, Cleveland, Ohio

ORLY VARDENY, PharmD
Assistant Professor, School of Pharmacy,
University of Wisconsin, Madison, Wisconsin

JAVAID H. WANI, MD, PhD
Endocrine Fellow, Tulane University Health
Sciences Center, New Orleans, Louisiana

M. GERARD WATERS, PhD
Merck & Co., Inc., Rahway, New Jersey

STEPHEN D. WIVIOTT, MD
Assistant Physician, Cardiovascular Division,
Brigham Women's Hospital, Boston; and
Assistant Professor of Medicine, Harvard
Medical School, Investigator, TIMI Study
Group, Boston, Massachusetts

Contents

> The identification of patients at high risk for cardiovascular events is imperative in the reduction of cardiovascular mortality and morbidity. Although coronary artery disease, peripheral arterial disease, cerebrovascular disease, hypertension, and diabetes mellitus contribute to the risk of developing cardiovascular events, we are now faced with emerging fronts because of an increase in life expectancy and the epidemic of hypertension, obesity, metabolic syndrome, and diabetes. Recent data emphasize the beneficial role of renin-angiotensin-aldosterone system (RAAS) blockers. This article addresses the role of RAAS activation in the high-risk metabolic milieu and the role of angiotensin receptor blockers in targeting and inhibiting the RAAS for cardiovascular protection.

> Aliskiren, the first in a new class of orally effective direct renin inhibitors (DRIs) was recently approved for the treatment of hypertension. In this review, we discuss the history of the development of DRIs and available data regarding the effects of DRIs in the treatment of hypertension and related target organ damage.

> Despite tremendous progress made in the management of CHD, a significant number of fatal and nonfatal CHD events still occur, which leads researchers to target other modifiable risk factors for CHD including low HDL-c (high density lipoprotein cholesterol). Although the torcetrapib experience was a major blow to CETP inhibition and indeed to the entire field of HDL-targeted therapeutics, it was not fatal. The off-target effects of torcetrapib appear to be substantial and may have overridden any potential cardiovascular benefit. Despite continued uncertainty regarding the cardiovascular implications of genetic CETP deficiency and pharmacologic CETP inhibition, there remain reasons to believe in the mechanism and the possibility that clean CETP inhibitors will not only improve plasma lipids but also reduce cardiovascular risk.

Treatment with niacin effectively improves multiple lipid parameters and cardiovascular outcomes. Widespread use of niacin, however, is limited by flushing, which is mediated primarily by prostaglandin D_2 (PGD_2). Laropiprant is a selective PGD_2 receptor 1 (DP1) antagonist that reduces objective measures of niacin-induced flushing symptoms upon initiation of therapy and with more chronic use. Results from early dosing and formulation studies have culminated in the development of a combination extended-release (ER) niacin/laropiprant tablet aimed at providing the beneficial lipid-modifying effects of niacin, while reducing niacin-induced flushing. The improvement in the tolerability of niacin with ER niacin/laropiprant allows niacin dosing to initiate directly at 1 g and rapidly advance to a 2-g target dose. ER niacin/laropiprant generally is tolerated well and represents a new treatment option for dyslipidemia that offers the potential for more patients to receive the lipid-modifying and cardiovascular benefits of niacin.

Despite innovative medications and devices, heart failure (HF) continues to be the leading cause for admission to hospitals in the United States in patients older than 65 years. Many trials have succeeded in improving survival and many have failed. In this article, the authors briefly review the past, describe the present, and speculate about future HF trials.

This article reviews the results from several recent reports describing the safety and efficacy of statin therapy in the setting of heart failure. It additionally discusses the ongoing controversy regarding the lipid paradox and possible mechanisms responsible for potential benefit of statin therapy in heart failure.

Cyclooxygenase-2 (cox-2) inhibitors, also known as coxibs, were introduced with the promise that they would provide pain relief similar to that of traditional non-steroidal anti-inflammatory drugs (NSAIDs) but would be better tolerated with lower risk of gastrointestinal (GI) side effects. Although coxibs were associated with lower GI risk, experimental and observational data raised the specter of increased cardiovascular risk associated with this class of drugs. This article describes the pharmacologic and biologic basis of cardiovascular risk associated with coxibs, summarizes the evidence for cardiovascular risk associated with cox-2 inhibitors, and weighs the risks and potential benefits of pain management with these agents.

market, and another agent, vildagliptin (LAF237), is being used in Europe and else-where. This article is intended to evaluate the effectiveness of DPP-4 inhibitors as a therapeutic modality for managing type 2 diabetes. The authors conducted a liter-ature search of various databases to identify the clinical trials involving the DPP in-hibitors and concluded that the DPP-4 inhibitors, for example, sitagliptin and vildagliptin, are efficacious for managing diabetes as monotherapy or combination therapy.

Cardiology Clinics

THE CLINICS ARE NOW AVAILABLE ONLINE!

Access your subscription at:
www.theclinics.com

Foreword

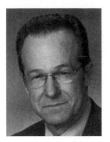

Michael H. Crawford, MD
Consulting Editor

Over the years the pendulum has swung between procedures/devices and drugs for the treatment of cardiovascular disease. We are just emerging from a long period of dominance of percutaneous interventions, stents, closure devices, implanted electrophysiologic devices, ablation, ventricular assist devises and minimally invasive surgery. New trials such as COURAGE are demonstrating the power of established drug therapy, and several promising new agents are now approved or close to being approved by the US Food and Drug Administration (FDA). The FDA is reorganizing to meet the challenge of recent complications from drugs, and proposing laws to impose more reasonable expectations for drug-related tort cases. In this milieu it seemed timely to review some of the newer pharmacologic agents and targeted disease areas for which newer drugs have made a big impact.

I was delighted that Dr. JoAnne Foody agreed to guest edit this issue. Dr. Foody is a general cardiologist whose practice emphasizes cardiovascular disease prevention. She has assembled a stellar group of experts to contribute to this issue of *Cardiology Clinics*.

Many of our new pharmacologic agents are designed for primary or secondary prevention. Truly successful prevention would eliminate the need for procedures and devices. Since cardiovascular disease is a world-wide problem now, drugs make a lot more sense for developing countries than do procedures and devices.

There are two types of articles in this issue: those that discuss a specific drug or family of drugs and those that discuss new pharmacologic approaches to specific diseases. The former includes articles on angiotension receptor blockers, direct renin inhibitors, cholesterol ester transfer protein inhibitors, niacin plus laropiprant, cyclooxygenase inhibitors, ranolazine, dipeptidyl peptidase-4, anticoagulants and prasugrel. Discussed disease areas include heart failure, coronary artery disease and hypertension. This issue will be of immense practical value to those in the front lines of cardiovascular disease prevention and management.

Michael H. Crawford, MD
Division of Cardiology
Department of Medicine
University of California
San Francisco Medical Center
505 Parnassus Avenue, Box 0124
San Francisco, CA 94143-0124, USA

E-mail address:
crawfordm@medicine.ucsf.edu (M.H. Crawford)

doi:10.1016/j.ccl.2008.09.001
0733-8651/08/$ – see front matter

Preface
Prevention as the Intervention

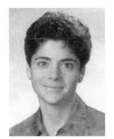

JoAnne M. Foody, MD
Guest Editor

Although cardiovascular mortality has recently been noted to be declining in the United States, it remains the number one cause of death in men and women. In the United States alone, cardiovascular disease (CVD) kills nearly 1 million people a year. This translates to a financial cost of between $50 and $100 billion per year (indirect and direct cost, ie, treatment and lost wages cost). These statistics are likely to worsen as the current epidemics of hypertension, obesity, metabolic syndrome, diabetes, heart failure, and atrial fibrillation collide with increased life expectancy worldwide.

Numerous clinical trials have demonstrated that CVD is largely preventable through the modification of risk factors. There is mounting evidence that controlling hypertension and diabetes mellitus, improving lipid profiles, and modifying the coagulation cascade can reduce the risk of a first or subsequent heart attack. As a result of this evidence, there has been a paradigm shift toward a targeted, early, and aggressive modification of individual risk and toward delaying or stopping the development of clinical atherosclerotic disease (primary prevention) and treating individuals after the manifestation of symptomatic coronary artery disease (secondary prevention).

As the paradigm has shifted toward the concept of global risk and the interplay of multiple risk factors in the manifestations of CVD and the identification and prevention of risk factors, efforts have been made to better understand the underlying pathophysiology that contributes to atherosclerosis and to develop approaches to modify the disease at its most basic core.

The race continues for new medications to treat and prevent atherosclerosis, atherothrombosis, hypertension, hyperlipidemia, diabetes, and heart failure. Over the past year, new data supporting various new medications have emerged from clinical research studies. New cardiac drugs are being developed at a rapid pace. Several new drugs and classes of drugs, including angiotensin receptor blockers (ARBs), direct renin inhibitors, cholesteryl ester transfer protein inhibitors, laropiprant, cyclooxygenase inhibitors, ranolazine, and the new thienopyridine prasugrel, are reviewed in this issue. These concise yet comprehensive reviews should help cardiologists keep up to date with the latest drug information, the evidence supporting the use of the new drugs, and the opportunities for improvement in the care of patients who have or are at risk for cardiovascular disease.

With respect to cardiovascular events and morbidity, hypertension is associated with the greatest burden of disease worldwide. Its relationship with target organ damage, including stroke, coronary heart disease, heart failure, myocardial infarction (MI), atrial fibrillation, end-stage renal disease, peripheral vascular disease, and left ventricular hypertrophy, is well established. The control of hypertension with pharmacotherapy has the potential to reduce stroke, MI, and heart failure by one third. Although hypertension remains the most prevalent of all risk factors, its control remains poor, and various antihypertensive agents have been used. Recent data emphasize the beneficial role of renin-angiotensin-aldosterone system (RAAS) blockers, including angiotensin-converting

doi:10.1016/j.ccl.2008.07.004
0733-8651/08/$ – see front matter © 2008 Elsevier Inc. All rights reserved.

cardiology.theclinics.com

enzyme inhibitors (ACEIs) and ARBs, because of their favorable cardiovascular outcomes and the potential role of direct renin inhibitors in blood pressure control.

The Joint National Committee and the World Health Organization are in agreement that hypertension in most patients who are treated is controlled inadequately and that rates of cardiovascular morbidity remain high. Additional pharmacologic treatments have the potential to ameliorate this situation. The RAAS has been a highly successful pharmacologic target, because the system is strongly implicated in the development of hypertension-related target organ damage. Compensatory increases in plasma renin levels that lead to adjustments in angiotensin production and conversion may present limitations for existing RAAS inhibitors, however. The development of a small-molecule renin inhibitor, aliskiren, may address angiotensin production directly at its rate-limiting step. Studies in humans attest to an effective blood pressure–lowering effect, a side effect profile no different from AT_1 receptor blockers, and the option of combination therapies. Because angiotensin receptor blockade, ACE inhibition, calcium channel blockade, and diuretic therapy all lead to sharp increases in plasma renin activity, aliskiren offers a novel approach to this problem.

Epidemiologic data suggest that the prevalence of diabetes worldwide is expected to double in the next 20 years. The lifetime risk for developing diabetes among Americans born in this millennium is now nearly 40%. New treatment options exist for the management of diabetes. One promising modality is the inhibition of dipeptidyl peptidase IV (DPP-4). One problem in diabetes is a defect in the incretin-signaling pathway, the hormones that are released by cells in the gut to facilitate digestion and metabolism. The focus of research has been on the incretin hormone, glucagonlike peptide-1 (GLP-1), which guards against an excess increase in blood glucose and helps monitor the emptying of the stomach.

Sitagliptin (Januvia), the first in a new class of agents called dipeptidyl peptidase IV (DPP-4) inhibitors, received FDA approval recently for the treatment of patients who have type 2 diabetes. This once-daily oral therapy can be used as monotherapy or in combination with either metformin (Glucophage) or a thiazolidinedione (TZD). The DPP-4 inhibitors are not associated with hypoglycemia, a common side effect seen with many of the available antidiabetes drugs, especially at the beginning of treatment when insulin secretion is unregulated, even though the glucose level is dropping. Given the significant interplay of diabetes and cardiovascular risk and disease, the article reviewing DPP-4 as a new target of action for type 2 diabetes mellitus is important for all practicing cardiologists.

Coronary heart disease (CHD), the physical manifestation of atherosclerosis, is a major cause of death and disability. Of the 17 million deaths that occur from cardiovascular disease in the world each year, CHD is a significant contributor. Patients who have CHD often have atherosclerosis in other vascular beds, predisposing them to the risk for other occlusive events, such as ischemic stroke. Antiplatelet drugs, together with antihypertensive and lipid-lowering agents, form part of the panoply of drugs that are used in the management of patients who have experienced an episode of acute coronary syndrome. Although much attention is focused on atherosclerosis, atherothrombosis remains a major cause of morbidity and mortality. Therapies addressing the coagulation cascade at all points, including novel agents such as prasugrel, a new thienopyridine, hold the promise of reducing risk, albeit at the expense of increased bleeding rates. Acute coronary syndromes constitute a spectrum of disorders, including acute MI (heart attack) and unstable angina, which occur when activated platelets release substances at the site of plaque rupture that lead to platelet aggregation and thrombosis. Although antiplatelet drugs, such as aspirin and clopidogrel, help reduce the incidence of acute thrombus formation, there have always been acknowledged tradeoffs between fewer heart attacks, strokes, and cardiovascular deaths, and excess bleeding. Today, the holy grail of antithrombotic therapy remains the same—to find drugs that reduce the risk of cardiovascular events and death in heart patients without the associated risk for increased bleeding.

Heart failure, too, proves complex to many clinicians and therapies to address the morbidity and mortality associated with the condition are urgently needed. Less than one fourth of physicians specializing in geriatrics, internal or family medicine, or cardiology believe they can accurately predict whether patients who have heart failure are at risk for dying, new research finds. Fortunately, new therapies are on the horizon for addressing several aspects of heart failure. Selective aldosterone antagonists, such as eplerenone, address key challenges facing clinicians caring for patients who have heart failure. Previous studies had demonstrated that mortality remains high in post-MI systolic dysfunction patients, even when the patients are receiving optimal treatment through neurohormonal blockade with both ACE inhibitors and beta-blockers. In addition, although the Randomized Spironolactone Evaluation Study (RALES)[1] found a clear mortality benefit for adding the nonselective aldosterone antagonist spironolactone on top of optimal treatment, the drug's hormonal side effects rendered its use difficult or inappropriate in some patients. The EPHESUS[2] trial suggests that the addition of the selective aldosterone blocker eplerenone to patients who have post-MI systolic dysfunction results in substantial improvements in the clinical course, including significant reductions in morbidity and mortality. Of critical importance to the practicing physician is that these benefits of eplerenone were additive to the effects of other therapies known to improve the natural history of patients who have post-MI heart failure.

The evidence base for cardiology continues to expand, and novel therapies continue to be developed to combat cardiovascular disease, atherosclerosis, and atherothrombosis at their root. Numerous clinical trials have demonstrated that we have the potential to prevent cardiovascular disease through the application of preventive strategies. Our challenge is to implement consistently the wide array of therapies in those patients most likely to benefit so that we may achieve the full potential of these agents.

JoAnne M. Foody, MD, FACC, FAHA
Associate Professor
Harvard Medical School
Brigham and Women's/Faulkner Hospitals
1153 Centre Street, Suite 4930
Boston, MA 02130, USA

E-mail address:
jfoody@partners.org (J.M. Foody)

REFERENCES

1. Pitt B, Zannad F, Remme WJ, et al. The Randomized Aldactone Evaluation Study Investigators. The effect of spironolactone on morbidity and mortality in patients with severe heart failure. N Engl J Med 1999; 341(10):709–17.
2. Pitt B, White H, Nicolau J, et al. Eplerenone reduces mortality 30 days after randomization following acute myocardial infarction in patients with left ventricular systolic dysfunction and heart failure. J Am Coll Cardiol 2005;46(3):42–531.

Angiotensin Receptor Blockers: Novel Role in High-Risk Patients

Usman Javed, MD[a],
Prakash C. Deedwania, MD, FACC, FACP, FCCP, FAHA[a,b],*

KEYWORDS

- Angiotensin receptor blockers • RAAS blockade
- Cardioprotection • High risk hypertension
- Diabetes mellitus

The identification of patients at high risk for cardiovascular events is imperative in the reduction of cardiovascular mortality and morbidity. Cardiovascular disease is the leading cause of death in the United States with a cardiac death occurring every 60 seconds.[1] Although coronary artery disease (CAD), peripheral arterial disease, cerebro vascular disease, hypertension, and diabetes mellitus (DM) contribute to risk for developing cardiovascular events, we are now faced with emerging fronts because of an increase in life expectancy and the epidemic of hypertension, obesity, metabolic syndrome, and diabetes.

The prevalence of diabetes, worldwide, is expected to increase from 2.8% in 2000 to 4.4% by the year 2030.[2] The lifetime risk for developing diabetes among Americans born in the year 2000 is projected at 32.8% and 38.5% for men and women, respectively.[3] Currently it accounts for more than 10% of total United States health care expenditure.[1] Cardiovascular disease is the leading cause of mortality and morbidity in patients who have diabetes, with up to 50% to 65% of patients who have diabetes dying from cardiovascular complications.[4]

The increase in prevalence of type 2 diabetes mellitus (T2DM) is heralded by obesity and metabolic syndrome (MS).[5] Recent National Health and Nutrition Examination Survey data have shown that the prevalence of people who are overweight or obese with a body mass index (BMI) of 20 or greater increased from 56% in 1988 to 1994 to 64% in 1999 to 2000.[6] According to the National Cholesterol Education Program Adult Treatment Panel[7] MS is defined by objective clinical criteria with clustering of three or more risk factors. An increase in BMI seems to have a linear relationship with development of type II diabetes;[8] prevalence of T2DM is three to seven times greater in obese subjects and 20 times greater if BMI is greater than 35 kg/m^2.[9]

Hypertension still trumps all risk factors when it comes to cardiovascular events and related morbidity.[4] Its relationship with target organ damage, including stroke, coronary heart disease, heart failure (HF), myocardial infarction (MI), atrial fibrillation, end-stage renal disease, peripheral vascular disease, and left ventricular hypertrophy has been well established.[10] Blood pressure control through antihypertensive therapy reduces stroke, MI, and HF by 20% to 40%.[11]

A meta-analysis involving 29 randomized trials and a total of 162,341 patients conducted by the Blood Pressure Lowering Treatment Trialists' Collaboration confirmed that angiotensin-converting enzyme inhibitors (ACEIs) provide benefits in a broad range of patients with and without hypertension.[12] The authors of a recent meta-analysis of 127 randomized trials concluded that the effects of renin-angiotensin system inhibition with ACEIs or

[a] Cardiology Section, Cardiovascular Research, UCSF Fresno Medical Education Program, UCSF School of Medicine, 2615 East Clinton Avenue (111), Fresno, CA 93703, USA
[b] Stanford University, Palo Alto, CA, USA
* Corresponding author. Cardiology Section, Cardiovascular Research, UCSF Medical Education Program, UCSF School of Medicine, 2615 East Clinton Avenue (111), Fresno, CA 93703.
E-mail address: deed1@sbcglobal.net (P.C. Deedwania).

Cardiol Clin 26 (2008) 507–526
doi:10.1016/j.ccl.2008.07.001
0733-8651/08/$ – see front matter. Published by Elsevier Inc.

angiotensin receptor blockers (ARBs) were mainly the result of lowering blood pressure, however.[13]

Although individual risk factor identification is important, in clinical practice most patients have multiple cardiovascular risk factors.[1] An increased incidence of cardiovascular events with numerous risk factors[14] was clearly demonstrated in the Multiple Risk Factor Intervention Trial (MRFIT).[15] When taken into account, the risk for cardiovascular disease increased from 24.7/10,000 person-years in patients who did not have diabetes to 77.8/10,000 person-years in high-risk patients who had diabetes with up to three risk factors.[16] The risk for a cardiovascular event increases considerably in patients who have a history of a prior cardiovascular event, such as CAD, peripheral arterial disease, or cerebrovascular event. Prospective data[1,16] have shown that up to 44% of patients who had a previous stroke can develop coronary disease or cardiac failure, whereas 20% to 46% of patients who have peripheral arterial disease are predicted to develop stroke, cardiac failure, or CAD.[1]

Risk factors associated with cardiovascular disease in addition to those mentioned earlier include male gender, age 45 years or older, family history of premature CAD, physical inactivity, race (ethnicity, such as African American, Hispanic, Native American, Asian American, and Pacific Islanders), impaired glucose tolerance, history of gestational diabetes and hypertension, dyslipidemia (HDL cholesterol <35 mg/dL and triglyceride >250 mg/dL), and polycystic ovary syndrome.[14]

As the paradigm has shifted toward the identification of the high-risk state for future cardiovascular events and their treatment, clinical practice and pharmacotherapy have evolved a better understanding of the underlying pathophysiology and the need for an aggressive preventive strategy in this high-risk population. It includes prevention and control of traditional risk factors, such as hypertension and diabetes, with lifestyle changes and therapeutic intervention. Because hypertension remains the most prevalent of all risk factors, a variety of antihypertensive agents have been used.[11,17] Patients who have uncomplicated hypertension or those who have no specific indication for a particular antihypertensive agent are recommended to be treated with a diuretic agent for control of their blood pressure. Beta-blockers are no longer used as a primary or secondary antihypertensive agent in patients who do not have a specific indication for these drugs because of worsening glycemic control and an unfavorable impact on the risk for stroke (especially with atenolol), particularly in elderly patients. Recent data emphasize the beneficial role of renin-angiotensin-aldosterone system (RAAS) blockers, including ACEIs and ARBs, because of their favorable cardiovascular outcomes.[18] ARBs or ACEIs, alone or in combination when used in high-risk patients, not only control blood pressure but also have shown cardiovascular benefit beyond blood pressure control.[19–21] This article addresses the role of RAAS activation in the high-risk metabolic milieu and the role of ARBs in targeting and inhibiting the RAAS for cardiovascular protection.

IMPORTANCE OF THE RENIN-ANGIOTENSIN-ALDOSTERONE SYSTEM PATHWAY AND SIGNIFICANCE OF ANGIOTENSIN RECEPTOR TYPE I

It is now well establish that the activation of the RAAS plays a critical role in the initiation and progression of hypertension, diabetes, vascular remodeling, and cardiovascular changes leading to target organ damage.[22] Several experimental and clinical studies have shown that RAAS blockade results in a paramount yet multifaceted effect with benefits beyond control of hypertension including reduction of new-onset T2DM, prevention of progression of nephropathy to renal failure, and modulation of signaling pathways involved in cardiovascular cascade contributing to the increased cardiovascular events.[23–26]

The RAAS is an in-step neuroendocrine cascade that controls cardiovascular, renal, adrenal, and sympathetic function by numerous mechanisms, including control of body fluid and electrolyte balance. Angiotensin II (ang II) is the primary mediator of the RAAS that elicits a wide range of effects through angiotensin II type 1 (AT1) receptor. These include vasoconstriction, sodium and water retention, and sympathetic activation leading to hypertension and vascular and cardiac remodeling, which if uninterrupted can lead to HF. Angiotensin II (ang II) formation occurs from angiotensinogen through a series of steps.[27] Renin, which is secreted by the juxtaglomerular apparatus in the kidney, catalyzes the conversion of angiotensinogen to angiotensin I (ang I). Ang I is subsequently converted to ang II by ACE. ACE-induced conversion accounts for about 60% of ang II. Alternate pathways also exist that convert angiotensinogen directly to angiotensin II. These include serine proteinases, such as chymase and cathepsin G, and tissue plasminogen activator–dependent pathways that contribute to significant production of ang II in diseased vessels and heart (eg, post-MI).[28,29]

Angiotensin II mediates its effects by acting on AT1 and type II (AT2) receptors (**Fig. 1**). AT1 receptors are widespread throughout the tissues and lead to deleterious effects, which include vasoconstriction, aldosterone release, increased sodium

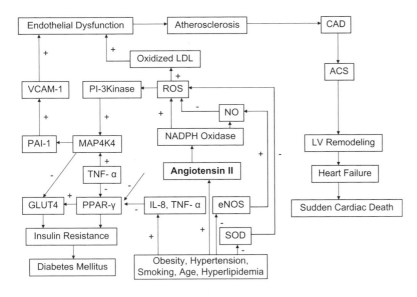

Fig. 1. Clinicopathological sequelae associated with angiotensin II type I receptor overexpression. ACS, acute coronary syndrome; CAD, coronary artery disease; eNOS, endothelial nitric oxide synthase; GLUT, glucose uptake transporter; IL-1, interleukin; LDL, low density lipoprotein; MAP4K4, mitogen-activated protein kinase; NADPH, nicotinamide adenine dinucleotide phosphatase; NO, nitric oxide; PAI-1, plasminogen activator inhibitor; PI-3, phosphatidyl-inositol-3; PPAR, peroxisome proliferator-activated receptor; ROS, reactive oxygen species; SOD, superoxide dismutase; TNF, tumor necrosis factor; VCAM-1, vascular cell adhesion molecule.

retention, and cellular hypertrophy of vessel wall and myocardium. The genomic effects of ATI result from an enhanced intracellular activation of transcription factors, such as nuclear factor-κB and activator protein 1, monocyte chemoattractant protein–1 (MCP-1), vascular cell adhesion molecule, plasminogen activator inhibitor, and the release of the cytokines interleukin-6 (IL-6) and tumor necrosis factor (TNF-α). The result is an increased oxidative stress and level of transforming growth factor (TGF) leading to a proinflammatory, atherogenic, and prothrombotic environment.[30–35] The function of the AT2 receptor, which is up-regulated in response to tissue injury, is not well understood but seems to mediate beneficial effects that include vasodilatation, inhibition of cell growth and proliferation, and cell differentiation. While blocking the AT1 receptor, most ARBs have an intrinsic AT2 receptor-stimulating property attributable to increased levels of ang II secondary to the RAAS feedback loop. Valsartan has been shown to reduce cardiac remodeling, coronary arterial thickness, and perivascular fibrosis by way of AT2 receptor stimulation. In vitro studies have also demonstrated that the renin, ACE, and AT1 receptor genes are significantly up-regulated in obese patients who have hypertension, which might explain the high risk for cardiovascular disease in these patients.[25–36]

The cardiovascular risk factors, such as diabetes, smoking, and dyslipidemia, increase the levels of ang II, which in turn might trigger the progression to atherosclerosis plaque destabilization, left ventricular hypertrophy, cardiac apoptosis, and increased arrhythmogenicity.[31] The net result

is the loss of cardiac muscle mass, left ventricle remodeling, progressing to HF, end-stage cardiomyopathy, and increased risk for sudden cardiac death.

RENIN-ANGIOTENSIN-ALDOSTERONE SYSTEM INHIBITION AND CARDIOVASCULAR PROTECTION

RAAS blockade has beneficial effects on inflammation, oxidative stress, and endothelial function. RAAS blockade attenuates hyperglycemia-induced endothelial dysfunction and reduces the release of proinflammatory cytokines that may mediate the development of cardiovascular disease in high-risk patients who have diabetes.[37] Lisinopril has been shown to reduce cardiovascular oxidative stress, cardiomyocyte hypertrophy, and loss of cardiac function in rats with streptozotocin-induced diabetes and preserve the elastin/collagen ratio in the aorta media (changes that are often associated with diabetes).[38]

Blockade of RAAS promotes insulin sensitivity by increasing the differentiation of preadipocytes and promoting the recruitment of preadipocytes. The result is an increase in small insulin-sensitive adipocytes, followed by a redistribution of lipids to adipose tissue and improved insulin sensitivity. In a fructose-fed rat model of metabolic syndrome, RAAS blockade with temocapril or olmesartan showed a significant improvement in insulin sensitivity and blood pressure and decrease in adipocyte size. This finding was later confirmed by in vitro study in primary cultured human preadipocytes that demonstrated inhibition of adipocyte differentiation with angiotensin II.[39–41]

Several small observational studies have shown an improvement in flow-mediated vasodilatation in patients who had hypertension, diabetes, and CAD associated with RAAS inhibition by ARBs. It is postulated to be mediated by increased production of endothelium-derived nitric oxide (NO) production. Beneficial effects of ARBs, such as increased superoxide dismutase activity and endothelial NO synthase activity, reduced vasoconstriction, and decreased blood pressure, may also contribute to improvement in endothelial function through increase in NO release and inhibition of NO degradation.[31] Further randomized controlled studies are needed to confirm the reduction of outcomes associated with improved endothelial function.

RENIN-ANGIOTENSIN-ALDOSTERONE SYSTEM AS A THERAPEUTIC TARGET IN HIGH-RISK PATIENTS: THE ROLE OF ANGIOTENSIN-CONVERTING ENZYME INHIBITORS

Although ACEIs were initially developed for treatment of hypertension, their use has been extended to HF, post-MI, and renal disease. In addition, ACEIs seem to have pleiotropic effects as documented by their vasodilating, anti-inflammatory, plaque stabilizing, antithrombotic, and antiproliferative properties. The net result is that their therapeutic effects go beyond blood pressure control leading to beneficial effects on vascular and cardiac remodeling, reduced incidence of diabetes, renal protection, and cerebral and cardiovascular protection. These properties of ACEIs have led to their use in primary and secondary prevention for cardiovascular disease.

Several clinical trials evaluating the efficacy of RAAS blockade with ACEIs or ARBs demonstrated reductions in new-onset diabetes and cardiovascular event rates following treatment with these agents. The Captopril Prevention Project (CAPPP) was a landmark trial that evaluated the effectiveness of captopril to reduce cardiovascular mortality and morbidity in more than 10,000 hypertensive patients. A subanalysis of CAPPP revealed that hypertensive patients who had diabetes receiving captopril had a 66% lower rate of fatal and nonfatal MI compared with conventional therapy with diuretics or beta-blockers ($P = .002$). Overall, fatal cardiovascular events were reduced by about 50% in patients receiving captopril compared with conventional therapy.[42]

The Heart Outcomes Prevention Evaluation (HOPE) was a pivotal study and a trendsetter in our current practice of cardiovascular medicine. During a 4.5-year follow-up, treatment with ramipril demonstrated significant reduction in cardiovascular events, mortality, and new-onset diabetes in high-risk patients.[43] The cardiovascular benefits of ramipril were unrelenting in the 2.6-year extension of the study, HOPE–The Ongoing Outcomes (HOPE-TOO).[44] Overall, during the 7.2 years of follow-up, patients receiving ramipril had a 3.6% absolute risk reduction in combined incidence of MI, stroke, and cardiovascular death compared with the placebo group ($P = .0002$); and 31% relative risk reduction (RRR) of new-onset DM in patients taking ramipril ($P = .0006$). Although it is somewhat debatable, the investigators concluded that cardiovascular protective effects of ramipril were primarily not related to their antihypertensive effects.

The European Trial on Reduction of Cardiac Events with Perindopril in Stable Coronary Artery Disease (EUROPA) extended the results seen in the HOPE trial.[45] In a large, well-treated patient population of stable CAD, perindopril showed a clear reduction in cardiovascular events and mortality versus placebo (8% versus 9.9%, $P < .0003$). The cardiovascular benefits of perindopril seemed to be beyond its antihypertensive properties because the drop in blood pressure was modest (5 versus 2 mmHg).

RENIN-ANGIOTENSIN-ALDOSTERONE SYSTEM AS A THERAPEUTIC TARGET IN HIGH RISK PATIENTS: THE ROLE OF ANGIOTENSIN RECEPTOR BLOCKERS

ARBs act by selectively blocking the binding of ang II to the AT1 receptor but not the AT2 receptor. ARBs have been shown to improve insulin-mediated glucose uptake, improve endothelial function, increase nitric oxide activation, reduce inflammatory response, and increase bradykinin levels (**Box 1**). Although many of these pleiotropic effect of ARBs have been well demonstrated in animal models, similar effect are yet to be established in human clinical studies.

ROLE OF ANGIOTENSIN RECEPTOR BLOCKERS IN ENDOTHELIAL IMPROVEMENT

ACEIs have already demonstrated their protective effects on cardiovascular, neurologic, and renal complications in high-risk patients. Better understanding of RAAS led to the realization that ACE inhibitors do not always provide complete blockade, however. As much as 40% of ang II formation occurs from alternative pathways leading to the concept described as ACE escape. Moreover, ACE inhibitors are not well tolerated in a significant fraction of patients because of associated angioedema and cough. Hence ARBs have emerged as an alternative and a potential adjunct to the ACEIs.

Box 1
Metabolic effects of angiotensin receptor blockers

Promote differentiation of adipocytes

Increase adipocyte uptake of glucose and lipid

Decrease glycogenolysis

Inhibit secretion of triglycerides into the circulation

Increase vasodilatation

Increase delivery of glucose and insulin to skeletal muscle

Inhibit apoptosis in pancreas

Decrease catecholamine release

ARBs are more selective than ACEIs in that they selectively antagonize AT1 receptors. A theoretic advantage of ARBs is that non-ACE sources of ang II are unable to activate AT1. Blockade of AT1 interrupts the negative feedback loop and increases circulating ang II levels. The result is unopposed AT2 stimulation because of heightened ang II levels resulting in vasodilatation and other beneficial effects. Despite these favorable effects of ARBs, an absolute effectiveness of benefits from this class of medication compared with the ACEIs is yet to be established, particularly in high-risk individuals.[22,27]

ARBs, like ACEIs, have an effect on the regulation of endothelial function. Ang II plays a significant role in endothelial dysfunction in general and in patients who have diabetes in particular. Insulin binds to tyrosine kinase, which leads to autophosphorylation of tyrosine residue turning on the insulin-signaling pathways, which enhances uptake of glucose by skeletal muscle. The second activated pathway is the mitogen-activated protein kinase, which promotes vascular smooth muscle cell proliferation and migration induced by insulin, thrombin, and platelet-derived growth factors. A third pathway is triggered that leads to activation of P70 S6 kinase, a regulator of protein synthesis.[45,46]

In animal models, valsartan has shown a reduction in the expression of proinflammatory markers, such as MCP-1, TNF, IL-6, and IL-1, and it inhibits migration of inflammatory cells into the injured arteries. Losartan has shown a decrease in reactive oxidants, increased NO production, and improved flow-mediated vasodilatation.[47–49] In humans, ARB treatment in patients who have essential hypertension decreases peripheral vascular resistance and radial arterial thickness and reduces left ventricular muscle mass.[50] These beneficial effects of ARBs have the potential to provide cardiovascular protection, especially in high-risk individuals.

CLINICAL STUDIES OF ANGIOTENSIN RECEPTOR BLOCKERS IN VARIOUS HIGH-RISK GROUPS

Several important questions remain concerning the role of RAAS inhibition and target end-organ protection. An intervention for lowering blood pressure alone reduces the progression of vascular and renal disease in high-risk patients. These individuals must be identified, however. Based on the results of several clinical trials, including HOPE, the Antihypertensive and Lipid-Lowering Treatment to Prevent Heart Attack trial, and the Losartan Intervention For Endpoint Reduction in Hypertension (LIFE) trial, the Seventh Report of the Joint National Committee on Prevention, Detection, Evaluation, and Treatment of High Blood Pressure (JNC 7) identified renal disease and diabetes as compelling indications for the use of more aggressive blood pressure (BP)–lowering treatment.[44,50–53] Also, in recognition of cardiovascular risk associated with BP elevation, JNC 7 categorized individuals who have systolic BP ranging from 120 to 139 mm Hg and diastolic BP ranging from 90 to 99 mm Hg as "prehypertensive." Although no pharmacologic intervention was recommended for the management of prehypertension, the stated expectation was that greater attention would be paid to nonpharmacologic approaches and lifestyle modification and an early recognition and intervention for a higher risk. Risk is set forth by the traditional factors described earlier; nonetheless, hypertension remains the most sensitive predictor of target organ damage.

The Trial of Preventing Hypertension (TROPHY) was a study designed to look at the implications of an early pharmacologic treatment with candesartan (an ARB) of prehypertension in preventing the development of hypertension. During the first 2 years, hypertension developed in 40.4% of subjects in the placebo group compared with only 13.6% of those in the candesartan group for a RRR of 66.3% ($P < .0001$). At 4 years, hypertension had developed in 63.0% in the placebo group versus 53.2% in the candesartan group (RRR 15.6%; $P < .0069$). The relative proportion of participants who were hypertension-free was 26.5% greater in the candesartan group.[54]

ANGIOTENSIN RECEPTOR BLOCKERS IN HIGH-RISK HYPERTENSIVES

LIFE was one of the initial clinical trials that compared the efficacy of an ARB in a high-risk population with evidence of target organ damage (left ventricular hypertrophy).[52] In patients who had advanced hypertension and left ventricular hypertrophy, losartan in comparison with atenolol showed reduction in composite cardiovascular mortality, MI, and stroke (11% losartan versus 13% atenolol, relative risk [RR] = 0.13; P = .021). The benefit was largely derived from the reduction in stroke (losartan 5% versus atenolol 7%). In the subgroup analysis of patients who did not have vascular disease, losartan reduced the primary composite endpoint of cardiovascular morbidity and mortality along with stroke (HR 0.18, P = .008). These beneficial effects of losartan were most evident in the diabetic subgroup. In the analysis of patients who had diabetes, losartan did reduce primary composite endpoint, cardiovascular mortality, and HF hospitalizations compared with atenolol (hazard ratio [HR] 0.77, P = .031), and mortality (HR 0.62, P = .002). In patients who had isolated systolic hypertension in the LIFE study, losartan reduced all-cause mortality (HR 0.72, P = .05) but failed to show a significant reduction in the primary composite endpoint of cardiovascular mortality and stroke compared with atenolol. In another subgroup analysis of the LIFE trial, losartan versus atenolol revealed that there was actually an increased risk for stroke, 8.9% versus 4.6% for African American patients (adjusted HR 2.18, P = .03). African American women derive similar benefit from ARBs as men. The subgroup of African American patients who had DM on losartan had a reduction in cardiovascular mortality but not a significant decrease in stroke.

Various other studies have evaluated the effects of ARBs on all-cause or cardiovascular mortality and morbidity in patients who have high cardiovascular risk (**Table 1**). The Morbidity and Mortality after Stroke, Eprosartan Compared with Nitrendipine for Secondary Prevention (MOSES) trial compared morbidity and mortality in treatment with eprosartan or nitrendipine.[55] The combined primary endpoint of all-cause mortality, and cardiovascular and cerebrovascular events in patients who had hypertension and history of stroke was compared with nitrendipine. The combined primary endpoint was significantly reduced with eprosartan compared with nitrendipine, with an incidence density of 13.25% versus 16.71%, respectively, and an incidence ratio (IDR) of 0.79 (95% CI 0.66–0.96; P = .014). The incidence was also significantly reduced with eprosartan for fatal and nonfatal stroke (IDR 0.75, 95% CI 0.55–0.97; P = .025). This difference in the primary outcome is seen despite similar reduction in blood pressure in the two treatment groups. This trial also

revealed that patients treated with eprosartan had significantly fewer cerebrovascular events compared with patients treated with nitrendipine.

The Valsartan Antihypertensive Long-term Use Evaluation (VALUE) study compared valsartan to the amlodipine in patients who had hypertension and high cardiovascular risk.[56] This large, multicenter, randomized trial enrolled 15,245 patients who had treated or untreated hypertension who were at high risk for cardiac events. During the mean follow-up of 4.2 years, there was no difference in all-cause mortality between the two groups (11.0% for valsartan, 10.8% for amlodipine; HR 1.04, 95% CI 0.94–1.14; P = .45%). Overall cardiac mortality was similar but fatal and nonfatal MI reached significance (4.8% versus 4.1%, adjusted HR 1.19, 95% CI 1.02–1.38, P = .02).

ARBs have also been shown to be beneficial in improving chronic cerebral ischemia. Administration of candesartan has been shown to improve cerebral artery media thickness, improve cerebral blood flow, and reduce the expression of c-Fos and c-Jun proteins in the brain that are associated with chronic neurodegenerative diseases.[57] Recent studies suggest that RAAS blockade may also reduce the incidence of cerebrovascular events in high-risk groups; for example, the risk for stroke was reduced with ramipril in the HOPE trial, which also included patients who had prior transient ischemic attack (TIA) or stroke.[43]

ANGIOTENSIN RECEPTOR BLOCKERS IN POST–MYOCARDIAL INFARCTION PATIENTS

Although there have been no head-to-head or placebo-controlled trials evaluating the effects of ARBs in patients who have had a recent MI, ARBs are often used in clinical practice to prevent the development or progression of HF and to reduce mortality in such patients irrespective of the presence of HF. This use is largely extrapolated from two clinical trials of ARB in post–MI patients (**Table 2**).

The Optimal Trial in Myocardial Infarction with the Angiotensin II Antagonist Losartan (OPTIMAAL) compared losartan with captopril in patients who had post-MI HF.[58] It failed to show non-inferiority of losartan to captopril in reducing all-cause mortality in patients. In the intent-to-treat analysis, the upper one-sided 95% confidence boundary for the relative risk for death from any cause was 1.28, which did not satisfy the non-inferiority criterion (upper boundary 1.10). Also, significantly fewer cardiovascular deaths and sudden cardiac deaths were observed in the captopril group. There was no difference in the incidence of MI. Consistent with previous trials, losartan was

Table 1
Clinical studies of angiotensin receptor blockers in hypertension

Trial	Condition	n	Follow-up	ARB	Outcome	Results
TROPHY	Prehypertension	809	4 y	Candesartan versus placebo for 2 y, followed by no therapy	Hypertension	66.3% RRR at 2 y and 15.6% RRR at 4 y
LIFE	Hypertension	9,193	5 y	Losartan versus atenolol	Composite, CV death, stroke, MI	13% RRR
VALUE	Hypertension	15,245	4.2 y	Valsartan versus amlodipine	Composite endpoint	No difference
SCOPE	Hypertension, elderly	4,964	3.7 y	Candesartan versus diuretic versus beta-blocker	Composite, CV death, nonfatal MI, and non fatal stroke	No difference in composite endpoint, 28% RRR in nonfatal stroke
MOSES	Hypertension, stroke	1,405	2.5 y	Eprosartan versus nitrendipine	Composite, all-cause mortality, CV, and cerebrovascular	IDR for composite endpoints 0.79 (P = .014), for stroke 0.75 (P = .03)

Abbreviations: CV, cardiovascular; IDR, incidence ratio; MOSES, Morbidity and Mortality after Stroke, Eprcsartan Compared with Nitrendipine for Secondary Prevention trial; SCOPE, The Study on Cognition and Prognosis in the Elderly; VALUE, Valsartan Antihypertensive Long-term Use Evaluation.

Table 2
Clinical studies of angiotensin receptor blockers in diabetes and nephropathy

Trial	Condition	n	Follow-up	ARB	Outcome	Results
OPTIMAAL	Acute MI and HF	5,477	6 mo	Losartan versus captopril	All-cause mortality, nonfatal MI, SCD	No difference, ↑ mortality with losartan
VALIANT	Acute MI and HF	14,703	2.1 y	Valsartan versus captopril or both	All-cause mortality, CV death, MI & CHF hospitalization	No difference
ValHeFT	CHF	5,010	4 y	Valsartan versus placebo	All-cause mortality	No change in mortality, ↓ hospitalization
ELITE II	CHF	3,152	1.6 y	Losartan versus captopril	Composite	No difference
CHARM-Added	CHF	2,548	3.4 y	Candesartan versus placebo	Composite	15% RRR
CHARM-Alternate	CHF	2,028	2.8 y	Candesartan versus placebo	Composite	23% RRR
CHARM-Preserved	CHF	3,023	3 y	Candesartan versus placebo	CV death	11% RRR
CHARM overall	CHF	7,601	2 y	Candesartan versus placebo	All-cause mortality	17% RRR
ONTARGET	CAD, diabetes, hypertension	25,620	4.8 y	Telmisartan versus ramipril or both	Composite, CV death, stroke, MI, hospitalization	Non-inferiority to ramipril, ↑ adverse effects with combination

Abbreviations: CHARM, Candesartan in Heart Failure: Assessment of Reduction in Mortality and Morbidity; CHF, congestive heart failure; ELITE, Evaluation of Losartan in the Elderly trial; ONTARGET, Telmisartan Alone and in combination with Ramipril Global Endpoint Trial; OPTIMAAL, Optimal Trial in Myocardial Infarction with the Angiotensin II Antagonist Losartan; SCD, sudden cardiac death; ValHeFT, Valsartan Heart Failure Trial; VALIANT, Valsartan In Acute Myocardial Infarction Trial.

better tolerated than captopril, with fewer patients discontinuing study medication for any reason.

In the Valsartan In Acute Myocardial Infarction Trial (VALIANT), valsartan was shown to be as effective as captopril in reducing all-cause mortality and morbidity in patients who had recent MI and were at high risk for further coronary events (P = .004). After a mean follow-up of 24.7 months, survival was similar in the valsartan, valsartan and captopril, and captopril monotherapy groups.[59] The non-inferiority analysis confirmed that valsartan was no less effective than captopril. Likewise, the secondary endpoint of cardiovascular death, MI, or hospitalization for HF was similar in the three groups (**Fig. 2**). Captopril and valsartan were equally well tolerated. Cough, taste disturbance, and rash were more common with captopril, whereas hypotension and renal dysfunction were more common in the valsartan group. The combination of valsartan and captopril did not provide any advantage over monotherapy with either and it was poorly tolerated and had higher discontinuation rate. Based on the results of the VALIANT, valsartan is now approved for use in post-MI setting.

ANGIOTENSIN RECEPTOR BLOCKERS IN HEART FAILURE

Although treatment with ACEIs is now well established as first-line therapy for all patients who have HF, it is also recognized that some patients may not tolerate ACEIs and others might still be symptomatic despite optimal doses of ACEIs. It has been postulated that ARBs can be a suitable alternative and can provide additional benefits because of blockade of ang II produced by the alternate pathway. There is now good evidence that valsartan and candesartan are beneficial in patients who have HF who are unable to tolerate therapy with an ACEI. This evidence is based on evaluation of treatment with ARBs in several large clinical trials in patients who had HF (see **Table 2**).

The Evaluation of Losartan in the Elderly trial (ELITE II) was designed to compare the effects of losartan with those of captopril on mortality, morbidity, safety, and tolerability in patients who have symptomatic HF (New York Heart Association [NYHA] class II–III, mean left ventricular ejection fraction [LVEF] <35%).[60] In this high-risk cohort, 60% percent had a history of MI, 50% had hypertension, and about one third had atrial fibrillation. On analysis, a 13% reduction in mortality was observed in patients treated with captopril. There was no difference in hospitalizations (P = .45). Losartan was better tolerated than captopril because of more frequent cough in the captopril arm. Because ELITE II was a superiority trial and losartan was not superior to captopril, it remains unclear whether losartan is more effective in this setting. A major critique of the study

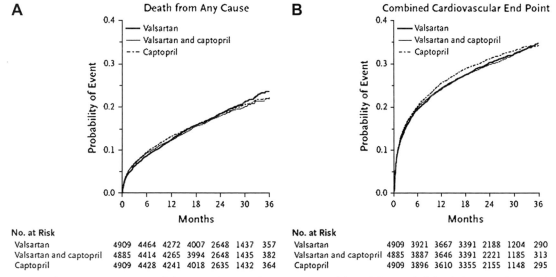

Fig. 2. Kaplan-Meier estimates of the rate of death from any cause (A) and the rate of death from cardiovascular causes, reinfarction, or hospitalization for HF (B), according to treatment group. (*From* Pfeffer MA, McMurray JJV, Velazquez EJ, et al, for the Valsartan in Acute Myocardial Infarction Trial Investigators. Valsartan, captopril, or both in myocardial infarction complicated by heart failure, left ventricular dysfunction, or both. N Engl J Med 2003;349:1898; with permission. Copyright © 2003, Massachusetts Medical Society.)

is the lower dose of losartan (50 mg/d) that is believed to be insufficient compared with captopril (150 mg/d).

In the Valsartan Heart Failure Trial (ValHeFT), valsartan was evaluated in patients who had a history of HF (NYHA class II–IV) and an ejection fraction less than 40% who were still symptomatic on standard therapy with diuretic, digoxin, and ACEI.[61] The co-primary outcomes were mortality and the combined endpoint of mortality and morbidity. Patients were assigned to receive valsartan or placebo in addition to background therapy, including ACEIs in 93%. There was no difference in mortality between the two groups. A subgroup analysis revealed that patients not receiving an ACE inhibitor at baseline (7.3%, n = 366) derived the greatest benefit from valsartan with a 44% reduction in the combined endpoint of mortality and morbidity. Significantly more patients receiving valsartan discontinued therapy (9.9% versus 7.2%; P < .001) because of common adverse effects. Subgroup analysis from ValHeFT suggested that an ARB might be appropriate in patients unable to tolerate an ACEI, but also raised questions about the safety of the combination of an ACEI, β-blocker, and ARB.

The Randomized Evaluation of Strategies for Left Ventricular Dysfunction (RESOLVD) trial compared candesartan with enalapril or the combination of candesartan and enalapril.[62] Primary outcomes included the distance on 6-minute walk, ventricular function as assessed by ejection fraction, end-diastolic and end-systolic volumes, blood pressure, quality of life, and levels of aldosterone and brain natriuretic peptide. Over a 43-week follow-up, this study showed that candesartan and enalapril resulted in similar improvements in exercise tolerance, ventricular function, NYHA functional class, and quality of life. In addition, blood pressure, aldosterone, and brain natriuretic peptide levels decreased significantly more in the combination therapy group. Candesartan and enalapril were found equally effective with respect to the primary endpoints and tolerability.

The Candesartan in Heart Failure: Assessment of Reduction in Mortality and Morbidity (CHARM) program had three parallel, independent, integrated, and randomized, double-blind, placebo-controlled clinical trials comparing candesartan with placebo in patients who had symptomatic HF.[63] The primary endpoint for each arm was to determine whether candesartan would reduce the risk for cardiovascular death or hospital admission for HF compared with standard therapy alone. CHARM-Alternative[64] is important because it compared candesartan with placebo in patients who had left ventricular dysfunction and a history of intolerance to ACEIs. The most common reason for ACEI intolerance was cough, accounting for more than 70% of subjects, whereas 4% of patients had documented angioedema. A total of 59% of patients treated with candesartan and 73% of the placebo group reached the target dose. In the candesartan group, 334 patients had primary endpoints (cardiovascular death and hospitalization for HF) versus 406 patients in the placebo group (RRR 23%, P = .0004). There was no statistically significant difference in cardiovascular or total mortality. Hospital admissions for worsening HF were reduced by 32% (P < .0001) in patients treated with candesartan. Candesartan was discontinued more often than placebo for renal dysfunction, hyperkalemia, and hypotension. Results from CHARM-Alternative study suggest that patients who cannot tolerate an ACEI should be treated with candesartan, with the prospect of reduction in HF decompensation but not in mortality and risk for MI.

CHARM-Preserved[65] was the second arm that enrolled patients who had HF with preserved LVEF (>40%). Sixty percent of patients in each group had NYHA class II symptoms and nearly 40% had class III symptoms. Subjects had a higher number of underlying risks for cardiovascular events: hypertension in 65%, MI in 45%, diabetes and angina in 27%, and stroke in 9%. The primary outcome, including MI, cardiovascular death, and noncardiovascular death, was similar in the two treatment groups. Hospitalization for HF was lower in the candesartan group than in the placebo group but overall admissions were similar (P = .79). In a high-risk population of patients who had presumed diastolic HF, candesartan reduced hospital admission for HF but did not attenuate mortality, MI, or total hospital admissions.

The results of the CHARM-Added[66] study suggested that adding candesartan at the relatively high mean dose of 24 mg on top of standard therapy with a beta-blocker and an ACEI in NYHA HF class II–III patients who have reduced LVEF reduces cardiovascular mortality by 17% and HF hospitalization by 17%. Overall, in the CHARM program, the mortality rate was 23% in candesartan group and 25% in patients receiving placebo (P = .032). Fewer cardiovascular deaths and hospital admissions for congestive heart failure (CHF) were observed in the candesartan group. Pooled analyses of the CHARM studies demonstrated that RRR of mortality was 12% with candesartan. The composite outcome of cardiovascular death and nonfatal MI was reduced by 13% (P = .012).

ANGIOTENSIN RECEPTOR BLOCKERS IN NEPHROPATHY

The renoprotective effect of the ARBs is the constellation of improved renal blood flow and endothelial function, usually by reducing intraglomerular pressure and preserving NO activity. This finding has been confirmed in animal and human studies. In rat models, the use of valsartan reduced albuminuria and chronic allograft rejection. AT1 receptor blockade leads to an increase in circulating ang II, which stimulates the unblocked AT2 receptor. The result is pressure natriuresis and vasodilatation because of an increased NO and bradykinin production.

The role of the renin-angiotensin axis and its interaction with endothelium and insulin-signaling pathways seems to have potential in prevention of diabetes and end-stage renal disease in using agents that block the RAAS. Clinical trials have shown the effects of ARBs on renal disease progression in high-risk patients (**Table 3**). ARBs reduce or eliminate microalbuminuria, an early sign of renal damage. The benefit of ARB therapy has also been demonstrated in patients who have nondiabetic nephropathy.

In the Reduction of Endpoints in NIDDM with the Angiotensin II Antagonist Losartan (RENAAL) study,[67] losartan compared with placebo significantly reduced serum creatinine, end-stage renal disease, and death in patients who had diabetic nephropathy (RR = 0.84; P = .02, number needed to treat [NNT] = 28). A new subgroup analysis of most cardiovascular outcomes showed no significant differences, but favored irbesartan over placebo for HF (P = .048.)

In two other studies, irbesartan was studied in patients who had diabetic nephropathy. In the Irbesartan in Diabetic Nephropathy Trial (IDNT),[68] when compared with amlodipine irbesartan showed significant reduction of overt proteinuria, end-stage renal disease, and doubling of serum creatinine (RR = 0.80, P = .02, NNT = 16). In the Irbesartan in Patients with Type 2 Diabetes and Microalbuminuria trial (IRMA),[69] therapy with 150 mg or 300 mg of irbesartan was compared with placebo. The primary endpoint of the study was the onset of overt nephropathy, which was defined as urinary albumin excretion rate greater than 200 μg/min and at least 30% higher than baseline. Irbesartan showed RRR of 44% and 68% (150 mg and 300 mg of irbesartan, respectively) versus conventional therapy.

The Combination Treatment of Angiotensin II Receptor Blocker and Angiotensin-Converting Enzyme Inhibitor in Nondiabetic Renal Disease (COOPERATE)[70] study evaluated the combination of losartan and trandolapril in patients who had nondiabetic nephropathy and showed significant reduction in composite endpoint of doubling of the serum creatinine or end-stage renal disease compared with either treatment alone (RRR 62% and 60% for losartan and trandolapril, respectively). These results not only emphasize the role of ARB in nondiabetic nephropathy but also demonstrate the benefit of combination therapy with ACEIs and ARBs. In the Irbesartan in the Management of Proteinuric Patients at High Risk for Vascular Events trial (IMPROVE),[71] combination of ramipril and irbesartan compared with ramipril showed a greater reduction in onset of overt proteinuria but did not achieve statistical significance (46% versus 42%, P not significant). This finding has led to the suggestion of using monotherapy with RAAS blockers in early-stage renal disease and relatively low albumin excretion, and combination therapy in patients who have heavier proteinuria who have failed monotherapy.

PREVENTION OF DIABETES MELLITUS WITH ANGIOTENSIN RECEPTOR BLOCKERS
Pathophysiologic Basis

In obese patients who are diabetic, there is a potential inhibition of the differentiation of the human preadipocytes into mature adipocytes. This inhibition is in part attributable to an up-regulation of angiotensinogen and angiotensin II receptor overexpression in the adipose tissue.[72–74] This phenomenon is supported by the promotion of preadipocyte differentiation in vitro by the ARBs. An overexpression of angiotensin receptors in obesity leads to inhibition of peroxisome proliferator-activated receptor (PPAR)–γ activity, which might lead to insulin resistance.[73–75] Activation of this nuclear receptor might have a significant role in diabetes prevention. Irbesartan and telmisartan have been shown to enhance PPAR-γ activation in vitro and to increase adiponectin secretion by adipocytes, both of which might result in improved insulin sensitivity and lead to prevention of diabetes and atherogenicity.[76,77] BMI has been shown to have a positive correlation with increasing circulating plasma ang II and TNF-α levels. A positive relation has also been demonstrated between hyperinsulinemia, TNF-α levels, and ang II secretion from the adipose tissue. Higher levels of circulating ang II are known to be associated with hypertension and hyperinsulinemia. They are also considered a proinflammatory factor, leading to expression of inflammatory genes in vascular smooth muscle cells.[78,79]

Table 3
Clinical studies of angiotensin receptor blockers in coronary heart disease and heart failure

Trial	Condition	n	Follow-up	ARB	Outcome	Results
DETAIL	T2DM	250	5 y	Telmisartan versus enalapril	Decline in GFR; ESRD; all cause mortality	Non-inferiority to enalapril
CALM	HTN, T2DM, microalbuminuria	199	3 mo	Candesartan, lisinopril or both	Change in BP and UA/Cr	Combination: decrease in BP and UA/Cr > versus candesartan or lisinopril
IMPROVE	HTN, microalbuminuria	405	5 mo	Irbesartan, ramipril, or both	Reduction in urine albumin excretion	Combination 46% ↓; ramipril 42% ↓ (*P* not significant)
COOPERATE	Nondiabetic nephropathy	263	2.9 y	Losartan, trandolapril, or both	Time to doubling of serum creatinine, ESRD	RRR 62% combination versus trandolapril; 60% versus losartan
IRMA-2	Diabetic nephropathy	590	3 mo	Irbesartan versus placebo	Albuminuria, overt proteinuria	24% ↓ with 150 mg and 38% with 300 mg, 70% ↓ in proteinuria
IDNT	Diabetic nephropathy	1715	2.6 y	Irbesartan versus amlodipine versus placebo	ESRD, doubling of serum creatinine	23% RRR versus placebo, 20% versus amlodipine
RENAAL	Diabetic nephropathy	1513	3.4 y	Losartan versus placebo	Composite, ESRD, 2X serum creatinine, death	16% RRR composite, 25% ↓ in 2X serum creatinine, no change in death
MARVAL	Diabetic nephropathy, HTN	332	6 mo	Valsartan versus amlodipine	Urinary albumin excretion rate	29.6% ↓ with valsartan versus 17.2%, ↑ with amlodipine

Abbreviations: CALM, Candesartan And Lisinopril Microalbuminuria trial; COOPERATE, Combination Treatment of Angiotensin II Receptor Blocker and Angiotensin-Converting Enzyme Inhibitor in Nondiabetic Renal Disease Trial; DETAIL, Diabetics Exposed to Telmisartan and Enalapril; ESRD, end-stage renal disease; GFR, glomerular filtration rate; HTN, hypertension; IDNT, Irbesartan in Diabetic Nephropathy Trial; IMPROVE, Irbesartan in the Management of Proteinuric Patients at High Risk for Vascular Events trial; IRMA, Irbesartan in Patients with Type 2 Diabetes and Microalbuminuria trial; MARVAL, Microalbuminuria Reduction With Valsartan; RENAAL, Reduction of Endpoints in NIDDM with the Angiotensin II Antagonist Losartan trial; UA/Cr, uric acid/creatinine ratio.

Another proposed pathway to insulin resistance in obese patients who have diabetes is the ang II–mediated phosphorylation of insulin signaling cascade. Significant vasoconstrictive effects of ang II on pancreatic vasculature hasten islet cell apoptosis. Increased oxidative stress secondary to RAAS activation has also been related to beta cell destruction. RAAS inhibition attenuates this negative response in the islet cells. Furthermore, unaffected bradykinin and NO production from ARBs improves blood flow to the skeletal muscle leading to enhanced insulin-mediated glucose disposal. In part, glucose use is increased by overexpression of GLUT 4.[80,81]

Clinical Evidence

Numerous studies have validated that ARBs, like ACEIs, may also reduce the onset of diabetes in high-risk patients (**Table 4**). Earlier data from the Antihypertensive Treatment and Lipid Profile in a North of Sweden Efficacy study (ALPINE)[82] showed that candesartan in comparison to hydrochlorothiazide significantly decreased new onset of diabetes (RR = 0.13; CI = 0.02–0.97; $P = .03$). In the CHARM study, candesartan again showed a 19% reduction in the new onset of diabetes (RR = 0.81; CI = 0.66–0.97) compared with placebo in patients who had chronic HF.

Similar results have been reported in the VALUE trial, suggesting a 23% reduction (RR = 0.77; CI = 0.69–0.86; $P < .001$) in new onset of diabetes in a hypertensive population with valsartan in comparison to amlodipine. The CHARM program showed that incidence of developing diabetes showed a 22% reduction in patients receiving candesartan compared with placebo.

In a recent comprehensive meta-analysis, assessment was made pertaining to the onset of diabetes in patients treated with ACEI or ARB.[83] Thirteen randomized trials were included that had enrolled 93,451 high-risk patients who did not have diabetes, of whom 42,780 patients received an ACEI or an ARB. These patients had either hypertension, left ventricular dysfunction, or vascular disease. A total of 2989 new cases of type II diabetes were observed in patients treated with the RAAS-blocking agent (7.12%) compared with 4528 events in 50,671 patients in the control group (8.95%), with an absolute risk reduction of 1.85% ($P < .001$). The number needed to treat to prevent one new case of diabetes averaged 46 over a 4- to 5-year period. Diabetes developed in 6.5% of patients randomized to ACEIs compared with 8.4% in placebo (odds ratio [OR] = 0.73; $P < .001$) and 8.2% in ARBs compared with 10.5% in placebo (OR = 0.73; $P < .001$).

There are multiple limitations in recommending ARBs for prevention of diabetes, however. First, the aforementioned studies had different baseline characteristics. Second, the use of thiazide diuretics and beta-blockers has been variable within all studies, because both agents have deleterious effects on glycemic control. Third, none of the studies have addressed new onset of diabetes as a primary endpoint and most of the data are based on post hoc analyses. Furthermore, the negative results of the Diabetes Reduction Assessment with Ramipril and Rosiglitazone Medication (DREAM) study have also raised doubts about the role of RAAS blockade for prevention of diabetes.

COMBINATION THERAPY WITH ANGIOTENSIN-CONVERTING ENZYME INHIBITORS AND ANGIOTENSIN RECEPTOR BLOCKERS IN HIGH-RISK GROUPS

When we re-evaluate the RAAS, we know that ACEIs block formation of ang II and degradation of bradykinin, whereas ARBs directly inhibit binding of ang II to AT1 receptors. As mentioned before, ACEIs may not completely block alternate pathways involved in the formation of ang II. Studies have shown that circulating ang II levels return to normal or may even increase with chronic ACE inhibition. This phenomenon, so-called "ACE escape," suggests poor long-term inhibition of RAAS with ACEIs. It has been suggested that a more comprehensive RAAS blockade with ACEI and ARB combination may be synergistic because of different sites and mechanisms of action. Recent observations, however, have provided mixed results with combination therapy as an effective option for rendering cardioprotective benefits.

Because of the synergistic effect, combination therapy with an ACE inhibitor and ARB seems more effective than monotherapy for treating hypertension. In a small study of 177 patients who had hypertension, losartan plus enalapril more effectively reduced diastolic blood pressure than either losartan or enalapril alone ($P = .012$ and $P = .002$, respectively).[23]

The Candesartan And Lisinopril Microalbuminuria (CALM)[84] study evaluated the effects of a combination of candesartan and lisinopril on blood pressure and urinary albumin excretion in a high-risk population with microalbuminuria, hypertension, and type 2 diabetes. The combined regimen reduced diastolic blood pressure 16.3 mm Hg compared with 10.4 mm Hg for candesartan and 10.7 mm Hg for lisinopril alone ($P < .001$). The combination therapy reduced the urinary

Table 4
Angiotensin receptor blocker trials of prevention of type 2 diabetes mellitus by renin-angiotensin-aldosterone inhibition

Study	Treatment Arm: Subjects who had New DM	Treatment Arm: Subjects who did not have DM	Control Arm: Subjects who had New DM	Control Arm: Subjects who did not have DM	Relative Risk (RR)	CI	P-value Favoring Treatment Arm
LIFE (2002)	241	4006	319	3592	0.75	0.63–0.88	$P = .001$
SOLVD (2003)	9	153	31	138	0.26	0.13–0.53	$P < .001$
ALPINE (2003)	1	196	8	196	0.13	0.02–0.97	$P = .03$
SCOPE (2003)	93	2160	115	2170	0.75	0.62–1.06	NS
CHARM (2003)	163	2715	202	2721	0.81	0.66–0.97	$P < .001$
VALUE (2004)	690	5267	845	5152	0.77	0.69–0.86	$P < .0001$

Abbreviation: NS, not significant; SCOPE, The Study on Cognition and Prognosis in the Elderly; SOLVD, Studies Of Left Ventricular Dysfunction.

albumin/creatinine ratio by 50% compared with 24% for candesartan and 39% for lisinopril alone (*P* < .001). In another study of 108 patients who had progressive chronic renal disease,[85] the combination of valsartan and benazepril significantly reduced systolic and diastolic blood pressures (*P* < .001). This combination also resulted in a −0.82 ± 1.63 change in the proteinuria/creatinuria ratio from baseline to the end of the study compared with valsartan alone (*P* = .047). The benefits of combination therapy with ACEI and ARB in patients who have HF have been described previously. ValHeFT and CHARM-Added studies clearly showed beneficial effects, with CHARM-Added showing significant reduction in cardiovascular mortality and morbidity in patients who had HF.

THE ONTARGET STUDY

The Telmisartan Alone and in combination with Ramipril Global Endpoint Trial (ONTARGET)[86] was a landmark trial that evaluated the cardioprotective properties of telmisartan, ramipril, or their combination. This study compared the effectiveness of 80 mg of telmisartan versus 10 mg of ramipril versus combinations of the two in 25,620 high-risk patients. Baseline characteristics included controlled blood pressure, age 55 years or older with a history of CAD, peripheral arterial disease, stroke, or TIA within a week to less than a year, or complicated patients who had diabetes with end-organ damage. Overall, the study population in the ONTARGET was similar to that enrolled in the HOPE trial.[43] The primary outcome was the composite endpoint of cardiovascular mortality, stroke, acute MI, and hospitalization for CHF. Secondary outcomes include newly diagnosed CHF, a revascularization procedure, newly diagnosed diabetes, development of cognitive decline or dementia, new onset of atrial fibrillation, and nephropathy. The study results showed that mean blood pressure was lowered in the telmisartan group (a 0.9/0.6 mm Hg greater reduction than ramipril) and the combination therapy group (a 2.4/1.4 mm Hg greater reduction than ramipril). At a median follow-up of 56 months, the primary events had occurred in 1412 (16.5%), 1423 (16.7%), and 1386 (16.3%) patients, respectively, in the ramipril, telmisartan, and combination groups (RR 1.01 and 0.99 for the telmisartan and combination arms, respectively), showing no difference between the treatment arms. There was no significant difference in other primary or secondary outcomes. None of the secondary outcomes were achieved. When compared with the ramipril group, the telmisartan group had lower rates of cough and angioedema but higher rates

of hypotensive symptoms. In the combination group, there was higher risk for hypotensive symptoms (4.8% versus 1.7%, *P* < .001), syncope (0.3% versus 0.2%, *P* = .03), and renal dysfunction (13.5% versus 10.2%, *P* < .001). This study established the non-inferiority of telmisartan to ramipril. There was no additional benefit of combination therapy because of additive adverse effects (see **Fig. 3**).

Although in a different group of patients, the results of ONTARGET are in accordance with VALIANT,[59] which compared the effects of dual-agent RAAS blockade in patients who had signs of HF with depressed left ventricular function. Likewise, the non-inferiority of ARB (valsartan) to ACEI (captopril) was confirmed; however, no additional cardiovascular benefit was observed with combined therapy. In ONTARGET and VALIANT, combination therapy was associated with higher rate of side effects and discontinuation rates. Based on these results, there does not seem to be any rationale for the use of combination therapy with ACEIs and ARBs in high-risk hypertensive and post-MI patients. Such a combination is indeed beneficial in patients who have HF, however.

FUTURE DIRECTIONS

Given the essential contribution of angiotensin II in regulating blood pressure and endothelial function and vascular and cardiac remodeling, RAAS blockade has been inculcated as inevitable part of cardiovascular therapeutics in various conditions. Studies are under way to determine whether doses greater than those used in the previous trials

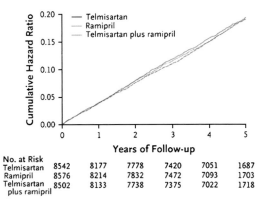

No. at Risk						
Telmisartan	8542	8177	7778	7420	7051	1687
Ramipril	8576	8214	7832	7472	7093	1703
Telmisartan plus ramipril	8502	8133	7738	7375	7022	1718

Fig. 3. Kaplan-Meier curves for the primary outcome in the three study groups. The composite primary outcome was death from cardiovascular causes, MI, stroke, or hospitalization for HF. (*From* ONTARGET Investigators, Yusuf S, Teo KK, Pogue J, et al. Telmisartan, ramipril, or both in patients at high risk for vascular events. N Engl J Med 2008;358:1553; with permission. Copyright © 2008, Massachusetts Medical Society.)

or combination of ARB and ACEI therapy will provide more extensive RAAS inhibition and greater protection from end-organ damage in various high-risk groups.

The Telmisartan Randomized Assessment Study in ACE-Intolerant Subjects with Cardiovascular Disease (TRANSCEND) trial[87] is evaluating telmisartan in reducing cardiovascular risk independent of blood pressure reduction. The Irbesartan in Heart Failure with Preserved Systolic Function (I-PRESERVE)[88] trial will evaluate irbesartan therapy in elderly patients (>60 years of age) who have a clinical diagnosis of HF with preserved systolic function. The largest secondary stroke prevention trial undertaken to date, Prevention Regimen for Effectively Avoiding Second Strokes (PROFESS),[89] is currently comparing the efficacy and safety of aspirin plus extended-release dipyridamole with clopidogrel, and of telmisartan with placebo, in preventing recurrent strokes. Finally, ROADMAP[90] is a large-scale trial to assess renoprotective effects of olmesartan. This study will assess the onset of microalbuminuria in patients who have type 2 diabetes.

SUMMARY

When extrapolating results from various clinical studies of the ARBs it should be noted that most ARB trials compared the efficacy of the ARB with another drug. The ValHeft and CHARM studies addressed the specified outcomes comparing the combination therapy with ARBs versus placebo on all-cause mortality or cardiovascular events in HF. None of the trials compared one ARB to another. As a group, these studies do not provide useful information to compare the effectiveness of different ARBs specifically in patients who have high blood pressure and no other compelling indications.

The available level of evidence establishes RAAS blockade as a strategic therapeutic option for high-risk patients because it regulates blood pressure, vascular response to injury, and cardiac and vascular remodeling. Future strategies for treating high-risk patients will focus on early interventions that prevent or delay end-organ damage. The role of ACE inhibitors is well established in this regard; however, there is now substantive evidence that this can be equally achieved with ARBs, which also effectively lower BP and prevent end-organ damage. As our understanding of the pharmacotherapeutics of ARBs improves, the combination RAAS blockade may be reserved for special patient groups, such as those who have diabetic nephropathy or HF. With close consideration of safety and tolerability, individualizing

treatment by using ARBs that have proven efficacy for specific disease states will be the key to this approach.

REFERENCES

1. Kannel WB. Hazards, risks, and threats of heart disease from the early stages to symptomatic coronary heart disease and cardiac failure. Cardiovasc Drugs Ther 1997;11(Suppl 1):199–212.
2. Wild S, Roglic G, Green A, et al. Global prevalence of diabetes: estimates for the year 2000 and projections for 2030. Diabetes Care 2004;27:1047–53.
3. Narayan KM, Boyle JP, Thompson TJ, et al. Lifetime risk for diabetes mellitus in the United States. JAMA 2003;290:1884–90.
4. Lewington S, Clarke R, Qizilbash N, et al. Age-specific relevance of usual blood pressure to vascular mortality: a meta-analysis of individual data for one million adults in 61 prospective studies. Lancet 2002;360:1903–13.
5. Steinberger J, Daniels SR. Obesity, insulin resistance, diabetes, and cardiovascular risk in children: an American Heart Association scientific statement from the Atherosclerosis, Hypertension, and Obesity in the Young Committee (Council on Cardiovascular Disease in the Young) and the Diabetes Committee (Council on Nutrition, Physical Activity, and Metabolism). Circulation 2003;107:1448–53.
6. Hedley A, Ogden C, Johnson C, et al. Prevalence of overweight and obesity among US children, adolescents, and adults, 1999–2002. JAMA 2004;291:2847–50.
7. Third report of the National Cholesterol Education Program (NCEP) expert panel on detection, evaluation and treatment of high blood cholesterol in adults (adult treatment panel III). National cholesterol education program, National Heart, Lung, and Blood Institute, National Institutes of Health. Circulation 2002;106:3143–421.
8. Sowers JR. Obesity as a cardiovascular risk factor. Am J Med 2003;115(Suppl 8A):37S–41S.
9. McFarlane SI, Jacober SJ, Winer N, et al. Control of cardiovascular risk factors in patients with diabetes and hypertension at urban academic medical centers. Diabetes Care 2002;25:718–23.
10. Williams B, Poulter N, Brown M, et al. British hypertension society guidelines for hypertension management (BHS-IV): summary. BMJ 2004;328:634–40.
11. Neal B, Macmahon S, Chapman N. Effects of ACE inhibitors, calcium antagonists, and other blood-pressure lowering drugs: results of prospectively designed overviews of randomized trials. Blood Pressure Lowering Treatment Trialists' Collaboration. Lancet 2000;356:1955–64.
12. Effects of different regimens to lower blood pressure on major cardiovascular events in older and younger

adults: meta-analysis of randomized trials. Blood Pressure Lowering Treatment Trialists' Collaboration. BMJ 2008;336:1121–3.

13. Casas J, Chua W, Loukogeorgakis S, et al. Effect of inhibitors of the renin-angiotensin system and other antihypertensive drugs on renal outcomes: systematic review and meta-analysis. Lancet 2005;366: 2026–33.

14. Kempler P. Learning from large cardiovascular clinical trials: classical cardiovascular risk factors. Diabetes Res Clin Pract 2005;68(Suppl 1):S43–7.

15. Stamler J, Vaccaro O, Neaton JD, et al. Diabetes, other risk factors, and 12-yr cardiovascular mortality for men screened in the multiple risk factor intervention trial. Diabetes Care 1993;16:434–44.

16. Centers for Disease Control and prevention. National diabetes fact sheet: general information and national estimates on diabetes in the United States, 2005. Atlanta (GA): US Department of Health and Human Services, Centers for Disease Control and Prevention; 2005.

17. Seventh report of the joint national committee on prevention, detection, and treatment of high blood pressure. Hypertension 2003;42:1206–52.

18. Lip GY, beevers DG. More evidence on blocking the renin-angiotensin-aldosterone system in cardiovascular disease and the long-term treatment of hypertension: data from recent clinical trials (CHARM, EUROPA, ValHeFT, HOPE-TOO and SYST-EUR2). J Hum Hypertens 2003;17:747–50.

19. Khaper N, Singal PK. Modulation of oxidative stress by a selective inhibition of angiotensin II type 1 receptors in MI rats. J Am Coll Cardiol 2001;37:1461–6.

20. Leiter LA, Lewanczuk RZ. Of the renin-angiotensin system and reactive oxygen species type 2 diabetes and angiotensin II inhibition. Am J Hypertens 2005;18:121–8.

21. Watanabe S, Tagawa T, Yamakawa K, et al. Inhibition of the renin-angiotensin system prevents free fatty acid–induced acute endothelial dysfunction in humans. Arterioscler Thromb Vasc Biol 2005;25: 2376–80.

22. Unger T, Culman J, Gohlke P. Angiotensin II receptor blockade and end-organ protection: pharmacological rationale and evidence. J Hypertens 1998; 16(Suppl 7):S3–9.

23. Andraws R, Brown DL. Effect of inhibition of the renin-angiotensin system on development of type 2 diabetes mellitus (meta-analysis of randomized trials). Am J Cardiol 2007;99:1006–12.

24. McCall KL, Craddock D, Edwards K. Effect of angiotensin-converting enzyme inhibitors and angiotensin II type 1 receptor blockers on the rate of new-onset diabetes mellitus: a review and pooled analysis. Pharmacotherapy 2006;26:1297–306.

25. Tsouli SG, Liberopoulos EN, Kiortsis DN, et al. Combined treatment with angiotensin-converting enzyme inhibitors and angiotensin II receptor blockers: a review of the current evidence. J Cardiovasc Pharmacol Ther 2006;11:1–15.

26. Luno J, Praga M, de Vinuesa SG. The renoprotective effect of the dual blockade of the renin angiotensin system (RAS). Curr Pharm Des 2005; 11:1291–300.

27. Chung O, Stoll M, Unger T. Physiologic and pharmacologic implications of AT_1 versus AT_2 recpetors. Blood Press 1996;5(Suppl 2):47–52.

28. Johnston CI, Risvanis J. Preclinical pharmacology of angiotensin II receptor antagonists: update and outstanding issues. Am J Hypertens 1997;10: 306S–10S.

29. Timmermans PB, Wong PC, Chiu AT, et al. Angiotensin II receptors and angiotensin II receptor antagonists. Pharmacol Rev 1993;45:205–51.

30. Drexler H, Hornig B. Endothelial dysfunction in human disease. J Mol Cell Cardiol 1999;31:51–60.

31. Britten MB, Zeiher AM, Schachinger V. Clinical importance of coronary endothelial vasodilator dysfunction and therapeutic options. J Intern Med 1999;245:315–27.

32. Fishel RS, Eisenberg S, Shai SY, et al. Glucocorticoids induce angiotensin-converting enzyme expression in vascular smooth muscle. Hypertension 1995;25:343–9.

33. Brown NJ, Agirbasli MA, Williams GH, et al. Effect of activation and inhibition of the rennin-angiotensin system on plasma PAI-1. Hypertension 1998;32: 965–71.

34. Gainer JV, Morrow JD, Loveland A, et al. Effect of bradykinin-receptor blockade on the response to angiotensin-converting enzyme inhibitor in normotensive and hypertensive subjects. N Engl J Med 1998;339:1285–92.

35. Hornig B, Kohler C, Drexler H. Role of bradykinin in mediating vascular effects of angiotensin-converting enzyme inhibitors in humans. Circulation 1997;95: 1115–8.

36. Diet F, Pratt RE, Berry GJ, et al. Increased accumulation of tissue ACE in human atherosclerotic coronary artery disease. Circulation 1996;94:2756–67.

37. Willemsen JM, Westerink JW, Dallinga-Thie GM, et al. Angiotensin II type 1 receptor blockade improves hyperglycemia-induced endothelial dysfunction and reduces proinflammatory cytokine release from leukocytes. J Cardiovasc Pharmacol 2007;49:6–12.

38. Fiordaliso F, Cuccovillo I, Bianchi R, et al. Cardiovascular oxidative stress is reduced by an ACE inhibitor in a rat model of streptozotocin-induced diabetes. Life Sci 2006;79:121–9.

39. Nascimben L, Bothwell JH, Dominguez DY, et al. Angiotensin II stimulates insulin-independent glucose uptake in hypertrophied rat hearts. [abstract]. J Hypertens 1997;15(Suppl 4):S84.

40. Lyon CJ, Law RE, Hsueh WA. Minireview: adiposity, inflammation, and atherogenesis. Endocrinology 2003;144:2195–200.

41. Moule KS, Denton RM. Multiple signaling pathways involved in the metabolic effects of insulin. Am J Cardiol 1997;80:41A–9A.

42. Hansson L, Lindholm LH, Niskanen L, et al. Effect of angiotensin-converting-enzyme inhibition compared with conventional therapy on cardiovascular morbidity and mortality in hypertension: the Captopril Prevention Project (CAPPP) randomised trial. Lancet 1999;353:611–6.

43. Yusuf S, Sleight P, Pogue J, et al. Effects of an angiotensin-converting-enzyme inhibitor, ramipril, on cardiovascular events in high-risk patients. The Heart Outcomes Prevention Evaluation Study Investigators. N Engl J Med 2000;342:145–53.

44. Effects of long-term vitamin E supplementation on cardiovascular events and cancer: a randomized controlled trial. The HOPE and HOPE-TOO Trial Investigators. JAMA 2005;293:1338–47.

45. Fox KM. Efficacy of perindopril in reduction of cardiovascular events among patients with stable coronary artery disease: randomised, double-blind, placebo-controlled, multicentre trial (the EUROPA study). Lancet 2003;362:782–8.

46. Schorb W, Peeler TC, Madigan NN, et al. Angiotensin II-induced protein tyrosine phosphorylation in neonatal rat. J Biol Chem 1994;269:19626–32.

47. Wan J, Kurosaki T, Huant XY, et al. Tyrosine kinases in activation of the MAP-kinase cascade by G protein-coupled receptors. Nature 1996;380:541–4.

48. Saad MJ, Velloso LA, Carvalho CR. Angiotensin II induces tyrosine phosphorylation of insulin receptor substrate 1 and its association with phosphatidylinositol 3-kinase in rat heart. Biochem J 1995;310:741–4.

49. Bernobich E, de Angelis L, Lerin C, et al. The role of the angiotensin system in cardiac glucose homeostasis: therapeutic implications. Drugs 2002;62:1295–314.

50. Higashi Y, Chayama K, Yoshizumi M. Angiotensin II Type I receptor blocker and endothelial function in humans: role of nitric oxide and oxidative stress. Curr Med Chem 2005;3:133–48.

51. The ALLHAT Officers and Coordinators for the ALLHAT Collaborative Research Group. Major outcomes in high-risk hypertensive patients randomized to angiotensin-converting enzyme inhibitor or calcium channel blocker vs diuretic: the antihypertensive and lipid-lowering treatment to prevent heart attack trial (ALLHAT). JAMA 2002;288(23):2981–97.

52. Dahlof B, Devereux RB, Kjeldsen SE, et al. Cardiovascular morbidity and mortality in the losartan intervention for endpoint reduction in hypertension study (LIFE): a randomized trial against atenolol. Lancet 2002;359:995–1003.

53. Seventh report of the joint national committee on prevention, detection, and treatment of high blood pressure. U.S. Department of Health and Human Services. National Institutes of Health. National Heart, Lung, and Blood Institute. NIH Publication No. 04-5230; 2004.

54. Julius S, Nesbitt SD, Egan BM, et al. The Trial of Preventing Hypertension (TROPHY) Study Investigators. Feasibility of treating prehypertension with an angiotensin-receptor blocker. N Engl J Med 2006;354(16):1685–97.

55. Schrader J, Luders S, Kulschewski A, et al. Morbidity and mortality after stroke, eprosartan compared with nitrendipine for secondary prevention: principal results of a prospective randomized controlled study (MOSES). Stroke 2005;36:1218–26.

56. Julius S, Kjeldsen SE, Weber M, et al. Outcomes in hypertensive patients at high cardiovascular risk treated with regimens based on valsartan or amlodipine: the VALUE randomised trial. Lancet 2004;363:2022–31.

57. Ikejima H, Imanishi T, Tsujioka H, et al. Effects of telmisartan, a unique angiotensin receptor blocker with selective peroxisome proliferator-activated receptor-gamma-modulating activity, on nitric oxide bioavailability and atherosclerotic change. J Hypertens 2008;2:964–72 [My paper].

58. Dickstein K, Kjekshus J. OPTIMAAL Steering Committee of the OPTIMAAL Study Group. Effects of losartan and captopril on mortality and morbidity in high-risk patients after acute myocardial infarction: the OPTIMAAL randomized trial. Optimal trial in myocardial infarction with angiotensin II antagonist losartan. Lancet 2002;360(9335):752–60.

59. Pfeffer MA, McMurray JJ, Velazquez EJ, et al. for the Valsartan in Acute Myocardial Infarction Trial Investigators. Valsartan, captopril, or both in myocardial infarction complicated by heart failure, left ventricular dysfunction, or both. N Engl J Med 2003;349:1893–906.

60. Pitt B, Poole-Wilson PA, Segal R, et al. Effect of losartan compared with captopril on mortality in patients with symptomatic heart failure: randomized trial – the Losartan Heart Failure Survival Study ELITE II. Lancet 2000;355(9215):1582–7.

61. Krum H, Carson P, Farsang C, et al. Effect of valsartan added to background ACE inhibitor therapy in patients with heart failure: results from Val-HeFT. Eur J Heart Fail 2004;6:937–45.

62. McKelvie RS, Yusuf S, Pericak D, et al. Comparison of candesartan, enalapril, and their combination in congestive heart failure: randomized evaluation of strategies for left ventricular dysfunction (RESOLVD) pilot study. Circulation 1999;100:1056–64.

63. Pfeffer MA, Swedberg K, Granger CB, et al. Effects of candesartan on mortality and morbidity in patients with chronic heart failure. Lancet 2003;362:759–66.

64. Granger CB, McMurray JJ, Yusuf S, et al. Effects of candesartan in patients with chronic heart failure and reduced left-ventricular systolic function intolerant to angiotensin-converting-enzyme inhibitors: the CHARM-Alternative trial. Lancet 2003;362:772–6.

65. Yusuf S, Pfeffer MA, Swedberg K. Effects of candesartan in patients with chronic heart failure and preserved left-ventricular systolic function taking angiotensin-converting-enzyme inhibitors: the CHARM-Preserved trial. Lancet 2003;362:777–81.

66. McMurray JJ, Ostergen J, Swedberg K, et al. Effects of candesartan in patients with chronic heart failure and reduced left-ventricular systolic function taking angiotensin-converting-enzyme inhibitors: the CHARM-Added trial. Lancet 2003;362:767–71.

67. Breener BM, Cooper ME, de Zeeuw D, et al. Effects of losartan on renal and cardiovascular outcomes in patients with type 2 diabetes and nephropathy. N Engl J Med 2001;345:861–9.

68. Lewis EJ, Hunsicker LG, Clarke WR, et al. Renoprotective effect of the angiotensin-receptor antagonist irbesartan in patients with nephropathy due to type 2 diabetes. N Engl J Med 2001;345:851–60.

69. Parving HH, Lehnert H, Brochner-Mortensen J, et al. The effect of irbesartan on the development of diabetic nephropathy in patients with type 2 diabetes. N Engl J Med 2001;345:870–8.

70. Nakao N, Yoshimura A, Morita H, et al. Combination treatment of angiotensin-II receptor blocker and angiotensin-converting-enzyme inhibitor in non-diabetic renal disease (COOPERATE): a randomised controlled trial. Lancet 2003;361:117–24 [erratum in: Lancet 2003;361:1230].

71. Bakris GL, Ruilope L, Locatelli F, et al. Treatment of microalbuminuria in hypertensive subjects with elevated cardiovascular risk: results of the IMPROVE trial. Kidney Int 2007;72:879–85.

72. Sharma AM, Janke J, Gorzelniak K, et al. Angiotensin blockade prevents type 2 diabetes by formation of fat cells. Hypertension 2002;40(5):609–11.

73. Furuhashi M, Ura N, Takizawa H, et al. Blockade of the rennin-angiotensin system decreases adipocyte size with improvement in insulin sensitivity. J Hypertens 2004;22(10):1977–82.

74. Kingston R. Blockade of the renin-angiotensin system decreases adipocyte size with improvement in insulin sensitivity. J Hypertens 2004;22:1867–8.

75. Jandeleit-Dahm KA, Tikellis C, Reid CM, et al. Why blockade of the renin-angiotensin system reduces the incidence of new-onset diabetes. J Hypertens 2005;23(3):463–73.

76. Mazzone T. Strategies in ongoing clinical trials to reduce cardiovascular disease in patients with diabetic mellitus and insulin resistance. Am J Cardiol 2004;93(11A):27C–31C.

77. Aranda JM Jr, Conti R. Angiotensin II blockade: a therapeutic strategy with wide applications. Clin Cardiol 2003;26:500–2.

78. Hsueh WA, Quinones MJ. Role of endothelial dysfunction in insulin resistance. Am J Cardiol 2003;92:10J–7J.

79. Carlsson PO, Bernie C, Jansson L. Angiotensin II and the endocrine pancreas; effects on islet blood flow and insulin secretion in rats. Diabetologia 1998;41(2):127–33.

80. Henriksen EJ, Jacob S. Angiotensin converting enzyme inhibitors and modulation of skeletal muscle insulin resistance. Diabetes Obes Metab 2003;5(4):214–22.

81. Henriksen EJ, Jacob S, Kinnick TR, et al. ACE inhibition and glucose transport in insulin resistant muscle: roles of bradykinin and nitric oxide. Am J Physiol 1999;277(1 Pt. 2):R332–6.

82. Lindholm LH, Persson M, Alaupovic P, et al. Metabolic outcome during 1 year in newly detected hypertensives: results of the antihypertensive treatment and lipid profile in a north of Sweden efficacy evaluation (ALPINE study). J Hypertens 2003;21(8):1563–74.

83. Azizi M, Linhart A, Alexander J, et al. Pilot study of combined blockade of the renin-angiotensin system in essential hypertensive patients. J Hypertens 2000;18:1139–47.

84. Mogensen CE, Neldam S, Tikkanen I, et al. Randomised controlled trial of dual blockade of renin-angiotensin system in patients with hypertension, microalbuminuria, and non-insulin dependent diabetes: the candesartan and lisinopril microalbuminuria (CALM) study. BMJ 2000;321:1440–4.

85. Ruilope LM, Aldigier JC, Ponticelli C, et al. Safety of the combination of valsartan and benazepril in patients with chronic renal disease. European Group for the Investigation of Valsartan in Chronic Renal Disease. J Hypertens 2000;18(1):89–95.

86. ONTARGET Investigators, Yusuf S, Teo KK, Pogue J, et al. Telmisartan, ramipril, or both in patients at high risk for vascular events. N Engl J Med 2008;358:1547–59.

87. Teo K, Yusuf S, Sleight P, et al. ONTARGET/TRANSCEND Investigators. Rationale, design, and baseline characteristics of 2 large, simple, randomized trials evaluating telmisartan, ramipril, and their combination in high-risk patients: the Ongoing Telmisartan Alone and in Combination with Ramipril Global Endpoint Trial/Telmisartan Randomized Assessment Study in ACE intolerant subjects with cardiovascular disease (ONTARGET/TRANSCEND) trials. Am Heart J 2004;148:52–61.

88. Diener HC, Sacco R, Yusuf S, et al. Steering Committee; PRoFESS Study Group. Rationale, design and baseline data of a randomized, double-blind, controlled trial comparing two antithrombotic

regimens (a fixed-dose combination of extended-release dipyridamole plus ASA with clopidogrel) and telmisartan versus placebo in patients with strokes: the prevention regimen for effectively avoiding second strokes trial (PRoFESS). Cerebrovasc Dis 2007;23:368–80.

89. McMurray JJ, Carson PE, Komajda M, et al. Heart failure with preserved ejection fraction: clinical characteristics of 4133 patients enrolled in the I-PRESERVE trial. Eur J Heart Fail 2008;10: 149–56.

90. Haller H, Viberti GC, Mimran A, et al. Preventing microalbuminuria in patients with diabetes: rationale and design of the Randomised Olmesartan and Diabetes Microalbuminuria Prevention (ROADMAP) study. J Hypertens 2006;24(2):403–8.

Renin Inhibitors: Novel Agents for Renoprotection or a Better Angiotensin Receptor Blocker for Blood Pressure Lowering?

Eduardo Pimenta, MD[a],*, Suzanne Oparil, MD[b]

KEYWORDS
- Hypertension • Renin inhibitors
- Renin-angiotensin-aldosterone system

The renin-angiotensin-aldosterone system (RAAS) is an important modulator of blood pressure (BP) and volume regulation in both normotensive and hypertensive persons.[1] The development of pharmacologic antagonists to its various components has proved useful in the treatment of hypertension and related target-organ damage. Renin, which is synthesized and released predominately from the juxtaglomerular granular epithelioid cells in the kidney, catalyzes the formation of angiotensin (Ang) I from angiotensinogen. Ang I, in turn, is processed by angiotensin-converting enzyme (ACE) and other proteases to form Ang II (**Fig. 1**). Renin is required for the production of Ang I and II.

Renin is synthesized as a preprohormone that contains a signal peptide that leads the inactive molecule to the exterior of the cell.[2] Prorenin is rendered enzymatically active by both proteolytic and nonproteolytic processes. Proteolytic activation occurs via the actual removal of the pro-peptide chain. Most proteolytic activation of prorenin occurs within the juxtaglomerular cells.[3] Nonproteolytic activation is a 2-step process that allows prorenin that has been secreted from the juxtaglomerular cells into the circulation to acquire enzymatic activity without removal of the pro-segment. While both prorenin and active renin are secreted from the juxtaglomerular cells into the circulation, prorenin is the predominant circulating form, accounting for approximately 90% of total renin in normal human plasma and for an even greater portion of the total in diabetic patients.[4–6]

The major physiologic and pathophysiologic effects of the RAAS are mediated by the octapeptide Ang II. Ang II has a variety of biological actions that lead to hypertension and related target organ damage. It is a potent vasoconstrictor and

Dr. Pimenta has no conflicts. Dr. Oparil has received grants-in-aid from Abbott Laboratories, Astra Zeneca, Boehringer Ingelheim, Bristol Myers-Squibb, Daiichi-Sankyo, Forest Laboratories, GlaxoSmithKline, Novartis, Merck & Co, Pfizer, Sankyo, Sanofi-Aventis, and Schering-Plough; and has served as a consultant for Bristol Myers-Squibb, Daiichi Sankyo, Merck & Co, Novartis, Pfizer, Sanofi Aventis, and The Salt Institute.

[a] Department of Hypertension and Nephrology, Dante Pazzanese Institute of Cardiology, Av. Dr. Dante Pazzanese, 500, Sao Paulo, SP, Brazil, 04012-909.
[b] Vascular Biology and Hypertension Program, University of Alabama at Birmingham, 703 19th Street South, ZRB 1034, Birmingham, AL 35294-2041, USA
* Corresponding author.
E-mail address: espimenta@hotmail.com (E. Pimenta).

Cardiol Clin 26 (2008) 527–535
doi:10.1016/j.ccl.2008.06.003

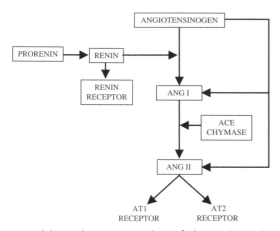

Fig. 1. Schematic representation of the renin-angiotensin-aldosterone system. ACE, angiotensin-converting enzyme; Ang, angiotensin; AT1, angiotensin II type 1 receptor; AT2, angiotensin II type 2 receptor.

stimulates sodium retention directly via renal vascular and tubular effects and indirectly by increasing aldosterone synthesis and release, thirst, and antidiuretic hormone release. Ang II also increases sympathetic outflow from the brain and norepinephrine release from peripheral sympathetic nerve terminals. In addition, Ang II is a potent growth hormone and mitogen, inducing both cell hyperplasia and hypertrophy. Importantly, Ang II inhibits renin release via a feedback mechanism that tends to stabilize BP in the normal range in normotensive individuals.

The actions of Ang II can be antagonized by blocking Ang II at the AT1 receptor site or by reducing the generation of Ang II. β-blockers (BB) inhibit the β-adrenergic receptor-mediated release of renin from the kidney, thus reducing plasma renin activity (PRA).[7,8] However, renin secretion from the juxtaglomerular cells is also regulated by chloride transport across the renal macula densa cells. Ang II receptor activity and renal perfusion pressure play important roles in renin release as well. β-adrenergic blockade alone

can therefore only partially decrease the secretion of renin and reduce the generation of Ang II.

ACE inhibitors and angiotensin receptor blockers (ARB) lower BP and prevent target organ damage and cardiovascular disease events by blocking the RAAS. ACE inhibitors were first developed as an unintended consequence of the search for an explanation for the drop in BP induced by the venom of a pit viper.[9] The discovery in the venom of the snake *Bothrops jararaca* of a peptide that blocked kininase II led to the synthesis of the ACE inhibitors.[10,11] ACE inhibitors are potent orally active inhibitors of the enzyme that converts the inactive decapeptide Ang I into the active octapeptide Ang II. Although ACE inhibitors decrease Ang II generation, they stimulate PRA by blocking feedback inhibition of renin release (**Table 1**). ARBs are selective antagonists of the AT1 receptor of Ang II that also stimulate PRA via blockade of Ang II–mediated feedback inhibition of renin release.

More recently, aliskiren, the first in a new class of orally effective direct renin inhibitors (DRIs) was approved for the treatment of hypertension. In this review, we discuss the history of the development of DRIs and available data regarding the effects of DRIs in the treatment of hypertension and related target organ damage.

HISTORY

Renin was discovered in 1898 by Tigerstedt and Bergman[12] with the observation that extracts of renal tissues increase BP. Since then numerous attempts have been made to inhibit renin and thus lower BP. The concept of renin inhibition for managing hypertension by blocking the RAAS pathway at its point of activation is very attractive since the renin-angiotensinogen reaction is the first and rate-limiting step in the synthesis of Ang II. It has been postulated that blocking the RAAS by inhibiting the catalytic action of renin directly would be potentially more efficacious in treating hypertension and associated with fewer adverse

Table 1
Effects of antihypertensive agents on targets of the renin-angiotensin-aldosterone system pathway

	Angiotensin I	Angiotensin II	Renin Concentration	Plasma Renin Activity
Direct renin inhibitors	↓	↓	↑	↓
Angiotensin receptor blockers	↑	↑	↑	↑
Angiotensin-converting enzyme inhibitors	↑	↓	↑	↑

↑ increased; ↓ decreased.
Data from Staessen JA, Li Y, Richart T. Oral renin inhibitors. Lancet 2006;368:1449–56; with permission.

effects than blocking downstream components of the RAAS.[13]

While the concept of inhibiting renin directly is appealing, the development of effective orally active DRIs has been technically challenging. First, preclinical studies of DRIs designed for human use must be performed in primates, such as marmosets, or in transgenic models expressing both human renin and angiotensinogen genes, because of the species specificity of the renin-angiotensinogen reaction.[14] The sequence of renin differs greatly among species, such that human renin will not cleave heterologous angiotensinogen and inhibitors designed for human renin will not inhibit the activity of heterologous renin. Second, the reagents used in the first attempts to inhibit human renin, renin antibodies, and synthetic analogs of the prosegment of prorenin, proved unsatisfactory for a variety of reasons.[15,16] These proteins had short half lives when administered parenterally, were inactive when administered orally, and led to immunologic complications such as the development of autoantibodies. Accordingly, developmental efforts shifted toward a search for effective small molecule renin inhibitors.

The first successful small molecule inhibitor of renin was pepstatin, an aspartyl protease inhibitor.[17] While pepstatin successfully inhibited renin in vitro, it had a variety of disadvantages, including lack of selectivity for renin and poor solubility in water. Structural derivatives of pepstatin increased its solubility and selectivity for renin, but none of these compounds was ever used clinically because of low efficacy in vivo, lack of oral bioavailability, and high cost of synthesis.[18–20]

The first clinical experience with a selective renin inhibitor was obtained with the angiotensinogen analog renin inhibitor peptide (RIP).[21] Although RIP effectively reduced BP during intravenous administration in humans, it was abandoned because of evidence of a direct cardiodepressant effect unrelated to the renin inhibition.

Subsequent efforts to develop small molecule renin inhibitors were directed toward synthesizing peptide analogs of the N-terminal amino acid sequence of angiotensinogen that contained amino acid substitutions at the renin cleavage site (scissile bond). These peptide inhibitors had limited potency (micromolar range) and were replaced with noncleavable analogs that had the advantages of greater potency (nanomolar range) and oral bioavailability.[13] Some of those peptide-like analogs, eg, remikiren, enalkiren, and zankiren, reduced PRA and increased plasma renin concentration after oral administration in humans, indicating renin inhibition.[22–25] However, these

drugs had a weak BP lowering effect when administered orally.[25,26] Oral administration of remikiren and parenteral infusion of enalkiren in healthy salt-restricted volunteers did not lower BP or alter heart rate, but did evoke dose-dependent decreases in PRA, Ang I, and Ang II that were rapidly reversed after termination of the treatments.[27,28] High-dose intravenous boluses of enalkiren did reduce BP in hypertensive patients when salt-depleted, while heart rate remained unchanged.[29] A comparison of placebo, enalaprilat (1.25 mg intravenously), and enalkiren (0.03 to 1.00 mg/kg intravenously) in hypertensive patients pretreated with hydrochlorothiazide (HCTZ) to activate the RAAS showed that enalkiren produced decreases in systolic BP (SBP) and diastolic BP (DBP) that were statistically significant compared with placebo but less robust than seen with enalaprilat.[30] Similarly, both orally and intravenously administered remikiren (Ro 42-5892) produced significant decreases in SBP, PRA, and circulating Ang II in hypertensive subjects.[31] Oral administration of another compound, CGP-38560A, was compared with captopril, at what were considered to be maximal doses: 0.25 mg/kg of the renin inhibitor and 50 mg of captopril.[32] BP decreased markedly after captopril (15.3 mm Hg), but not after renin inhibitor (6.4 mm Hg) administration.

The peptidomimetic renin inhibitors failed as antihypertensive medications because of their large molecular size and lipophilicity, which resulted in poor intestinal absorption and considerable first-pass hepatic metabolism, significantly limiting oral bioavailability.[23] In addition, their short duration of action and weak BP-lowering activity, as well as the successful marketing of ACE inhibitors and ARBs in the 1980s and 1990s contributed to the failure of the first-generation DRIs.[33]

ALISKIREN

Aliskiren is a low molecular weight (MW 552, free base) nonpeptidic renin inhibitor that consists of a substituted octanamide (**Fig. 2**). The extended peptide-like backbone that characterized earlier peptidomimetic renin inhibitors was eliminated. The addition of various alkylether aromatic side chains promoted interaction with the S3sp subpocket of the active site of renin and dramatically enhanced the affinity of aliskiren for renin and its selectivity over other aspartic peptidases. Retrosynthesis analysis was used to simplify the synthetic process and reduce the high cost of manufacture.[13]

Aliskiren, the only orally active renin inhibitor approved for the treatment of hypertension in humans, is a competitive transition state analog

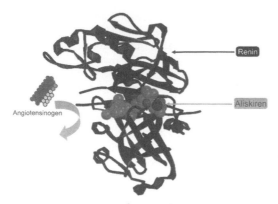

Fig. 2. Representation of the 3-dimensional structure of aliskiren. (*From* Gradman AH, Kad R. Renin inhibition in hypertension. J Am Coll Cardiol 2008; 51:519–28; with permission.)

and selective inhibitor of human renin. It has a therapeutic potential similar to that of other antagonists of the RAAS.[34] In humans, the plasma concentration of aliskiren increases dose-dependently after oral administration in doses of 40 to 640 mg/day, peaking after 3 to 6 hours.[35] The average plasma half-life is 23.7 hours, ranging from 20 to 45 hours, making aliskiren suitable for once-daily administration (**Table 2**). The oral bioavailability of aliskiren in humans is limited (2.7%).[35] Aliskiren is 47% to 51% protein bound and the steady-state plasma concentration is reached after 5 to 8 days of treatment. The main elimination route of aliskiren is via biliary excretion as unmetabolized drug.[35]

Aliskiren is more potent and selective for human renin than the other orally active DRIs, ie, remikiren and enalkiren. Aliskiren is not metabolized by cytochrome P450, and thus has low potential for significant interactions with other drugs, eg, warfarin, lovastatin, digoxin, valsartan, amlodipine, metformin, celecoxib, atenolol, atorvastatin, ramipril, and HCTZ.[36–39]

Aliskiren effectively blocks the RAAS. In a double-blind cross-over study in 18 healthy volunteers receiving a low-sodium diet, the effects of four oral doses of aliskiren (40, 80, 160, and 640 mg/day) compared with placebo and the ACE inhibitor enalapril (20 mg) on components of RAAS were evaluated.[35] Aliskiren reduced PRA in a dose-dependent manner after both a single oral dose and 8 days of repeated once-daily dosing. The highest doses of aliskiren reduced Ang II levels by a maximum of 89% and 75% on days 1 and 8, respectively, compared with placebo, and aliskiren $\geq$ 80 mg/day decreased plasma and urinary aldosterone levels by 40% and 50%, respectively. Enalapril reduced Ang II levels similarly to aliskiren, but also increased PRA 15-fold.

The hormonal effects of dual RAAS blockade with aliskiren and the ARB valsartan were evaluated in 12 mildly sodium-depleted normotensive individuals in a double-blind crossover-designed study.[40] Participants received aliskiren 300 mg, valsartan 160 mg, a combination of aliskiren 150 mg plus valsartan 80 mg, or placebo. Valsartan monotherapy increased PRA, Ang I, and Ang II, while PRA, Ang I, and Ang II levels with combination therapy were similar to placebo, indicating that the addition of aliskiren to valsartan eliminates the compensatory increase in PRA and Ang caused by ARBs.

RENOPROTECTIVE EFFECTS OF ALISKIREN

Renoprotective effects of aliskiren have been demonstrated in double transgenic rats (dTGR) that express genes for both human renin and angiotensinogen. Aliskiren has been compared with valsartan in preventing target-organ damage in dTGR. Matched 6-week-old dTGR received either no treatment, low-dose or high-dose aliskiren, or low-dose or high-dose valsartan.[14] Untreated dTGR showed severe hypertension, albuminuria, and increased serum creatinine by week 7, with a 100% mortality rate by week 9. In

Table 2
Pharmacokinetic properties of oral renin inhibitors

	Bioavailability, %	IC$_{50}$, nmol/L	Plasma Half Life, h (SD)
Aliskiren	2.7	0.6	23.7 (7.6)
CGP 38560	<1.0	0.7	1.1
Enalkiren	NA	14.0	1.6 (0.4)
Remilkiren	<1.0	0.8	9.4 (4.1)
Zankiren	NA	1.1	NA

IC$_{50}$ is the concentration needed for 50% inhibition of human renin. NA indicates data not available.
Data from Staessen JA, Li Y, Richart T. Oral renin inhibitors. Lancet 2006;368:1449–56; with permission.

contrast, both doses of aliskiren and high-dose valsartan lowered BP, reduced albuminuria and creatinine levels, and resulted in 100% survival at week 9. Treatment with aliskiren and high-dose valsartan also reduced left ventricular hypertrophy (LVH), and the magnitude of the aliskiren effect was somewhat dose-dependent.

Other animal studies showed that aliskiren protects the kidney by reducing renal inflammation and albuminuria. Administration of aliskiren or losartan to dTGR and control Sprague-Dawley rats reduced albuminuria and complement activation.[41] In another study performed in a rat model of advanced diabetic nephropathy, aliskiren reduced albuminuria and other markers of renal damage, including expression of transforming growth factor (TGF)-β and collagens III and IV.[42] When aliskiren was compared with ACE inhibitors or ARBs in these models, the renal and cardiac protective effects were approximately equal.[14,42]

Aliskiren also reduces albuminuria in humans. A study of 15 patients with type 2 diabetes and elevated urinary albumin/creatinine ratio (UACR > 30 mg g^{-1}) examined the effects on SBP and UACR of treatment with aliskiren 300 mg once daily and furosemide in a stable dose for 28 days, followed by a 4-week withdrawal period.[43] Both 24-hour SBP assessed by ambulatory BP monitoring and UACR decreased significantly with aliskiren. UACR decreased significantly (17%) in the first 2 to 4 days of treatment and reached a maximum reduction of 44% at the end of the treatment period (**Fig. 3**). UACR decreased progressively throughout the treatment period, whereas the 24-hour BP did not fall further after day 7. Five of the 15 patients had greater than 50% reduction in albuminuria at the end of treatment compared with baseline; 11 of the 15 had greater

than 25% reduction, and 13 had greater than 10% reduction. During posttreatment washout, UACR remained significantly below baseline for 12 days.

ALISKIREN IN THE TREATMENT OF HUMAN HYPERTENSION

Aliskiren, both as monotherapy and in combination with other agents, has been evaluated extensively in hypertensive patients. Aliskiren monotherapy has a dose-dependent antihypertensive effect that is significantly greater than placebo. In a randomized double-blind study, 652 patients with mild to moderate hypertension defined as DBP $\geq$ 95 and <110 mm Hg, were assigned to receive placebo, irbesartan 150 mg, or once-daily doses of aliskiren (150, 300, or 600 mg) for 8 weeks after a 2-week placebo run-in period.[44] Once-daily oral treatment with each of the three doses of aliskiren significantly decreased mean sitting SBP and DBP compared with placebo (**Fig. 4**). No additional BP reduction was obtained with aliskiren 600 mg. After 8 weeks of treatment, 21% and 50% ($P < .05$) of patients assigned to placebo and aliskiren 300 mg, respectively, achieved BP control defined as BP lower than 140/90 mm Hg.

In another randomized, double-blind, placebo-controlled trial, 672 hypertensive patients (mean sitting DBP 95 to 109 mm Hg) received placebo or aliskiren 150, 300, or 600 mg once daily.[45] After 8 weeks, aliskiren 150, 300, and 600 mg significantly reduced mean sitting BP (systolic/diastolic) by 13.0/10.3, 14.7/11.1, and 15.8/12.5 mm Hg from baseline, respectively, versus 3.8/4.9 mm Hg with placebo (all $P < .0001$ for SBP and DBP). Aliskiren significantly reduced mean 24-hour ambulatory BP and its BP-lowering effect persisted for up to 2 weeks after treatment withdrawal. Aliskiren 150, 300, and 600 mg reduced PRA (geometric

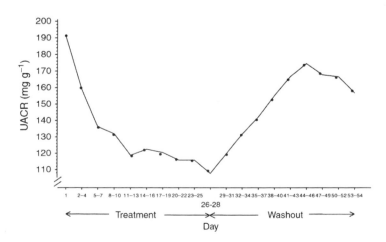

Fig. 3. Urinary albumin/creatinine ratio in diabetic patients with micro- or macroalbuminuria treated with aliskiren for 28 days followed by 28 days washout. (*From* Persson F, Rossing P, Schjoedt KJ, et al. Time course of the antiproteinuric and antihypertensive effects of direct renin inhibition in type 2 diabetes. Kidney Int 2008;73(12):1419–25; with permission).

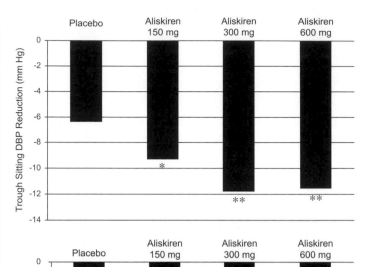

Fig. 4. Blood pressure reduction achieved with aliskiren compared with placebo. SBP, systolic blood pressure; DBP, diastolic blood pressure. *P < .01 compared with placebo; **P < .0001 compared with placebo.

mean change from baseline) by 79.5%, 81.1%, and 75.0%, respectively, whereas PRA increased by 19.5% from baseline in the placebo group. Aliskiren treatment resulted in dose-dependent increases from baseline in renin concentration. Aliskiren was well tolerated; overall adverse event rates were 40.1%, 46.7%, and 52.4% with aliskiren 150, 300, and 600 mg, respectively, compared with 43.0% with placebo.

A pooled analysis that included 8481 patients who participated in double-blind trials and received aliskiren monotherapy or placebo for 8 to 12 weeks showed that once-daily aliskiren, 150 or 300 mg, produced reductions in mean trough sitting DBP of 10.1 and 11.8 mm Hg, respectively, compared with 6.2 mm Hg for placebo (P < .0001).[46] Trough SBP was lowered by 12.5 and 15.2 mm Hg, compared with 5.9 mm Hg for placebo (P < .0001). There were no statistically significant differences in the magnitude of BP reduction in men versus women or in patients younger versus older than 65 years.

Aliskiren monotherapy has been compared with representatives of several different classes of anti-hypertensive medications and has been shown to produce comparable or greater reductions in BP. For example, in a double-blind study, 842 patients with hypertension (mean sitting DBP 95 to 109 mm Hg) were randomized to aliskiren 150 mg or the ACE inhibitor ramipril 5 mg.[47] Dose titration (to aliskiren 300 mg/ramipril 10 mg) and subsequent addition of hydrochlorothiazide (12.5 mg, titrated to 25 mg if required) were permitted at weeks 6, 12, 18, and 21 for inadequate BP control. The active treatment period was completed by 81.6% of patients. At week 26, aliskiren-based therapy produced greater mean reductions in SBP (17.9 versus 15.2 mm Hg, P = .0036) and DBP (13.2 versus 12.0 mm Hg, P = .025) and higher rates of SBP control (<140 mmHg; 72.5% versus 64.1%, P = .0075) compared with ramipril-based therapy. During withdrawal, BP increased more rapidly after stopping ramipril-based than aliskiren-based therapy.

When used in combination with a thiazide diuretic, aliskiren is more effective than either monotherapy in reducing BP. In an 8-week, double-blind, placebo-controlled trial, 2776 patients with mean sitting DBP 95 to 109 mm Hg were randomized to receive once-daily treatment with aliskiren (75, 150, or 300 mg), hydrochlorothiazide (HCTZ) (6.25, 12.5, or 25 mg), the combination of aliskiren and HCTZ, or placebo, in a factorial design.[48] Combination treatment was superior to both component monotherapies in reducing BP (maximum SBP/DBP reduction of 21.2/14.3 mm Hg from baseline with aliskiren/HCTZ 300/25 mg), and resulted in a higher responder rate (patients with DBP < 90 mm Hg and/or ≥ 10 mm Hg reduction) and a better control rate (patients achieving SBP/DBP < 140/90 mm Hg) than either monotherapy. Aliskiren monotherapy reduced PRA by up to 65% from baseline and when HCTZ was combined with aliskiren, decreases in PRA of 46.1% to 63.5% were observed.

Dual RAAS inhibition with maximum recommended doses of the DRI aliskiren and the ARB valsartan has shown greater antihypertensive efficacy than monotherapy with either agent. In a double-blind study, 1797 patients with hypertension (mean sitting DBP 95 to 109 mm Hg and 8-hour daytime ambulatory DBP ≥ 90 mm Hg) were randomly assigned to receive once-daily aliskiren 150 mg, valsartan 160 mg, a combination of aliskiren 150 mg and valsartan 160 mg, or placebo for 4 weeks, followed by forced titration to maximum recommended doses for another 4 weeks.[49] At week 8, the mean sitting SBP was lowered from baseline by 17.2, 12.8, 13.0, and 4.6 mm Hg, respectively, and mean sitting DBP was lowered from baseline by 12.2, 9.7, 9.0, and 4.1 mm Hg, respectively, with the combination of aliskiren

300 mg and valsartan 320 mg, valsartan 320 mg monotherapy, aliskiren 300 mg monotherapy, and placebo (P < .0001 combination compared with placebo or either monotherapy) (**Fig. 5**). The proportion of patients achieving a successful response to treatment at week 8 was significantly higher with the combination of aliskiren and valsartan (66%) than with aliskiren alone (53%; P = .0003) or valsartan alone (55%; P = .001). Valsartan monotherapy produced significantly greater increases in PRA from baseline than did placebo (160% versus 18%; P = .0003). By contrast, aliskiren alone significantly reduced PRA by 73% (P < .0001 versus placebo), while the combination of aliskiren and valsartan led to a 44% reduction in PRA (P < .0001 versus placebo). The combination of aliskiren and valsartan provided significantly greater reductions in plasma aldosterone concentration from baseline at week 8 than did placebo (−31% versus +7%; P < .0001). Valsartan alone also reduced aldosterone concentration (−25%; P = .0007 versus placebo), while aliskiren monotherapy had no significant effect on aldosterone concentration. The rates of adverse events and laboratory abnormalities were similar in all groups.

Some have hypothesized that reactive renin secretion may limit the effectiveness of DRIs.[50] Although aliskiren suppresses PRA, it causes major reactive increases in plasma renin concentration. If the system is at all leaky, allowing even a small percentage of the excess prorenin generated during DRI treatment to be activated, the antihypertensive effect of the DRI may be offset, limiting its utility as an antihypertensive agent. Further study and additional clinical experience with aliskiren and other DRIs, as they become available, are needed to validate or refute this hypothesis.

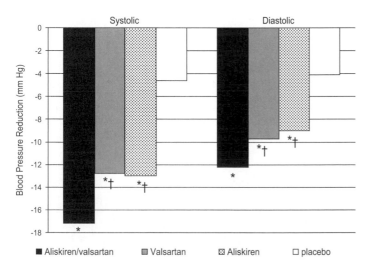

Fig. 5. Effect of study treatments on mean systolic and diastolic blood pressure. *P < .0001 compared with placebo; †P < .0001 compared with aliskiren/valsartan combination.

SUMMARY

Introduction of the DRI aliskiren has opened doors for newer possibilities in antihypertensive therapy. Aliskiren has antihypertensive efficacy comparable to other classes of antihypertensive medications, including diuretics, ACEinhibitors, ARBs, and calcium channel blockers and with a tolerability and safety profile similar to placebo. It also has additive antihypertensive effects when combined with these other drug classes. Preliminary studies of the effects of aliskiren on target organ damage demonstrate comparable or greater efficacy compared with other RAAS antagonists. Results of clinical outcome trials are needed to establish the role of this novel class of antihypertensive medication in the therapeutic armamentarium.

REFERENCES

1. Pimenta E, Oparil S. Etiology and pathogenesis of systemic hypertension. In: Crawford MH, DiMarco JP, Paulus WJ, editors. Cardiology, 3rd edition. London: Mosby, in press.

2. Danser AH, Denium J. Renin, pro-renin and putative (Pro)renin receptor. Hypertension 2005;46:1069–76.

3. Reudelhuber TL, Ramla D, Chiu L, et al. Proteolytic processing of human pro-renin in renal and non-renal tissues. Kidney Int 1994;46:1522–4.

4. Danser AH, Derkx FH, Schalekamp MA, et al. Determinants of interindividual variation of renin and pro-renin concentrations: evidence for a sexual dimorphism of (pro)renin levels in humans. J Hypertens 1998;16:853–62.

5. Luetscher JA, Kraemer FB, Wilson DM, et al. Increased plasma inactive renin in diabetes mellitus. A marker of microvascular complication. N Engl J Med 1985;312:1412–7.

6. Price DA, Porter LE, Gordon M, et al. The paradox of the low-renin state in diabetic nephropaty. J Am Soc Nephrol 1999;10:2382–91.

7. Bühler FR, Laragh JH, Vaughan ED, et al. Antihypertensive action of propranolol: specific anti-renin responses in high and normal renin forms of essential, renal, renovascular and malignant hypertension. Am J Cardiol 1973;32:511–22.

8. Michelakis AM, McAllister RG. The effect of chronic adrenergic receptor blockade on plasma renin activity in man. J Clin Endocrinol Metab 1972;34:386–94.

9. Ondetti MA. Design of specific inhibitors of angiotensin-converting enzyme: new class of orally active antihypertensive agents. Science 1977;196:441–4.

10. Ferreira SH. A bradykinin-potentiating factor present in the venom of Bothrops jararaca. Br J Pharmacol 1965;24:163–9.

11. Ferreira SH, Greene X. Isolation of bradykinin-potentiating peptides from Bothrops jararaca venom. Biochemistry 1970;9:2583–93.

12. Tigerstedt R, Bergman PG. Niere und Kreislauf. Skand Arch Physiol 1898;8:223–71.

13. Gradman AH, Kad R. Renin inhibition in hypertension. J Am Coll Cardiol 2008;51:519–28.

14. Pils B, Shagdarsuren E, Wellner M, et al. Aliskiren, a human renin inhibitor, ameliorates cardiac and renal damage in double-transgenic rats. Hypertension 2005;46:569–76.

15. Azizi M, Webb R, Nussberger J, et al. Renin inhibition with aliskiren: where are we now, and where are we going? J Hypertens 2006;24:243–56.

16. Michel JB, Galen FX, Guettier C, et al. Immunological approach to blockade of the renin-substrate reaction. J Hypertens 1989;7:S63–70.

17. Gross F, Lazar J, Orth H. Inhbition of the renin-angiotensinogen reaction by pepstatin. Science 1972;175:656.

18. Evin G, Gardes J, Kreft C, et al. Soluble pepstatins: a new approach to blockade in vivo of the renin angiotensin system. Clin Sci 1978;55:167s–71s.

19. Eid M, Evin G, Castro B, et al. New renin inhibitors homologous with pepstatin. Biochem J 1981;197:465–71.

20. Boger J, Lohr NS, Ulm EH, et al. Novel renin inhibitors containing the amino acid statine. Nature 1983;303:81–4.

21. Zusman RM, Burton J, Christensen D, et al. Hemodynamic effects of a competitive renin in inhibitory peptide in humans. Evidence for multiple mechanisms of action. Trans Assoc Am Physicians 1983;96:365–74.

22. Macfayden RJ, Jones CR, Doig JK, et al. Responses to an orally active renin inhibitor, remikiren (Ro 42-5892), after controlled salt depletion in humans. J Cardiovasc Pharmacol 1995;25:347–53.

23. Rongen GA, Lenders JW, Smits P, et al. Clinical pharamacokinetics and efficacy of renin inhibitors. Clin Pharmacokinet 1995;29:6–14.

24. Himmelmann A, Bergbrant A, Svensson A, et al. Remikiren (Ro 42-5892)—an orally active renin inhibitor in essential hypertension. Effects on blood pressure and the renin-angiotensin-aldosterone system. Am J Hypertens 1996;9:517–22.

25. Ménard J, Boger RS, Moyse DM, et al. Dose-dependent effects of the renin inhibitor zankiren HCl after a single oral dose in mildly sodium-depleted normotensive subjects. Circulation 1995;91:330–8.

26. Rongen GA, Lenders JW, Kleinbloesem CH, et al. Efficacy and tolerability of the renin inhibitor Ro 42-5892 in patients with hypertension. Clin Pharmacol Ther 1993;54:567–77.

27. Camenzind E, Nussberger J, Juillerat L, et al. Effect of the renin response during renin inhibition: oral Ro 42-5892 in normal humans. J Cardiovasc Pharmacol 1991;18:299–307.

28. Delabays A, Nussberger J, Porchet M, et al. Hemo-dynamic and humoral effects of the new renin inhib-itior enalkiren in normal humans. Hypertension 1989; 13:941–7.

29. Weber MA, Neutel JM, Essinger I, et al. Assessment of renin dependency of hypertension with a dipep-tide renin inhibitor. Circulation 1990;81:1768–74.

30. Neutel JM, Luther RR, Boger RS, et al. Immediate blood pressure effects of the renin inhibitor enalkiren and the ACE inhibitor enalaprilat. Am Heart J 1991; 122:1094–100.

31. Van den Meiracker AH, Admiraal PJ, Man in't Veld AJ, et al. Prolonged blood pressure reduction by orally active renin inhibitor RO-42-5892 in essen-tial hypertension. Br Med J 1990;301:205–10.

32. Jeunemaitre X, Menard J, Nussberger J, et al. Plasma angiotensin, renin and blood pressure during acute renin inhibition by GCP 38 560A in hypertensive patients. Am J Hypertens 1989;2: 819–27.

33. Staessen JA, Li Y, Richart T. Oral renin inhibitors. Lancet 2006;368:1449–56.

34. Nussberger J. Renin inhibitors. In: Oparil S, Weber MA, editors. Hypertension: a companion to Brenner and Rector's the kidney, 2nd edition. Phila-delphia: Elsevier; 2005. p. 754–64.

35. Nussberger J, Wuerzner J, Jensen C, et al. Angio-tensin II suppression in humans by the orally active renin inhibitor aliskiren (SPP100). Comparison with enalapril. Hypertension 2002;39:e1–e8.

36. Dieterle W, Corynen S, Vaidyanathan S, et al. Effect of the oral renin inhibitor aliskiren on the pharmaco-kinetics and pharmacodynamics of a single dose of warfarin in healthy subjects. Br J Clin Pharmacol 2004;58:433–6.

37. Dieterle W, Corynen S, Vaidyanathan S, et al. Pharma-cokinetic interactions of the oral renin inhibitor aliski-ren with lovastatin, atenolol, celecoxib and cimetidine. Int J Clin Pharmacol Ther 2005;43:527–35.

38. Dieterich H, Kemp C, Vaidyanathan S, et al. Pharma-cokinetic interaction of the oral renin inhibitor aliski-ren with hydrochlorothiazide in healthy volunteers. Clin Pharmacol Ther 2006;79:P12 [abstract].

39. Dieterich H, Kemp C, Vaidyanathan S, et al. Aliski-ren, the first in a new class or orally effective renin inhibitors, has no clinically significant drug interac-tions with digoxin in healthy volunteers. Clin Pharma-col Ther 2006;79:P64 [abstract].

40. Azizi M, Ménard J, Bissery A, et al. Pharmacologic demonstration of the synergistic effects of a combi-nation of the renin inhibitor aliskiren and the AT1 receptor antagonist valsartan on the angiotensin II-renin feedback interruption. J Am Soc Nephrol 2004;15:3126–33.

41. Shagdarsuren E, Wellner M, Braesen JH, et al. Com-plement activation in angiotensin II-induced organ damage. Circ Res 2005;97:716–24.

42. Kelly DJ, Zhang Y, Moe G, et al. Aliskiren, a novel renin inhibitor, is renoprotective in a model of advanced diabetic nephropaty in rats. Diabetologia 2007;50:2398–404.

43. Persson F, Rossing P, Schjoedt KJ, et al. Time course of the antiproteinuric and antihypertensive effects of direct renin inhibition in type 2 diabetes. Kidney Int 2008;73(12):1419–25.

44. Gradman AH, Schmieder RE, Lins RL, et al. Aliski-ron, a novel orally effective rennin inhibitor, provides dose-dependent antihypertensive efficacy and placebo-like tolerability in hypertensive patients. Circulation 2005;111:1012–8.

45. Oh BH, Mitchell J, Herron JR, et al. Aliskiren, an oral rennin inhibitor, provides dose-dependent efficacy and sustained 24-h blood pressure control in patients with hypertension. J Am Coll Cardiol 2007;49:1157–63.

46. Dahlöf B, Anderson DR, Arora V, et al. Aliskiren, a direct renin inhibitor, provides antihypertensive efficacy and excellent tolerability independent of age or gender in patients with hypertension. J Clin Hypertens 2007;9:A157 [abstract].

47. Andersen K, Weinberger MH, Egan B, et al. Com-parative efficacy and safety of aliskiren, an oral direct renin inhibitor, and ramipril in hypertension: a 6-month, randomized, double-blind trial. J Hyper-tens 2008;26:589–99.

48. Villamil A, Chysant SG, Calhoun D, et al. Renin inhi-bition with aliskiren provides additive antihyperten-sive efficacy when used in combination with hydrochlorothiazide. J Hypertens 2007;25:217–26.

49. Oparil S, Yarows SA, Patel S, et al. Efficacy and safety of combined use of aliskiren and valsartan in patients with hypertension: a randomized double-blind trial. Lancet 2007;370:221–9.

50. Sealey JE, Laragh JH. Aliskiren, the first renin inhib-itor for treating hypertension: reactive renin secre-tion may limit its effectiveness. Am J Hypertens 2007;20:587–97.

Cholesteryl Ester Transfer Protein (CETP) Inhibitors: Is There Life After Torcetrapib?

Hemanth Neeli, MD[a,b], Daniel J. Rader, MD[b,*]

KEYWORDS

• CETP • CETP inhibitors • Torcetrabip • HDL • Illuminate

Statins have revolutionized the prevention and treatment of coronary heart disease (CHD) for the last 15 years by targeting LDL-c (low density lipoprotein cholesterol), one of the major risk factors for CHD. Recent guidelines have recommended achieving even lower LDL-c levels especially in the high-risk patients[1] as this translates into improved clinical outcomes. Despite tremendous progress made in the management of CHD, a significant number of fatal and nonfatal CHD events still occur [2,3] that entail the need to target other modifiable risk factors for CHD including low HDL-c (high density lipoprotein cholesterol). Low HDL-c is an independent risk factor for CHD even in patients who have low LDL-c levels.[4] Large-scale population studies have demonstrated a strong independent inverse relationship between the HDL-c level and the risk of CHD,[5] which has propelled efforts to find novel therapies to increase HDL-c levels. One mg/dl increase in HDL-c lowers CHD risk by 2% in men and 3% in women.[6] Data from the landmark Framingham Heart Study showed that for a given level of LDL-c, the risk of CHD increases 10-fold as the HDL-c varies from high to low. Conversely, for a fixed level of HDL-c, the risk increases three-fold as LDL-c varies from low to high.

HDL METABOLISM AND MECHANISMS OF ATHEROPROTECTION

HDL particles and their major protein apolipoprotein A-I (apoA-I) are synthesized and secreted by both the liver and intestine. After apoA-I is secreted, it acquires phospholipids and unesterified cholesterol from the same organs via the transporter ATP binding cassette A1 (ABCA1) forming the discoid nascent HDL particle.[7,8] HDL and apoA-I promote a key process called "reverse cholesterol transport" (RCT) in which they serve as acceptors for cholesterol from peripheral tissues and then transport the cholesterol back to liver for excretion into bile eventually. Lipid-loaded macrophages in the arterial wall efflux free cholesterol to nascent HDL via ABCA1 and to mature HDL via ATP-binding cassette G1 (ABCG1) respectively.[9,10] Much of the free cholesterol is esterified by the enzyme lecithin:cholesterol acyl transferease (LCAT) forming spherical mature HDL. HDL returns cholesterol to the liver by at least two major pathways. One pathway is via scavenger receptor BI (SR-BI) in the liver, which mediates the "selective uptake" of cholesterol from HDL. This is an important pathway in rodents. The second pathway involves the transfer of cholesteryl ester (CE) facilitated by the cholesteryl ester transfer protein (CETP) to apoB containing lipoproteins that are eventually taken up by the liver via the LDL receptor. This is an important pathway for the hepatic uptake of HDL cholesterol in humans.[11]

CURRENT THERAPIES TARGETING HDL-C

Life style changes like daily exercise,[12] weight loss,[13] moderate consumption of alcohol,[14] and

[a] Section of Hospital Medicine, Temple University Hospital, 1316 West Ontario Street, Philadelphia, PA 19140, USA
[b] Institute for Translational Medicine and Therapeutics, University of Pennsylvania School of Medicine, 654 BRB II/III, 421 Curie Blvd, Philadelphia, PA 19104, USA
* Corresponding author.
E-mail address: rader@mail.med.upenn.edu (D.J. Rader).

Cardiol Clin 26 (2008) 537–546
doi:10.1016/j.ccl.2008.06.005

smoking cessation[15] can raise HDL-c levels. Moderate intensity exercise for more than 12 weeks raises HDL-c by 4.6%; weight loss of 1 kg increases HDL-c by 1%; moderate consumption of alcohol (30 grams per day) increases HDL-c by 8.3%. The National Cholesterol Education Program Adult Treatment Panel III update specifies that drug therapies to increase HDL-c may have a role in high-risk patients after their LDL-c and non-HDL-c level goals are met.[1] Statins can raise HDL-c by 6%–12%,[16–18] which may be in part through decreased CETP expression.[19]

Nicotinic acid (niacin) is the most effective drug currently available to raise HDL-c levels. A meta-analysis of all randomized trials with nicotinic acid have shown that it increases HDL-c by an average of 16%.[20] Niacin significantly decreased recurrent myocardial infarction (MI) and total mortality in the Coronary Drug Project (CDP).[21] Simvastatin-niacin combination in CHD patients who have low HDL-c and normal LDL-c has shown angiographic regression of the atherosclerotic plaque accompanied by 26% increase in HDL-c in the HDL-Atherosclerosis Treatment Study (HATS).[22] In the Arterial Biology for the Investigation of the Treatment Effects of Reducing Cholesterol (ARBITER) 2 trial, addition of extended-release niacin to statin therapy in patients who have CHD and moderately low HDL-c levels increased HDL-c by 21% and showed a trend towards decrease in the progression of atherosclerosis (as measured by change in carotid intima-media thickness [IMT]).[23] The Atherothrombosis Intervention in Metabolic Syndrome with Low HDL/High Triglycerides and Impact on Global Health Outcomes (AIM-HIGH) and Heart Protection Study 2 Treatment of HDL to Reduce the Incidence of Vascular Events (HPS2-THRIVE) will determine the long-term clinical benefit of extended release niacin when added to statin therapy.

Fibrates can increase HDL-c levels modestly. Meta-analysis of all randomized controlled trials with fibrates including the CDP, Bezafibrate Infarction Prevention (BIP) trial, Veterans Affairs HDL-c Intervention trial (VA-HIT)[24] and Helsinki Heart Study[25] have shown that fibrates increase HDL-c by an average of 10%.[20] However, the Fenofibrate Intervention and Endpoint Lowering in Diabetes (FIELD) trial, which randomized type II diabetic patients with and without CHD to micronized fenofibrate and placebo showed only a 1% increase in HDL-c.[26] Although several clinical trials with fibrates have shown efficacy regarding reduction in cardiovascular events, the FIELD trial did not achieve its primary endpoint, possibly due in part to statin drop-in,[26] and the benefits of fibrates are not proven to be related to HDL raising. The Action to Control Cardiovascular Risk in Diabetes (ACCORD) trial,[27] an ongoing large clinical trial will determine if HDL-c raised by fenofibrate translates into improved clinical outcomes beyond the benefits offered by statins in a cohort of diabetes patients. Given the limitations and inconsistent outcomes of the available therapies that raise HDL-c, there is a growing need to develop novel therapies aimed at increasing HDL-c.

EVOLUTION OF CETP AS A NOVEL TARGET

CETP is a plasma protein that facilitates transfer of CE from HDL particles to apoB- containing particles in exchange for triglycerides.[28] CETP emerged as a potential target when it was found that a subset of the Japanese population with genetic deficiency of CETP had markedly elevated HDL-c.[29] The human CETP gene has been mapped to chromosome 16 and spans 25,000 base pairs including 16 exons.[29] Two CETP gene mutations that cause CETP deficiency are more common than the others: a G to A substitution in the 5′ splice donor site of intron 14 (Int14+1 G→A) and a missense mutation of exon 15 (D442G).[30,31] Homozygotes and compound heterozygotes for these loss-of-function mutations have little to no detectable CETP activity in the plasma and very high levels of HDL-c.[32] However, the association of CETP deficiency with coronary disease remains unclear.[33–35]

The human CETP gene is highly polymorphic and several single nucleotide polymorphism (SNP) have been characterized.[36,37] The TaqIB polymorphism is the most extensively studied in relation to its association with HDL-c level, CETP mass and even CHD risk. It accounts for about 6% of the variance in CETP levels.[38] The most common genotype B1B1 is associated with higher CETP mass/activity and lower HDL-c in various population studies.[37,39] The effects of the TaqIB polymorphism on the lipid parameters are influenced by gender, alcohol consumption, insulin levels, and body mass index.[37,40,41] The B2B2 genotype is associated with lower CETP, higher HDL-c, and in some studies a decreased CHD risk.[39,42] In the REGRESS (Regression Growth Evaluation Statin Study) Study[43] pravastatin slowed the progression of coronary atherosclerosis to a greater extent in individuals with the B1B1 than the B2B2 genotype.

Klerkx and colleagues[38] described a haplotype model with promoter mutations −629 C/A, −971 G/A and −2708 G/A in a cohort of CHD patients that explained the variation in CETP activity better than TaqIB. Later the same group showed in

REGRESS cohort that there is functional interaction between −629C/A, −971G/A and −1337C/T polymorphisms and CETP concentration.[44] McCaskie and colleagues[45] evaluated the effect of −629 C/A, −2708 G/A, and TaqIB in two community-based populations and a cohort of CHD patients in Australia; they found that the common haplotype AAB2 was consistently associated with decreased CETP activity and elevated HDL-c levels, but it was not associated with CHD risk. In a genetic substudy of PREVEND, Borggreve and colleagues[46] demonstrated that −629A, TaqIB B2 allele carriers had increased risk of CHD despite higher HDL-c levels. A recent meta-analysis of 132 studies involving approximately 200,000 subjects showed that the common CETP variants TaqIB, I405V and −629C/A are associated with modest decrease in CETP activity, modest increase in HDL-c levels, and weakly with reduced CHD risk.[47] Thus, although this issue has not been definitively settled, the weight of evidence suggests that genetic variants that reduce CETP activity and increase HDL-C are associated with modest protection against CHD.

Studies have also addressed the relationship between plasma CETP mass or activity and atherosclerosis and cardiovascular events. A small case-control study showed that patients who have MI and stroke were found to have higher CETP mass than healthy controls controlled for CETP gene mutations.[48] Elevated CETP mass is associated with atherogenic lipid profile[49] and rapid progression of angiographic coronary lesions[50] and carotid IMT.[49] A nested case-control study of the prospective EPIC-Norfolk study showed increased incidence of coronary events in subjects with elevated CETP mass.[51] However, a nested case-control study of Prevention of Renal and Vascular End-stage Disease (PREVENT) study showed the contrary.[52] The milieu in which CETP functions might modify its own function, explaining the above discrepant results. In the EPIC-Norfolk study, higher CETP mass increased the incidence of CHD only when the triglycerides were high, while in the PREVEND study higher CETP mass was associated with lower risk of CHD in the setting of low triglyceride levels.

Measures of CETP activity might be more informative than CETP mass, but the assays for CETP activity are cumbersome and not standardized. Only a few studies have looked into the CETP activity and its correlation to CHD. In patients who underwent diagnostic coronary angiography, higher CETP activity was found in patients who have significant CHD than those without significant CHD.[53] In another small study, diabetic patients had a higher CETP activity than nondiabetic controls, and the CETP activity was positively correlated to carotid IMT in both diabetic and control groups.[54] An observational study of all patients who have first MI showed that higher CETP activity was associated with earlier presentation of MI than lower CETP activity.[55] Thus the CETP mass and activity data, although not completely consistent, also generally support the concept that higher plasma levels of CETP are associated with increased cardiovascular risk.

CLINICAL EXPERIENCE WITH THE CETP INHIBITOR TORCETRAPIB

Torcetrapib, the most extensively studied CETP inhibitor to-date, selectively inhibits plasma CETP by causing a nonproductive complex between CETP and HDL.[56] Several early clinical trials were conducted to define the dose and change in lipid parameters, the kinetics of the drug and dynamics of HDL metabolism. Torcetrapib at 120 mg twice daily increased HDL cholesterol by 91% and decreased LDL cholesterol by 42% in healthy subjects.[57] In subjects with low HDL-c levels, torcetrapib increased HDL-c and decreased LDL-c levels, either when administered as monotherapy or combined with a statin.[58] Torcetrapib was shown to increase apoA-I concentrations modestly by decreasing the catabolism of apoA-I.[59] In a phase 2 trial, 162 subjects with below average HDL-c were randomized to torcetrapib 10, 30, 60, or 90 mg/day or placebo.[60] There was a dose-dependent increase in HDL-c from 9% to 55%. In another phase 2 multicenter, randomized, double-blinded trial, 174 patients who have low HDL-c either on statins or with LDL-c > 130 mg/dL who would be eligible for statins according to NCEP ATP III guidelines were randomized to varying doses of torcetrapib or placebo for 8 weeks after a run-in period with atorvastatin.[61] There was a dose-dependent increase in HDL-c from 8% to 40%, with additional decrease in LDL-c beyond that achieved with atorvastatin alone. In the same trial, torcetrapib/atorvastatin combination was shown to increase the large HDL2 subfractions and decrease the small LDL subfractions while increasing both HDL and LDL particle size.[62] In patients who have heterozygous familial hypercholesterolemia (HeFH) who lack LDL receptor, torcetrapib/atorvastatin combination not only raised HDL-c but also decreased LDL-c significantly when compared to atorvastatin alone.[63] In patients who have hypertriglyceridemia, torcetrapib/atorvastatin combination had an enhanced LDL lowering effect.[63] When fenofibrate and ezetimibe were administered with torcetrapib and atorvastatin in healthy subjects, there was no change in the pharmacokinetics of torcetrapib.[64,65]

Torcetrapib at the 60 mg dose was studied in three phase III atherosclerosis imaging trials. The Rating Atherosclerotic Disease Change by Imaging with a New CETP Inhibitor (RADIANCE) 1 and 2 trials were designed to determine the effect of torcetrapib on atherosclerosis progression in patients with HeFH and mixed dyslipidemia respectively.[66,67] After an initial run-in phase with atorvastatin, 850 patients were randomized to receive atorvastatin/torcetrapib combination or atorvastatin monotherapy. At the end of 2 years, despite significant rise in HDL-c and reduction in LDL-c levels, there was no difference in the progression of carotid IMT among the intervention and control groups in both RADIANCE 1 and 2.

The Investigation of Lipid Level Management Using Coronary Ultrasound to Assess Reduction of Atherosclerosis by CETP Inhibition and HDL Elevation (ILLUSTRATE) trial studied the effect of torcetrapib on coronary atherosclerosis progression. Patients who have CHD were pretreated with atorvastatin to reach an LDL goal of ≤of 100 mg/dL and then randomized to torcetrapib/atorvastatin or atorvastatin monotherapy.[63] All patients underwent intravascular ultrasonography (IVUS) at baseline and 77% of them had a repeat IVUS after 2 years. At the end of 2 years, there was no significant difference in the percent atheroma volume between the two groups. Posthoc analysis showed an inverse relationship between change in HDL-c level and both total atheroma volume and percent atheroma volume.[68]

Torcetrapib was also studied in a large phase III clinical outcome trial, the Investigation of Lipid Level Management to understand its Impact in Atherosclerotic Events (ILLUMINATE) trial.[69] ILLUMINATE randomized 15,067 patients who have CHD or CHD equivalents to torcetrapib/atorvastatin or atorvastatin after a run-in period with atorvastatin to reach an LDL goal of ≤100 mg/dL. The trial was terminated on December 2, 2006 because of increased mortality in the torcetrapib arm and the clinical development of torcetrapib was terminated. Interim analysis at 12 months showed a 72% increase in HDL-c and 25% decrease in LDL-c in due to torcetrapib. There were more cardiovascular (49 versus 35) and noncardiovascular (40 versus 20) deaths in the torcetrapib group than the atorvastain group. Cancer (24 versus 14) and infections (9 versus 0) were the most common cause of noncardiovascular death. There were significant increases in systolic blood pressure of 5.4 mm Hg, increases in serum sodium and bicarbonate levels, and decreases in serum potassium in the torcetrapib group. Posthoc analysis showed that the aldosterone levels in the torcetrapib arm were significantly elevated at 3 months when compared to the atorvastatin-only group despite being similar at the beginning of the trial. Cardiovascular events were inversely proportional to the increase in HDL-c above the median.

It is likely that off-target effects of torcetrapib contributed to the adverse outcome in ILLUMINATE.[70] All phase III imaging trials of torcetrapib also showed a significant increase in systolic blood pressure in the torcetrapib arm (2.8 mm Hg, 5.1 mm Hg, 4.6 mm Hg increase in RADIANCE 1, 2 and ILLUSTRATE respectively). In rats (both normotensive and spontaneously hypertensive models), which naturally lack CETP, torcetrapib increased blood pressure dose-dependently with a concomitant increase in gene expression of renin angiotensin system (RAS) and endothelin-1 from the adrenal glands as well as aorta (**Fig. 1**).[71] Torcetrapib caused an acute elevation in blood

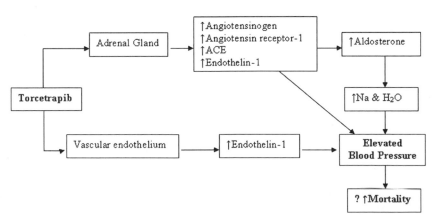

Fig. 1. Off-target effects of torcetrapib. ACE, angiotensin converting enzyme.

pressure through its interaction with adrenal glands in rats, rabbits and nonhuman primates despite the use of various receptor-blocking agents to counteract the increase in blood pressure.[72] Structural analogs of torcetrapib devoid of CETP inhibitory function still raised blood pressure in animal models suggesting that the blood pressure effect is not through CETP inhibition.[73] These studies suggest that the elevation in the blood pressure in the ILLUMINATE trial is molecule specific and not class specific. It is unclear whether the mechanisms leading to the blood pressure accounted for the adverse cardiovascular events in ILLUMINATE, but it is likely that off-target effects of torcetrapib at least contributed to the increased cardiovascular risk in this trial.[70]

POTENTIAL ADVERSE EFFECTS VERSUS BENEFITS OF CETP INHIBITION

Despite substantial increases in HDL-c levels, the impact of CETP inhibition with torcetrapib on atherosclerosis and CV events is disappointing.[63,67,69] As noted above, the off-target effects of torcetrapib undoubtedly played a role in the disappointing outcomes. However, this experience has focused increased attention on whether the mechanism of CETP inhibition is beneficial or could even be adverse despite increasing HDL-c levels. Specifically, it has been suggested that CETP inhibition might impair RCT by generating HDL particles that are less competent at promoting macrophage cholesterol efflux and/or by reducing the return of HDL-derived cholesterol to the liver for biliary excretion. Although earlier data suggested that HDL from CETP deficient subjects could be defective in promoting cholesterol efflux, more recent data suggests that CETP deficient HDL is as good or even better at promoting efflux, particularly via the ABCG1 pathway.[74] Furthermore, HDL from torcetrapib-treated subjects (120 mg daily) was also shown to increase macrophage cholesterol efflux primarily through ABCG1,[75] possibly enhanced by increased content of LCAT and apoE. Thus the concept that CETP inhibition impairs cholesterol efflux is not supported by experimental data; however, promotion of cholesterol efflux may require adequate increases in HDL-c levels.

The issue of whether CETP inhibition could impair RCT by slowing the return of HDL-derived cholesterol to the liver is more complex. It appears that in healthy normolipidemic humans, most HDL cholesteryl ester (CE) is shuttled back to the liver after transfer to apoB-containing lipoproteins via the CETP pathway.[11] Indeed, in wild-type mice, introduction of CETP expression promoted RCT from macrophages to feces, although in LDL receptor–deficient mice, CETP expression had the opposite effect,[76] suggesting that the effect of CETP inhibition on RCT may depend on the efficiency of hepatic uptake of apoB-containing lipoproteins. Torcetrapib did not change fecal cholesterol excretion or biomarkers of cholesterol or bile acid synthesis,[59] but these are crude markers of RCT and the effect of CETP inhibition on RCT in humans has yet to be definitively tested.

In addition to promoting RCT, HDL has several other properties including anti-inflammatory, antioxidant and antithrombotic properties, which confer added atheroprotection. The anti-inflammatory properties include inhibition of expression of adhesion molecules in endothelial cells, thereby decreasing monocyte recruitment in the arterial wall.[77] By its antioxidant property, it inhibits the oxidation of LDL.[77] HDL improves the milieu of endothelial cells by increased production of nitric oxide (NO) through up regulation of endothelial NO synthase and decreased apoptosis through SRB1 initiated signaling.[78,79] HDL also demonstrates antithrombotic effects by a variety of mechanisms including activation of prostacycline synthesis, attenuation of tissue factor expression, and decreased thrombin generation.[78]

CETP inhibition also has favorable effects on apoB-containing lipoproteins. As reviewed above, torcetrapib consistently reduced LDL-c levels by 20%–25%. Torcetrapib decreased the VLDL, IDL, and LDL apoB-100 pools by increasing clearance of apoB-100.[80] In the presence of atorvastatin, torcetrapib decreased VLDL apoB-100 by increasing clearance and LDL apoB-100 by decreasing its production.[80] Torcetrapib, significantly reduces the postprandial formation and accumulation of atherogenic triglyceride-rich subspecies including chylomicrons and VLDL-1, as well as reduces their core CE content.[81] Although most animal studies have suggested that CETP inhibition decreases the progression of atherosclerosis,[73,82,83] a recent study failed to show an effect beyond that achieved by atorvastatin alone.[84]

CETP INHIBITORS IN CLINICAL DEVELOPMENT

JJT-705 (Japan Tobacco, Tokyo, Japan), also called the RO4607381, was the first CETP inhibitor to report human phase I trials. JTT-705 has been shown to ubiquitously inhibit CETP activity in rabbits, hamsters, and marmosets while increasing HDL-c levels and decreased the ratio of non-HDL-c to HDL-c.[85] Inhibition of CETP activity by

JTT-705 in rabbits not only increased the quantity of HDL, but also favorably affected the size distribution of HDL subpopulations and increased apo-E levels as well as the enzyme activity of paraoxonase and platelet-activating factor acetylhydrolase in HDL.[86] In a phase II trial for 4 weeks, JJT-705, administered at a dose of 900 mg, increased HDL-c by 34% and decreased CETP activity by 37% in healthy subjects with mild hyperlipidemia without any significant adverse effects.[87] In a small, randomized, placebo-controlled study, type II hyperlipidemic patients on pravastatin were randomized to JJT-705 or placebo. At the end of 4 weeks, the drug was well tolerated with statins and there was 28% increase in HDL-c level and 30% decrease in CETP activity.[88] In-depth analysis of 5 phase II trials of RO4607381/JTT-705 that include patients who have type II dyslipidemia, CHD or CHD risk equivalents randomized to RO4607381/JTT-705 or placebo in combination with different statins have shown a favorable safety profile of the drug with no differences in the cardiac or vascular adverse effects among the active and placebo arm.[89,90] In preclinical studies, and in contrast with torcetrapib, RO4607381/JTT-705 had no impact on blood pressure or RAS gene expression.[71]

Anacetrapib is another CETP inhibitor in clinical development. Two phase I randomized double blinded trials were conducted: one to study the pharmacokinetics and pharmacodynamics of anacetrapib in patients who have dyslipidemia; and the other, to study the effect of anacetrapib on ambulatory blood pressure in healthy individuals.[91] In the first, 50 patients with LDL-c between 100–190 mg/dL underwent a 2–4 week washout of their lipid lowering therapy followed by a 2-week diet run-in period prior to randomization. They were randomized to receive one of four doses of anacetrapib — 10, 40, 150, and 300 mg — or placebo, administered once a day for 28 days with a meal. At the end of 4 weeks, there was a dose-dependent increase in HDL-c from 41% in the 10 mg group to 129% in the 300 mg group, an increase in apoA-1 from 24% to 41%, and a dose-dependent decrease in LDL-c from 5% to 38%. An ambulatory blood pressure study used a crossover design in which 22 healthy subjects were randomized to 150 mg of anacetrapib or matching placebo for 10 days followed by a 14-day washout period before the crossover treatment began. Continuous 24-hour ambulatory blood pressure was measured on day −1 and last day of the treatment periods. At the end of the trial, there was no difference in the systolic or diastolic pressure between the treatment and placebo group. In both of the studies, the drug was well tolerated with no differences in adverse effects among the study and placebo group. In preclinical studies, and in contrast with torcetrapib, anacetrapib did not cause elevation in blood pressure or plasma levels of adrenal corticosteroids.[72]

SUMMARY

Though the torcetrapib experience was a major blow to CETP inhibition and indeed the entire field of HDL-targeted therapeutics, it was not fatal. The off-target effects of torcetrapib appear to be substantial and may have overridden any potential cardiovascular benefit. Despite continued uncertainty regarding the cardiovascular implications of genetic CETP deficiency and pharmacologic CETP inhibition, there remain reasons to believe in the mechanism and the possibility that clean CETP inhibitors will not only improve plasma lipids, but that they will reduce cardiovascular risk. However, there will be substantial scrutiny of the CETP inhibitors in clinical development and the only hope of registration is a positive clinical endpoint trial with acceptable safety. Currently, there is still life after torcetrapib; future developments will determine just how long that life will last.

REFERENCES

1. Grundy SM, Cleeman JI, Merz CN, et al. Implications of recent clinical trials for the National Cholesterol Education Program Adult Treatment Panel III guidelines. Circulation 2004;110(2):227–39.
2. Cannon CP, Braunwald E, McCabe CH, et al. Intensive versus moderate lipid lowering with statins after acute coronary syndromes. N Engl J Med 2004; 350(15):1495–504.
3. LaRosa JC, Grundy SM, Waters DD, et al. Intensive lipid lowering with atorvastatin in patients with stable coronary disease. N Engl J Med 2005;352(14): 1425–35.
4. Ashen MD, Blumenthal RS. Clinical practice. Low HDL cholesterol levels. N Engl J Med 2005; 353(12):1252–60.
5. Gordon T, Castelli WP, Hjortland MC, et al. High density lipoprotein as a protective factor against coronary heart disease. The Framingham Study. Am J Med 1977;62:707–14.
6. Gordon DJ, Probstfield JL, Garrison RJ, et al. High-density lipoprotein cholesterol and cardiovascular disease. Four prospective American studies. Circulation 1989;79(1):8–15.
7. Timmins JM, Lee JY, Boudyguina E, et al. Targeted inactivation of hepatic Abca1 causes profound

hypoalphalipoproteinemia and kidney hypercatabo-lism of apoA-I. J Clin Invest 2005;115(5):1333–42.

8. Brunham L, Kruit JK, Pape TD, et al. Intestinal ABCA1 is a significant contributor to plasma HDL-C and apoB levels in vivo. J Clin Invest 2006; 116:1052–62.

9. Wang N, Lan D, Chen W, et al. ATP-binding cassette transporters G1 and G4 mediate cellular cholesterol efflux to high-density lipoproteins. Proc Natl Acad Sci U S A 2004;101(26):9774–9.

10. Kennedy MA, Barrera GC, Nakamura K, et al. ABCG1 has a critical role in mediating cholesterol efflux to HDL and preventing cellular lipid accumula-tion. Cell Metab 2005;1(2):121–31.

11. Schwartz CC, VandenBroek JM, Cooper PS. Lipo-protein cholesteryl ester production, transfer, and output in vivo in humans. J Lipid Res 2004;45(9): 1594–607.

12. Tordjman K, Bernal-Mizrachi C, Zemany L, et al. PPARalpha deficiency reduces insulin resistance and atherosclerosis in apoE-null mice. J Clin Invest 2001;107(8):1025–34.

13. Yu-Poth S, Zhao G, Etherton T, et al. Effects of the National Cholesterol Education Program's Step I and Step II dietary intervention programs on cardio-vascular disease risk factors: a meta-analysis. Am J Clin Nutr 1999;69(4):632–46.

14. Chu NF, Makowski L, Hotamisligil GS, et al. Stability of human plasma leptin concentrations within 36 hours following specimen collection. Clin Biochem 1999;32(1):87–9.

15. Maeda K, Noguchi Y, Fukui T. The effects of cessation from cigarette smoking on the lipid and lipoprotein profiles: a meta-analysis. Prev Med 2003;37(4):283–90.

16. Edwards JE, Moore RA. Statins in hypercholestero-laemia: a dose-specific meta-analysis of lipid changes in randomised, double blind trials. BMC Fam Pract 2003;4:18.

17. Nissen SE, Tuzcu EM, Schoenhagen P, et al. Effect of intensive compared with moderate lipid-lowering therapy on progression of coronary atherosclerosis: a randomized controlled trial. JAMA 2004;291(9): 1071–80.

18. Jukema JW, Liem AH, Dunselman P, et al. LDL-C/HDL-C ratio in subjects with cardiovascular disease and a low HDL-C: results of the RADAR (Rosuvastatin and Atorvastatin in different Dosages And Reverse cholesterol transport) study. Curr Med Res Opin 2005;21(11):1865–74.

19. de Haan W, van der Hoogt CC, Westerterp M, et al. Atorvastatin increases HDL cholesterol by reducing CETP expression in cholesterol-fed APOE*3-Leiden.CETP mice. Atherosclerosis 2008;197(1): 57–63.

20. Birjmohun RS, Hutten BA, Kastelein JJ, et al. Efficacy and safety of high-density lipoprotein cholesterol-increasing compounds: a meta-analysis of randomized controlled trials. J Am Coll Cardiol 2005;45(2):185–97.

21. Canner PL, Berge KG, Wenger NK, et al. 15 year mortality in Coronary Drug Project patients - long-term benefit with niacin. J Am Coll Cardiol 1986; 8(6):1245–55.

22. Brown BG, Zhao XQ, Chait A, et al. Simvastatin and niacin, antioxidant vitamins, or the combination for the prevention of coronary disease. N Engl J Med 2001;345(22):1583–92.

23. Taylor AJ, Sullenberger LE, Lee HJ, et al. Arterial Biology for the Investigation of the Treatment Effects of Reducing Cholesterol (ARBITER) 2: a double-blind, placebo-controlled study of extended-release niacin on atherosclerosis progression in secondary prevention patients treated with statins. Circulation 2004;110(23):3512–7.

24. Rubins HB, Robins SJ, Collins D, et al. Gemfibrozil for the secondary prevention of coronary heart disease in men with low levels of high-density lipo-protein cholesterol. N Engl J Med 1999;341:410–8.

25. Frick MH, Elo O, Haapa K, et al. Helsinki Heart Study: primary-prevention trial with gemfibrozil in middle-aged men with dyslipidemia. Safety of treatment, changes in risk factors, and incidence of coronary heart disease. N Engl J Med 1987;317: 1237–45.

26. Keech A, Simes RJ, Barter P, et al. Effects of long-term fenofibrate therapy on cardiovascular events in 9795 people with type 2 diabetes mellitus (the FIELD study): randomised controlled trial. Lancet 2005;366(9500):1849–61.

27. Ginsberg HN, Bonds DE, Lovato LC, et al. Evolution of the lipid trial protocol of the Action to Control Cardiovascular Risk in Diabetes (ACCORD) trial. Am J Cardiol 2007;99(12A):56i–67i.

28. Lewis GF, Rader DJ. New insights into the regulation of HDL metabolism and reverse cholesterol trans-port. Circ Res 2005;96(12):1221–32.

29. Inazu A, Brown ML, Hesler CB, et al. Increased high-density lipoprotein levels caused by a common cholesteryl-ester transfer protein gene mutation. N Engl J Med 1990;323:1234–8.

30. Brown ML, Inazu A, Hesler CB, et al. Molecular basis of lipid transfer protein deficiency in a family with increased high-density lipoproteins. Nature 1989; 342(6248):448–51.

31. Inazu A, Jiang XC, Haraki T, et al. Genetic cholesteryl ester transfer protein deficiency caused by two prevalent mutations as a major determinant of increased levels of high density lipoprotein cholesterol. J Clin Invest 1994;94(5):1872–82.

32. Nagano M, Yamashita S, Hirano K, et al. Molecular mechanisms of cholesteryl ester transfer protein deficiency in Japanese. J Atheroscler Thromb 2004;11(3):110–21.

33. Hirano K, Yamashita S, Nakajima N, et al. Genetic cholesteryl ester transfer protein deficiency is extremely frequent in the Omagari area of Japan. Marked hyperalphalipoproteinemia caused by CETP gene mutation is not associated with longevity. Arterioscler Thromb Vasc Biol 1997;17(6):1053–9.

34. Zhong S, Sharp DS, Grove JS, et al. Increased coronary heart disease in Japanese-American men with mutations in the cholesteryl ester transfer protein gene despite increased HDL levels. J Clin Invest 1996;97:2687–8.

35. Moriyama Y, Okamura T, Inazu A, et al. A low prevalence of coronary heart disease among subjects with increased high-density lipoprotein cholesterol levels, including those with plasma cholesteryl ester transfer protein deficiency. Prev Med 1998; 27(5 Pt 1):659–67.

36. Drayna D, Lawn R. Multiple RFLPs at the human cholesteryl ester transfer protein (CETP) locus. Nucleic Acids Res 1987;15(11):4698.

37. Corbex M, Poirier O, Fumeron F, et al. Extensive association analysis between the CETP gene and coronary heart disease phenotypes reveals several putative functional polymorphisms and gene-environment interaction. Genet Epidemiol 2000; 19(1):64–80.

38. Klerkx A, Tanck M, Kastelein JJ, et al. Haplotype analysis of the CETP gene: not TaqIB, but the closely linked -629C→A polymorphism and a novel promoter variant are independently associated with CETP concentration. Hum Mol Genet 2003;12(2): 111–23.

39. Ordovas JM, Cupples LA, Corella D, et al. Association of cholesteryl ester transfer protein-TaqIB polymorphism with variations in lipoprotein subclasses and coronary heart disease risk: the Framingham study. Arterioscler Thromb Vasc Biol 2000; 20(5):1323–9.

40. Jungers P, Massy ZA, Khoa TN, et al. Incidence and risk factors of atherosclerotic cardiovascular accidents in predialysis chronic renal failure patients: a prospective study. Nephrol Dial Transplant 1997; 12(12):2597–602.

41. Hannuksela ML, Johanna Liinamaa M, Antero Kesaniemi Y, et al. Relation of polymorphisms in the cholesteryl ester transfer protein gene to transfer protein activity and plasma lipoprotein levels in alcohol drinkers. Atherosclerosis 1994;110(1):35–44.

42. Brousseau ME, O'Connor JJ Jr, Ordovas JM, et al. Cholesteryl ester transfer protein TaqI B2B2 genotype is associated with higher HDL cholesterol levels and lower risk of coronary heart disease end points in men with HDL deficiency: Veterans Affairs HDL Cholesterol Intervention Trial. Arterioscler Thromb Vasc Biol 2002;22(7):1148–54.

43. Kuivenhoven JA, Jukema JW, Zwinderman AH, et al. The role of a common variant of the cholesteryl ester transfer protein gene in the progression of coronary atherosclerosis. N Engl J Med 1998;338(2):86–93.

44. Frisdal E, Klerkx AHEM, Goff WL, et al. Functional interaction between -629C/A, -971G/A and -1337C/T polymorphisms in the CETP gene is a major determinant of promoter activity and plasma CETP concentration in the REGRESS Study. Hum Mol Genet 2005;14(18):2607–18.

45. McCaskie PA, Beilby JP, Chapman CM, et al. Cholesteryl ester transfer protein gene haplotypes, plasma high-density lipoprotein levels and the risk of coronary heart disease. Hum Genet 2007; 121(3-4):401–11.

46. Borggreve SE, Hillege HL, Wolffenbuttel BH, et al. An increased coronary risk is paradoxically associated with common cholesteryl ester transfer protein gene variations that relate to higher high-density lipoprotein cholesterol: a population-based study. J Clin Endocrinol Metab 2006;91(9):3382–8.

47. Thompson A, Di Angelantonio E, Sarwar N, et al. Association of cholesteryl ester transfer protein genotypes with CETP mass and activity, lipid levels, and coronary risk. JAMA 2008;299(23):2777–88.

48. Lu B, Budoff MJ, Zhuang N, et al. Causes of interscan variability of coronary artery calcium measurements at electron-beam CT. Acad Radiol 2002; 9(6):654–61.

49. de Grooth GJ, Smilde TJ, van Wissen S, et al. The relationship between cholesteryl ester transfer protein levels and risk factor profile in patients with familial hypercholesterolemia. Atherosclerosis 2004;173(2):261–7.

50. Klerkx A, de Grooth GJ, Zwinderman AH, et al. Cholesteryl ester transfer protein (CETP) concentration is associated with progression of atherosclerosis and response to pravastatin in men with coronary artery disease (REGRESS). Eur J Clin Invest 2004; 34:21–8.

51. Boekholdt SM, Kuivenhoven JA, Wareham NJ, et al. Plasma levels of cholesteryl ester transfer protein and the risk of future coronary artery disease in apparently healthy men and women: the prospective EPIC (European Prospective Investigation into Cancer and nutrition)-Norfolk population study. Circulation 2004;110(11):1418–23.

52. Borggreve SE, Hillege HL, Dallinga-Thie GM, et al. High plasma cholesteryl ester transfer protein levels may favour reduced incidence of cardiovascular events in men with low triglycerides. Eur Heart J 2007;28(8):1012–8.

53. Hibino T, Sakuma N, Sato T. Higher level of plasma cholesteryl ester transfer activity from high-density lipoprotein to apo B-containing lipoproteins in subjects with angiographically detectable coronary artery disease. Clin Cardiol 1996;19(6):483–6.

54. de Vries R, Kerstens MN, Sluiter WJ, et al. Cellular cholesterol efflux to plasma from moderately

hypercholesterolaemic type 1 diabetic patients is enhanced, and is unaffected by simvastatin treatment. Diabetologia 2005;48(6):1105–13.

55. Zeller M, Masson D, Farnier M, et al. High serum cholesteryl ester transfer rates and small high-density lipoproteins are associated with young age in patients with acute myocardial infarction. J Am Coll Cardiol 2007;50(20):1948–55.

56. Clark RW, Ruggeri RB, Cunningham D, et al. Description of the torcetrapib series of cholesteryl ester transfer protein inhibitors, including mechanism of action. J Lipid Res 2006;47(3):537–52.

57. Clark RW, Sutfin TA, Ruggeri RB, et al. Raising high-density lipoprotein in humans through inhibition of cholesteryl ester transfer protein: an initial multidose study of torcetrapib. Arterioscler Thromb Vasc Biol 2004;24(3):490–7.

58. Brousseau ME, Schaefer EJ, Wolfe ML, et al. Effects of an inhibitor of cholesteryl ester transfer protein on HDL cholesterol. N Engl J Med 2004;350(15):1505–15.

59. Brousseau ME, Diffenderfer MR, Millar JS, et al. Effects of cholesteryl ester transfer protein inhibition on high-density lipoprotein subspecies, apolipoprotein A-I metabolism, and fecal sterol excretion. Arterioscler Thromb Vasc Biol 2005;25(5):1057–64.

60. Davidson MH, McKenney JM, Shear CL, et al. Efficacy and safety of torcetrapib, a novel cholesteryl ester transfer protein inhibitor, in individuals with below-average high-density lipoprotein cholesterol levels. J Am Coll Cardiol 2006;48(9):1774–81.

61. McKenney JM, Davidson MH, Shear CL, et al. Efficacy and safety of torcetrapib, a novel cholesteryl ester transfer protein inhibitor, in individuals with below-average high-density lipoprotein cholesterol levels on a background of atorvastatin. J Am Coll Cardiol 2006;48(9):1782–90 [Abstract].

62. Thuren T, Longcore A, Powell C, et al. Effect of torcetrapib combined with atorvastatin on HDL-C and LDL-C levels, particle size, and composition: a phase 2 dose-ranging clinical trial. Atheroscler Suppl 2006;7(3):550–550.

63. Nissen SE, Tardif J-C, Nicholls SJ, et al. Effect of torcetrapib on the progression of coronary atherosclerosis. N Engl J Med 2007;356(13):1304–16.

64. Diringer K, Gibbs MA, Amin N, et al. Lack of an effect of ezetimibe on the pharmacokinetics of torcetrapib/atorvastatin in healthy subjects. Clin Pharmacol Ther 2007;81:S110–1.

65. Terra SG, Diringer K. The pharmacokinetics of torcetrapib/atorvastatin are unaffected by co-administration of fenofibrate in healthy adult subjects. J Am Coll Cardiol 2007;49(9):365A–365A [Abstract].

66. Kastelein JJP, van Leuven SI, Burgess L, et al. Effect of torcetrapib on carotid atherosclerosis in familial hypercholesterolemia. N Engl J Med 2007;356(16):1620–30.

67. Bots ML, Visseren FL, Evans GW, et al. Torcetrapib and carotid intima-media thickness in mixed dyslipidaemia (RADIANCE 2 study): a randomised, double-blind trial. Lancet 2007;370(9582):153–60.

68. Nicholls SJ, Brennan DM, Wolski K, et al. Abstract 684: changes in levels of high density lipoprotein cholesterol predict the impact of torcetrapib on progression of coronary atherosclerosis: Insights from ILLUSTRATE. Circulation 2007;116:127 [Abstract].

69. Barter PJ, Caulfield M, Eriksson M, et al. Effects of torcetrapib in patients at high risk for coronary events. N Engl J Med 2007;357(21):2109–22.

70. Rader DJ. Illuminating HDL—Is it still a viable therapeutic target? N Engl J Med 2007;357(21):2180–3.

71. Stroes ES, Kastelein JJ, Benardeau A, et al. Absence of effect of R1658/JTT-705 on blood pressure and tissue expression of renin-angiotensin system-related genes in rats. J Am Coll Cardiol 2008;51(10):A322–322 [Abstract].

72. Forrest MJ, Bloomfield D, Briscoe RJ, et al. Torcetrapib-induced blood pressure elevation is independent of cholesteryl ester transfer protein inhibition and is accompanied by an increase in circulating aldosterone levels. Br J Pharmacol 2008;154:1465–73.

73. DePasquale M, Knight D, Loging W, et al. Mechanistic studies of hemodynamics with a series of cholesterol ester transfer protein inhibitors. Circ Res 2007;101(11):1209–10.

74. Matsuura F, Wang N, Chen WG, et al. HDL from CETP-deficient subjects shows enhanced ability to promote cholesterol efflux from macrophages in an apoE- and ABCG1-dependent pathway. J Clin Invest 2006;116(5):1435–42.

75. Yvan-Charvet L, Matsuura F, Wang N, et al. Inhibition of cholesteryl ester transfer protein by torcetrapib modestly increases macrophage cholesterol efflux to HDL. Arterioscler Thromb Vasc Biol 2007;27(5):1132–8.

76. Tanigawa H, Billheimer JT, Tohyama J, et al. Expression of cholesteryl ester transfer protein in mice promotes macrophage reverse cholesterol transport. Circulation 2007;116(11):1267–73.

77. Barter PJ, Nicholls S, Rye KA, et al. Antiinflammatory properties of HDL. Circ Res 2004;95(8):764–72.

78. Mineo C, Yuhanna IS, Quon MJ, et al. High density lipoprotein-induced endothelial nitric-oxide synthase activation is mediated by Akt and MAP kinases. J Biol Chem 2003;278(11):9142–9.

79. Yuhanna IS, Zhu Y, Cox BE, et al. High-density lipoprotein binding to scavenger receptor-BI activates endothelial nitric oxide synthase. Nat Med 2001;7(7):853–7.

80. Millar JS, Brousseau ME, Diffenderfer MR, et al. Effects of the cholesteryl ester transfer protein inhibitor torcetrapib on apolipoprotein B100 metabolism in

humans. Arterioscler Thromb Vasc Biol 2006;26(6): 1350–6.

81. Guerin M, Le Goff W, Duchene E, et al. Inhibition of CETP by torcetrapib attenuates the atherogenicity of postprandial TG-rich lipoproteins in type IIB hyperlipidemia. Arterioscler Thromb Vasc Biol 2008; 28(1):148–54.

82. Okamoto H, Yonemori F, Wakitani K, et al. A cholesteryl ester transfer protein inhibitor attenuates atherosclerosis in rabbits. Nature 2000;406(6792): 203–7.

83. Morehouse LA, Sugarman ED, Bourassa PA, et al. Inhibition of CETP activity by torcetrapib reduces susceptibility to diet-induced atherosclerosis in New Zealand White rabbits. J Lipid Res 2007; 48(6):1263–72.

84. de Haan W, de Vries-van der Weij J, van der Hoorn J, et al. Torcetrapib does not reduce atherosclerosis beyond atorvastatin and induces more proinflammatory lesions than atorvastatin. Circulation 2008;117(19):2515–22.

85. Okamoto H, Iwamoto Y, Maki M, et al. Effect of JTT-705 on cholesteryl ester transfer protein and plasma lipid levels in normolipidemic animals. Eur J Pharmacol 2003;466(1-2):147–54.

86. Zhang B, Fan P, Shimoji E, et al. Inhibition of cholesteryl ester transfer protein activity by JTT-705 increases apolipoprotein E-containing high-density lipoprotein and favorably affects the function and enzyme composition of high-density lipoprotein in rabbits. Arterioscler Thromb Vasc Biol 2004;24(10): 1910–5.

87. de Grooth GJ, Kuivenhoven JA, Stalenhoef AF, et al. Efficacy and safety of a novel cholesteryl ester transfer protein inhibitor, JTT-705, in humans: a randomized phase II dose-response study. Circulation 2002;105(18):2159–65.

88. Kuivenhoven JA, de Grooth GJ, Kawamura H, et al. Effectiveness of inhibition of cholesteryl ester transfer protein by JTT-705 in combination with pravastatin in type II dyslipidemia. Am J Cardiol 2005; 95(9):1085–8.

89. Steiner G, Kastelein JJ, Kallend D, et al. Cardiovascular safety of the cholesteryl ester transfer protein inhibitor R1658/JTT-705: results from phase 2 trials. J Am Coll Cardiol 2008;51(10):A333–333.

90. Stein EA, Kallend D, Buckley B. Safety profile of the cholesteryl ester transfer protein inhibitor R1658/ JTT-705 in patients with type II hyperlipidemia or coronary heart disease. J Am Coll Cardiol 2008;51(10): A333–4.

91. Krishna R, Anderson MS, Bergman AJ, et al. Effect of the cholesteryl ester transfer protein inhibitor, anacetrapib, on lipoproteins in patients with dyslipidaemia and on 24-h ambulatory blood pressure in healthy individuals: two double-blind, randomized placebo-controlled phase I studies. Lancet 2007; 370(9603):1907–14.

Extended-Release Niacin/Laropiprant: Reducing Niacin-Induced Flushing to Better Realize the Benefit of Niacin in Improving Cardiovascular Risk Factors

John F. Paolini, MD, PhD[a],*, Harold E. Bays, MD[b],
Christie M. Ballantyne, MD[c], Michael Davidson, MD[d],
Richard Pasternak, MD[a], Darbie Maccubbin, PhD[a],
Josephine M. Norquist, MS[e], Eseng Lai, MD, PhD[a],
M. Gerard Waters, PhD[a], Olga Kuznetsova, PhD[a],
Christine McCrary Sisk, BS[a], Yale B. Mitchel, MD[a]

KEYWORDS

- Cardiovascular risk • Extended-release niacin
- Flushing • Laropiprant • Prostaglandin D_2

A substantial body of experimental, epidemiologic, and clinical trial data demonstrates that increased plasma low-density lipoprotein cholesterol (LDL-C) is associated with the progression of atherosclerotic coronary heart disease (CHD), and lowering LDL-C levels reduces CHD risk. Thus, reducing LDL-C levels remains the primary lipoprotein treatment target for reducing the risk of CHD.[1–3]

Guidelines from regulatory bodies and expert panels have established different CHD risk categories and specific LDL-C treatment targets for each category.[1,4] Statin drugs are recommended as the initial therapy for lowering CHD risk, based on their LDL-C-lowering efficacy and favorable safety profile for most patients. Although relative risk reductions in major cardiovascular events

Merck & Company, Incorporated provided financial support for the conduct of the studies described in this article. John F. Paolini, Richard Pasternak, Darbie Maccubbin, Josephine M. Norquist, Eseng Lai, M. Gerard Waters, Olga Kuznetsova, Christine McCrary Sisk, and Yale B. Mitchel are employees of Merck & Company, Incorporated who may own stock and/or hold stock options in the company. Harold E. Bays, Christie M. Ballantyne, and Michael Davidson have served as clinical investigators for Merck & Company, Incorporated.

[a] Merck & Company, Incorporated, 126 East Lincoln Avenue, Rahway, NJ 07065, USA
[b] Louisville Metabolic and Atherosclerosis Research Center, 3288 Illinois Avenue, Suite 101, Louisville, KY 40213, USA
[c] Baylor College of Medicine and Methodist DeBakey Heart and Vascular Center, Section of Atherosclerosis and Vascular Medicine, One Baylor Plaza, Houston, TX 77030, USA
[d] Chicago Center for Clinical Research, 515 North State Street, Suite 2700, Chicago, IL 60654, USA
[e] Merck & Company, Incorporated, PO Box 1000, Upper Gwynedd, PA 19454-2505, USA
* Corresponding author.
E-mail address: john_paolini@merck.com (J.F. Paolini).

Cardiol Clin 26 (2008) 547–560
doi:10.1016/j.ccl.2008.06.007

from clinical outcomes trials of approximately 30% have been achieved with statin therapy, a substantial residual risk for clinical events (myocardial infarction [MI], coronary death, coronary revascularization, and stroke) remains for patients, even when well-treated for elevated LDL-C with a statin (**Table 1**), underscoring the need for therapies that target additional lipid risk factors.[5,6]

Vast experimental and epidemiologic data support an inverse association between HDL-C levels and CHD.[1,7] A meta-analysis of three clinical outcomes trials demonstrated that a 1 mg/dL higher level of HDL-C was associated with a 2% (men) or 3% (women) lower CHD risk.[7] Thus, raising HDL-C is a promising treatment target toward reducing CHD risk. HDL is hypothesized to participate in the transport of cholesterol from peripheral tissues (eg, that may be located in endothelial plaques) to the liver. Additionally, HDL may suppress vascular inflammation associated with atherosclerosis and have favorable antioxidative and antithrombotic effects.[8] In addition, several epidemiologic studies have provided evidence that elevated triglyceride (TG) levels are correlated with increased CHD risk.[9–12] This may be related, in part, to the inverse relationship between TG and HDL-C levels and the association between elevated TG levels and small dense low-density lipoproteins (LDL), which are believed to be especially atherogenic.

A joint statement released recently by the American Diabetes Association (ADA) and the American College of Cardiology (ACC) emphasizes the clinical importance of lipoprotein risk factors other than LDL-C in patients at high-risk for cardiovascular disease.[13] Citing evidence from epidemiologic studies and posthoc analyses of clinical trials that suggest non-HDL-C and Apo B are better predictors of cardiovascular risk than LDL-C, the ADA-ACC consensus statement recommended non-HDL-C goals of less than 100 and less than 130 mg/dL, respectively, and Apo B goals of less than 90 and less than 80 mg/dL, respectively, for high-risk patients without established heart disease and for highest risk patients who have heart disease or who have diabetes and other cardiovascular risk factors.[13]

NIACIN

Niacin (nicotinic acid) is a water-soluble B vitamin used to treat dyslipidemia for over 50 years.[14–16] Used in gram amounts, niacin has broad beneficial effects on the lipid profile, reducing plasma LDL-C and TG and increasing HDL-C levels.[17–19] The use of niacin and statin drugs together improves multiple key lipid/lipoprotein parameters known to impact CHD risk. Several clinical trials have shown that niacin produces cardiovascular benefit when used alone or together with statins (see **Table 1**).[20–22] The Coronary Drug Project, a large-scale placebo-controlled trial conducted between 1966 and 1975, demonstrated that niacin reduces CHD events: a 27% reduction in nonfatal MI and a 15% reduction in the combined endpoint of nonfatal MI and death were observed compared with placebo-treated patients.[20] A 15-year follow-up of the Coronary Drug Project revealed that patients in the niacin group had an 11% reduction in total mortality compared with those in the placebo group.[23] Two angiographic trials provided evidence that niacin coadministered with the bile acid sequestrant colestipol caused either regression or slowed progression of coronary stenosis or atherosclerosis.[24,25] Finally, in the HDL-Atherosclerosis Treatment Study (HATS), simvastatin plus slow-release niacin resulted in significant regression of coronary stenosis versus placebo and, consistent with this finding, a reduction in cardiovascular events.[21]

UNDERUTILIZATION OF NIACIN

Despite the acknowledged benefits in comprehensive lipid management and prevention of cardiovascular events, niacin is underutilized in clinical practice. A persistent, major impediment to the optimal use of niacin is the associated cutaneous flushing. Most patients who receive niacin, even at the 500 mg dose, experience flushing of the face and trunk.[26,27]

One approach to mitigate the flushing effects of immediate-release niacin, whose peak blood levels are attained 30 to 60 minutes after administration, has been through the development of niacin formulations that slow the release rate after oral administration.[28] Slow-release niacin has a dissolution time of over 12 hours and reduced flushing. Unfortunately, such agents are associated with increased hepatotoxicity. An extended-release (ER) niacin formulation (NIASPAN [Abbott Laboratories, North Chicago, IL] niacin ER tablets) has an absorption time (8 to 12 hours) between that of immediate-release and slow-release niacin and, as a result, reduced flushing compared with immediate-release niacin and an acceptable hepatic safety profile.[29,30] Amelioration of flushing with NIASPAN, however, requires a four-step, gradual titration regimen over 3 months to reach the efficacious 2 g dose. In the United States, patients begin with 0.5 g daily at bedtime and titrate the dose in 0.5 g increments every 4 weeks to 2 g. In the European Union and several Asian countries, the titration requires additional steps, initiating at

Table 1
Niacin and atherosclerosis: a positive effect on clinical outcomes

Trial	Study Population	Treatment (Mean Dose)	Number of Participants	Change in Lipids by Treatment Group					Findings
				PBO	T–C (%)	TG (%)	LDL-C (%)	HDL-C (%)	
CDP	Men (30–64 yrs) post-MI	Niacin (3 g/d)	1119	2789	↓ 10	↓ 19	NR	NR	↓ 27% Nonfatal MI (P < .0005) ↓ 11% All-cause mortality vs. placebo (P = .0004)
CLAS I	Men (40–59 yrs) post-CABG	Niacin (4.3 g/d) + colestipol (30 g/d)	80	82	↓ 26	↓ 21	↓ 43	↑ 37	Significant angiographic regression
CLAS II	Men (40–59 yrs) post-CABG, 2-yr extension to CLAS I	Niacin (4.3 g/d) + colestipol (30 g/d)	56	47	↓ 25	↓ 18	↓ 40	↑ 37	Angiographic regression continued at 4 yrs
FATS	Men <62 yrs with high Apo B, CAD + history of VD	Niacin (4 g/d) + colestipol (30 g/d)	36	46	↓ 23	↓ 29	↓ 32	↑ 42	Significant angiographic regression ↓ 80% clinical events[a] (P < .01)
HATS	Men/women with CHD, low HDL-C	Niacin (2.4 g/d) + simvastatin (13 mg/d)	33	34	↓ 31	↓ 38	↓ 43	↑ 29	Significant angiographic regression ↓ 60% clinical events[a] (P = .02)
Stockholm IHD	Men/women post-MI	Niacin (3 g/d) + clofibrate (2 g/d)	279	276	↓ 13	↓ 19	NR	NR	↓ 36% ischemic heart disease mortality (P <.01); ↓ 26% total mortality (P < .05)
ARBITER 2	Men/women with CHD + low HDL-C	ER Niacin (1 g/d) + ongoing statin	78	71	↓ 1	↓ 13	↓ 2	↑ 21	Slowed atherosclerosis progression at 12 months; no significant effect on CV events
ARBITER 3	Men/women with CHD + low HDL-C completing ARBITER 2	ER niacin (1 g/d) + ongoing statin	57	–	NR	↓ 22	↓ 9	↑ 24	Additional slowing of atherosclerosis progression at 24 months

Abbreviations: ARBITER, Arterial Biology for the Investigation of Treatment Effects of Reducing Cholesterol; CABG, coronary artery bypass graft; CAD, coronary artery disease; CDP, Coronary Drug Project; CHD, coronary heart disease; CLAS, Cholesterol-Lowering Atherosclerosis Study; CV, cardiovascular; ER, extended release; FATS, Familial Atherosclerosis Treatment Study; HATS, Atherosclerosis Treatment Study; HDL, high-density lipoprotein; LDL, low-density lipoprotein; MI, myocardial infarction; NR, not recorded; PBO, placebo; T–C, total cholesterol; TG, triglyceride; VD, vascular disease; vs, versus.

[a] Coronary death, stroke, revascularization, MI, worsening ischemia.

the 375 mg dose for the first week and titrating weekly to 500, 750, and 1000 mg in the fourth week. There is then further titration in 500 mg increments every 4 weeks up to 2 g at week 12.

Clinically meaningful lipid efficacy requires ER niacin doses of at least 1 g/d, and the 2 g/d dose provides twice the LDL-C reduction, twice the HDL-C elevation, and several times the TG reduction. However, the frequent ER niacin titration steps, along with persistent, episodic, bothersome, and unpredictable flushing episodes that sometimes have no obvious explanation limit dose escalation and patient acceptance and often lead to discontinuation of niacin therapy and the failure to achieve the optimal 2 g dose.

Three observational studies have elucidated the limitations in tolerability of ER niacin. These studies evaluated use and dosing patterns in clinical practice and the impact of flushing and other tolerability issues on suboptimal dosing and discontinuation.[31–34] The studies were conducted in the United States and Canada, where NIASPAN is the most frequently used prescription niacin formulation. Taken together, the results demonstrated poor persistency with ER niacin use and poor use of the 2 g dose in clinical practice, with flushing being the major reason.

The first study demonstrated in a chart review of clinical practices that at the 1-year time point after therapy initiation, only 14.6% of the original cohort of patients still filled prescriptions, the second highest discontinuation rate among lipid-modifying drug classes, second only to bile acid sequestrants (**Fig. 1**). Additionally, patients were not being titrated upwards to the efficacious lipid-altering doses. At 6 months, 39% of the patients persistent with ER niacin therapy still were receiving less than or equal to 500 mg/d (see **Fig. 1**),[31,32] a dose which

offers little to no therapeutic benefit. At the end of the 1-year follow-up, only 5.8% of the original cohort took 1000 mg, and only 2.2% received more than 1500 mg.

The second study elucidated that flushing symptoms were the principal reasons given for discontinuation in about 91% of patients who discontinued ER niacin, and 54.4% experienced severe or extreme flushing.[33] In addition to flushing, other niacin-related adverse effects (ie, headache, gastrointestinal [GI] symptoms, insomnia) were described.

In the third study, patients initiating niacin therapy were interviewed prospectively about flushing symptoms.[34] Preliminary results demonstrated a trend consistent with the first retrospective observational study. At 6 months of follow-up, 53% still took 500 mg of ER niacin; 37% took 1 g, and only 2% took 2 g. The results also showed that the use of aspirin to reduce flushing was suboptimal, with regard to both the proportion of patients using aspirin and the dosage being used. Fewer than half of the patients using niacin received instruction from their physicians to use medication to mitigate flushing, and only 50% of those instructed actually used medication.

FLUSHING PATHWAY INHIBITION SUPPORTS A NEW NIACIN-DOSING REGIMEN

Although the mechanism by which niacin induces flushing is not understood completely, several lines of evidence suggest that flushing is mediated largely through prostaglandins, primarily PGD_2. First, predosing with aspirin (at doses of 325 mg and higher) or indomethacin, which inhibits synthesis of all prostanoids,[35] modestly attenuates niacin-induced flushing.[36–42] Second, plasma levels

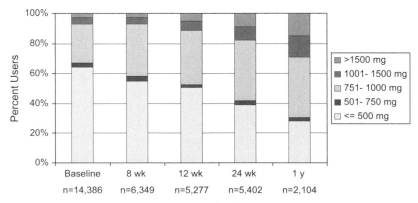

Fig. 1. Percentage of users of extended-release niacin at fixed time intervals by average daily dose. Includes patients with extended-release niacin prescription refills. Index prescription that identified patient's index date was recorded from a database as a 30-day supply. Sample size at baseline is therefore equal at 4 weeks (30 days). (*From* Kamal-Bahl S, Burke T, Watson D. Dosage, titration, and gaps in treatment with extended-release niacin in clinical practice. Curr Med Res Opin 2008;24:1819; with permission.)

of 9a, 11β-PGF_2, a metabolite of PGD_2, dramatically increases (430- to 800-fold) following a single oral dose of 500 mg niacin, peaking from 12 to 45 minutes after the dose and returning to baseline by 2 to 4 hours.[37] Importantly, niacin dosing does not increase histamine metabolites and modestly increases PGE_2[43,44] or a prostacyclin metabolite.[37] Third, intravenous infusion of PGD_2 is associated with intense facial flushing and nasal congestion.[45]

A study in a mouse model of niacin-induced vasodilation demonstrated that niacin-induced vasodilation is mediated in part by PGD_2 acting through one of the prostaglandin D type 1 receptors, called DP1.[46] Importantly, selective antagonism of DP1 with laropiprant produced significant dose-dependent suppression of PGD_2- and niacin-induced vasodilation.[46] Taken together, these observations suggest that blockade of the PGD_2 receptor, specifically the subtype 1 (DP1), may suppress the flushing symptoms associated with niacin. Moreover, although the flushing effects of niacin are mediated by the niacin receptor, they appear to be independent of the lipid-modifying effects of niacin.[14]

LAROPIPRANT

Laropiprant, a selective antagonist of DP1 (Ki 0.57 nM and 190-fold less potent at the thromboxane A2 receptor, TP), was examined in a series of clinical studies to determine its ability to reduce flushing and improve the tolerability of niacin. A clinical proof-of-concept study demonstrated that laropiprant significantly suppressed vasodilation induced by ER niacin and improved patient-reported flushing symptoms (using a rudimentary 11-point symptom severity scale) to a degree greater than that provided by aspirin before treatment.[47] The symptomatic improvement with laropiprant correlated with a reduction in the skin vasodilation induced by ER niacin, as quantitated with laser Doppler perfusion imaging.[47] Laropiprant was tolerated well, having been studied alone or coadministered with niacin in long-term preclinical animal chronic toxicity studies, as well as clinical pharmacology multiple-dose studies using up to 10 times the exposure used in subsequent human studies.[47]

MEASURING NIACIN-INDUCED FLUSHING: THE FLUSHING SYMPTOM QUESTIONNAIRE

Existing tools that report flushing adverse experiences and discontinuations were not considered sufficiently objective, precise, or robust to support a rigorous clinical development program. Thus, a quantitative Flushing Symptom Questionnaire (FSQ, Merck & Company, Incorporated, Whitehouse Station, New Jersey) was developed that consisted of an 11-item diary, assessing aspects of the frequency, severity, duration, and bother of niacin-induced flushing (including symptoms of redness, warmth, tingling, and/or itching).[48] The content of the FSQ was developed with input from patients taking niacin and clinicians experienced in treating patients with niacin to address four key objectives:

1. Accurately measure the magnitude and severity of niacin-induced flushing
2. Define the key treatment windows/endpoints in which niacin use is problematic to patients and for which a flushing pathway inhibitor provides value
3. Quantify the response to therapy and improvements in tolerability.
4. Provide a measure sufficiently precise and robust to support the requirements of dose-ranging and clinical impact studies

In addition to the questions that characterized the individual flushing symptoms (redness, warmth, itching, and tingling), a question of the FSQ, termed the Global Flushing Severity Score (GFSS), assessed aggregated flushing severity of all four symptoms (Overall, during the past 24 hours, how would you rate your flushing symptoms? [including redness, warmth, tingling, or itching of your skin] 0 = did not have, 1–2 = mild, 4–6 = moderate, 7–9 = severe, 10 = extreme). The FSQ items concerning the severity, bother, and individual flushing symptoms use a discretized analog response scale that combines both verbal descriptors and a 0 to 10 numerical rating, key design elements shared with other well-validated disability measures.[49]

A validation study was conducted to determine the most appropriate endpoints for assessing niacin-induced flushing associated with initiation and maintenance of therapy.[48] The results supported the measurement properties and validity of the FSQ. The GFSS item alone performed as well as or better than the four individual flushing symptoms. Finally, this study identified two specific time periods (and efficacy endpoints) of interest to measure niacin-induced flushing: the initiation phase (maximum GFSS during the first week of therapy) and maintenance phase (frequency of moderate or greater flushing during chronic 2 g dosing).

LAROPIPRANT IN PHASE II

Based on the validation data, the FSQ, administered by means of an eDiary (ie, patient self-reported flushing symptoms recorded in a PalmPilot device), was employed in Phase II to quantify the effects of ER niacin/laropiprant on niacin-induced flushing.[50] An 8-week, placebo-controlled, parallel group study was designed to determine the dose–response relationship of laropiprant-mediated inhibition of flushing during the initiation phase of treatment (week 1) and during the maintenance phase (defined as weeks 6 to 8 for this study) using the FSQ eDiary GFSS question.[50] Patients were randomized to NIASPAN 1 g alone (used as a formulation of ER niacin available at the time) or coadministered with laropiprant 18.75 to 150 mg or double placebo. After 4 weeks, all doses were doubled to achieve 2 g niacin and laropiprant 37.5 to 300 mg for an additional 4 weeks.

Coadministration of laropiprant with NIASPAN produced a significant reduction in niacin-induced flushing compared with ER niacin alone in dyslipidemic patients at initiation of treatment (**Fig. 2**) and with chronic maintenance of therapy. The beneficial effects of niacin on lipids were not affected. In this first study, all laropiprant doses were sufficient to significantly attenuate flushing with the 1 g initiation dose of niacin and the 2 g maintenance dose.

Laropiprant administered at 37.5 mg (rounded to 40 mg and given as two 1 g/20 mg tablets) was found to be the minimum dose that maximally protects against flushing associated with the expected patterns of chronic use of niacin

at the 2 g dose (compliant use and after missed doses). Similarly, the amount of laropiprant in the single 1 g tablet (20 mg) provides maximum protection against the flushing associated with the one-tablet starting dose of 1 g niacin (to be given as 1 g/20 mg).

Selection of an ER niacin formulation (Merck & Company, Incorporated) to be combined with laropiprant was based on various assessments, including pharmacokinetic profile, pharmaceutical properties, flushing profile (intrinsic flushing and response to laropiprant), lipid-altering efficacy, and safety/tolerability. The new ER niacin formulation demonstrated an acceptable safety and tolerability profile, with efficacy comparable to that of NIASPAN on HDL-C, LDL-C, and TG at the 2 g dose.

The results of the dosing and formulation studies culminated in the development of ER niacin/laropiprant, a combination agent aimed at providing the beneficial lipid-modifying effects of niacin, while offering improved tolerability. A two-step dose advancement regimen (1 g/20 mg for 4 weeks followed by 2 g/40 mg for chronic maintenance) was selected for subsequent studies of ER niacin/laropiprant. This new dosing regimen overcomes the limitations inherent in the 12-week gradual dose titration regimen believed to be a critical impediment to achieving the optimal 2 g dose with currently available ER niacin formulations. ER niacin/laropiprant ensures that patients receive a minimally therapeutic 1 g dose of niacin at the

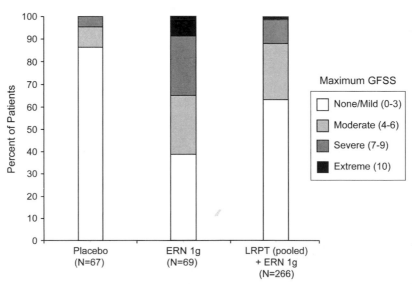

Fig. 2. Maximum Global Flushing Severity Score (GFSS) in week 1 in study 011, presented as percent of patients. *Abbreviations:* ERN, extended-release niacin; GFSS, Global Flushing Severity Score; LRPT, laropiprant. (*From* Paolini JF, Mitchel YB, Reyes R, et al. Effects of laropiprant on nicotinic acid-induced flushing in dyslipidemic patients. Am J Cardiol 2008;101:626; with permission.)

initiation of therapy, an important advance considering that 500 mg NIASPAN is a titration dose with nonsignificant LDL-C-lowering and that approximately one third of patients never titrate upward beyond 500 mg.[31]

PHASE III CLINICAL STUDIES WITH LAROPIPRANT

Two distinct sets of efficacy endpoints were evaluated in the ER niacin/laropiprant Phase III program: those related to lipid effects and those related to reducing niacin-induced flushing at initiation and with chronic maintenance of therapy. Another equally important objective of these studies was the assessment of the safety and tolerability profile of ER niacin/laropiprant, particularly with regard to the novel 1 g starting dose and the 1g → 2 g dose advancement regimen.

EFFECTS ON LIPIDS

Two pivotal Phase III clinical trials (studies 020 and 022) evaluated the lipid efficacy of ER niacin/laropiprant,[51,52] with the primary lipid endpoint being the percent change from baseline in LDL-C levels. In a randomized, placebo-controlled study (020), dyslipidemic patients (67% on statins) were randomized to ER niacin/laropiprant (n = 800), ER niacin (n = 543), or placebo (n = 270). Treatment with ER niacin/laropiprant and ER niacin was initiated at 1 g. After 4 weeks, the dose was advanced to 2 tablets per day (2 g for active treatment) for 20 additional weeks. ER niacin/laropiprant 2 g/40 mg produced significant and durable reductions in plasma LDL-C levels (−18.4%) relative to placebo in the overall study population (**Table 2**). Importantly, the LDL-C lowering efficacy of ER niacin/laropiprant was similar whether it was administered as monotherapy (ie, without statin background treatment, −17.4%) or as

combination therapy with statins (−18.9%). These similarities in LDL-C lowering with or without previous statin therapy were observed despite the large differences in baseline LDL-C levels in these two subgroups (approximately 95 vs. approximately 150 mg/dL; this difference was expected due to disparity in enrollment criteria based on statin use and risk category). Similarly, baseline HDL-C and TG levels did not influence the LDL-C lowering efficacy of ER niacin/laropiprant. Finally, the lipid effects of ER niacin/laropiprant and ER niacin were nearly identical, confirming earlier observations that laropiprant alone does not affect lipid levels.

The results of Study 020 generally were corroborated in a factorial study designed to evaluate the lipid-modifying efficacy of ER niacin/laropiprant plus simvastatin, compared with the monotherapy of each (Study 022). After a 6- to 8-week washout and a 4-week diet/placebo run-in, 1398 patients were randomized equally to ER niacin/laropiprant 1 g/20 mg, simvastatin (10, 20, or 40 mg), or ER niacin/laropiprant 1 g/20 mg plus simvastatin (10, 20, or 40 mg) once daily for 4 weeks. At week 5, treatment doses were doubled in all groups except simvastatin 40 mg (unchanged) and ER niacin/laropiprant 1 g/20 mg plus simvastatin 40 mg (switched to ER niacin/laropiprant 2 g/40 mg plus simvastatin 40 mg). Significantly larger reductions in LDL-C levels were evident with the coadministration of ER niacin/laropiprant 2 g/40 mg plus simvastatin (pooled across simvastatin doses of 20 mg and 40 mg) compared with ER niacin/laropiprant or simvastatin (pooled across simvastatin doses of 20 mg and 40 mg) (**Table 3**). In addition, when evaluating the lipid effects of ER niacin/laropiprant 2 g/40 mg plus simvastatin, all individual dose comparisons were significantly different from the respective monotherapy doses.

Table 2
Lipid efficacy from study 020

Lipid Parameter	Least Squares Mean (95% CI) % Change from Baseline in Lipids Across Weeks 12 Through 24[a]		
	Extended Release Niacin/Laropiprant 2 g	Placebo	Difference
Low-density lipoprotein (LDL)−C	−18.9 (−21.0, −16.8)	−0.5 (−3.3, 2.4)	−18.4 (−21.4, −15.4)
High-density lipoprotein (HDL)−C	18.8 (17.2, 20.4)	−1.2 (−3.4, 1.0)	20.0 (17.7, 22.3)
Triglycerides, median	−21.7 (−23.9, −19.5)	3.6 (−0.5, 7.6)	−25.8 (−29.5, −22.1)
Non HDL−C	−19.0 (−20.8, −17.2)	0.8 (−1.6, 3.3)	−19.8 (−22.4, −17.3)
Apo B	−16.4 (−18.0, −14.7)	2.5 (0.2, 4.7)	−18.8 (−21.2, −16.5)
Apo AI	11.2 (10.1, 12.4)	4.3 (2.7, 5.9)	6.9 (5.3, 8.6)

[a] Patients with at least one post-titration measurement included in the analysis.

Table 3
Lipid efficacy from study 022

Least Squares Mean Percent Changes in Lipid Parameters from Baseline to Week 12			
Treatment Group	LDL−C	TGª	HDL−C
ER niacin/laropiprant 2 g/40 mg	−17.0	−21.6	23.4
Simvastatin 20 mg	−34.7	−13.4	4.2
Simvastatin 40 mg	−38.2	−15.1	6.8
Pooled simvastatin 20 and 40 mg	−37.0	−14.7	6.0
ER niacin/laropiprant 2 g/40 mg + simvastatin 20 mg	−45.7[b,e]	−30.9[b,e]	27.7[c,e]
ER niacin/laropiprant 2 g/40 mg + simvastatin 40 mg	−48.9[b,e]	−33.6[b,e]	27.4[c,e]
Pooled ER niacin/laropiprant 2 g/40 mg + simvastatin	−47.9[b,d]	−33.3[b,d]	27.5[c,d]

Abbreviations: ER, extended release; HDL−C, high-density lipoprotein cholesterol; LDL−C, low-density lipoprotein cholesterol; TG, triglycerides.
[a] Expressed as median percent change.
[b] $P < .001$ versus ER niacin/laropiprant.
[c] $P < .050$ versus ER niacin/laropiprant.
[d] $P < .001$ versus pooled simvastatin.
[e] $P < .001$ versus corresponding dose of simvastatin alone.

In both studies, the kinetics of the response showed a tendency for the LDL-C lowering to plateau after 8 to 12 weeks of treatment (4 to 8 weeks at 2 g) and remain stable for the duration of the studies (12 to 24 weeks). Significant effects of ER niacin/laropiprant 1 g/20 mg alone or coadministered with simvastatin also were observed at the 4-week time point.

Although niacin is effective at reducing LDL-C levels, it also effectively raises HDL-C. In the factorial study (Study 022), ER niacin/laropiprant produced significant increases of 23% to 28% in HDL-C, whether administered alone or with simvastatin (see **Table 3**). These effects were observed irrespective of baseline LDL-C, HDL-C, or TG levels. Similar increases in HDL-C also were observed in Study 020.

Reductions in TG levels followed a similar pattern to the beneficial changes in LDL-C and HDL-C with ER niacin/laropiprant alone or coadministered with simvastatin, producing significantly larger reductions than the individual components (see **Table 3**).

Overall, the treatment effects of ER niacin/laropiprant on lipid parameters observed in the phase III studies were consistent across patient subgroups, including those defined by age, gender, race, baseline lipid values (high and low LDL-C, HDL-C, and TG), and diabetes mellitus status. Consistent treatment effects also were observed across subgroups of patients on different types of statins (simvastatin, atorvastatin, or other statins) and in patients taking statins and ezetimibe concomitantly.

EFFECTS ON NIACIN-INDUCED FLUSHING

Prespecified endpoints in the phase III studies evaluated the flushing profile of ER niacin/laropiprant during initiation of therapy when flushing is believed to be most intense and during chronic maintenance therapy when patients may experience intermittent, sometimes unpredictable flushing. These studies also assessed the tolerability of the abbreviated 1 g → 2 g dosing regimen of ER niacin/laropiprant relative to the 12-week gradual titration regimen of NIASPAN in a head-to-head study (Study 054), in which the use of aspirin was permitted to mitigate flushing symptoms.

The initiation phase is defined as the first week of niacin treatment, and the maintenance phase refers to the period after the first week of treatment, including the period after patients advance to the maintenance dose (2 g/40 mg of ER niacin/laropiprant or 2 g of niacin). In each study, ER niacin/laropiprant (administered according to the 1 g → 2 g dosing regimen) was compared with ER niacin alone, either according to the same 1 g → 2 g regimen (using Merck's ER niacin formulation) or to the usual regimen of conservative titration, starting at 500 mg and increasing in 500 mg increments every 4 weeks until reaching the 2 g dose (using NIASPAN).

INITIATION OF THERAPY AND ADVANCEMENT TO 2 G MAINTENANCE DOSE

The ability of laropiprant to mitigate flushing associated with the initiation of therapy was a primary objective in Study 020. ER niacin/laropiprant and ER niacin were administered according to the simplified ER niacin/laropiprant dosing regimen (a 1 g initial dose advanced to 2 g after 4 weeks). During the initiation of therapy (week 1), patients treated with ER niacin/laropiprant experienced significantly less flushing than did patients receiving ER niacin, as measured by the distribution of patients experiencing maximal flushing across the intensity categories of none/mild, moderate, severe, and extreme. Overall, fewer patients experienced moderate, severe, or extreme flushing with ER niacin/laropiprant 1 g versus ER niacin 1 g during week 1 (31% vs. 56%; $P < .001$), with a 65% reduction in the odds of experiencing such flushing. Similarly, fewer patients experienced severe or extreme flushing with ER niacin/laropiprant versus ER niacin (14% vs. 33%, $P < .001$). These results provide support for the concept of using an abbreviated dosing regimen with ER niacin/laropiprant, in which the starting dose is 1 g of ER niacin.

MAINTENANCE PHASE

On the basis of anecdotal reports, it has been ascertained that people develop tolerance with compliant dosing of niacin. An important objective of the ER niacin/laropiprant development program was to rigorously assess the chronic flushing response to niacin in a long-term study, by the objective use of a validated flushing tool. In Study 020, patients in the ER niacin/laropiprant and ER niacin groups remained at the 2 g dose for 20 weeks of treatment, making this study ideal for assessing flushing with therapy maintenance. After week 6, patients treated with ER niacin continued to report episodes of moderate, severe, or extreme flushing, while the flushing signal in patients treated with ER niacin/laropiprant gradually subsided to a level that approximated placebo. During the maintenance phase, the ER niacin/laropiprant group experienced significantly less flushing than the ER niacin group as measured by days per week with moderate or greater flushing, and the difference was consistent throughout the entire 24-week treatment period. At the end of the treatment period, patients in the ER niacin/laropiprant group had 0.2 days per week with moderate, severe, or extreme flushing versus 0.7 days per week in the ER niacin group (approximately 1 day per month vs. approximately 1 day per week, respectively). This flushing profile was not driven by a minority of patients experiencing high degrees of flushing; rather, approximately 60% of patients receiving ER niacin 2 g reported at least one episode of moderate or greater flushing throughout the period between weeks 6 and 24.

These data show that moderate or greater flushing is persistent in a large percentage of patients and that tolerance to this level of flushing is incomplete over at least a 6-month period. This is consistent with data illustrating a high rate of discontinuation from ER niacin use because of flushing over 1 year.[32]

COMPARISON WITH GRADUALLY TITRATED NIASPAN

NIASPAN typically is titrated gradually over a 12-week period in an attempt to address dose-related flushing symptoms. Thus, a phase III, head-to-head study (Study 054) was conducted to assess the novel 1 g → 2 g ER niacin/laropiprant abbreviated dosing regimen compared with NIASPAN. Each treatment was administered for 16 weeks, according to its standard dosing regimen. ER niacin/laropiprant 1 g was given for 4 weeks then advanced to 2 g for the remaining 12 weeks. NIASPAN 0.5 g was given for 4 weeks, then increased every 4 weeks in 0.5 g increments to 2 g for the final 4 weeks. Patients were instructed to take study therapy in the evening with food. According to the discretion of the patient, preadministration of aspirin (or other nonsteroidal anti-inflammatory drugs [NSAIDs]) 30 minutes before study medication was allowed to specifically mitigate flushing symptoms.

Patients treated with rapidly advanced ER niacin/laropiprant experienced significantly ($P < .001$) less flushing than those treated with gradually titrated NIASPAN, as measured by the number of days per week with moderate, severe, or extreme flushing (GFSS greater than or equal to 4) across the treatment period categorized as 0, greater than 0 and less than or equal to 0.5, greater than 0.5 and less than or equal to 1, greater than 1 and less than or equal to 2, greater than 2 and less than or equal to 3, and greater than 3 days per week. Overall, more than twice as many patients had no episodes of moderate, severe, or extreme flushing (GFSS greater than or equal to 4) with ER niacin/laropiprant versus NIASPAN (47% vs. 22%, respectively) across the 16-week treatment period. Importantly, clinically significant changes were identified across the entire scale, not only categorically but also numerically, and without the need for specific GFSS cut points.

The time profile of flushing across the entire treatment period was evaluated by means of by-week plots of the following: the number of days per week with moderate, severe, or extreme flushing in each week, and the percentage of patients who had moderate, severe, or extreme flushing in each week (**Fig. 3**). Despite the dose of ER

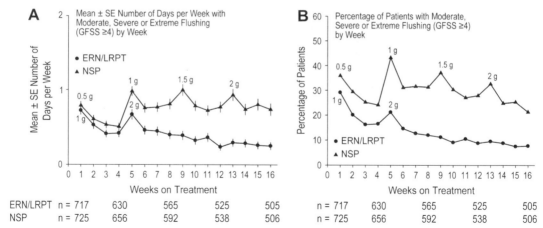

Fig. 3. Time profile of flushing in study 054: (*A*) Mean ±SE days per week with moderate, severe, or extreme flushing (GFSS greater than or equal to 4), by week. (*B*) Percentage of patients with moderate, severe, or extreme flushing (GFSS greater than or equal to 4), by week. *Abbreviations:* ERN, extended-release niacin; GFSS, Global Flushing Severity Score; LRPT, laropiprant; NSP, NIASPAN.

niacin/laropiprant (1 g) being double that of NIA-SPAN (0.5 g) during the first 4 weeks, the groups were similar with regard to the number of days per week with moderate, severe, or extreme flushing. Although the flushing signal gradually declined after week 5 in the ER niacin/laropiprant group, it remained elevated in the group treated with NIA-SPAN, with increases in the signal at each titration week. ER niacin/laropiprant patients experienced fewer days per week with moderate, severe or extreme flushing relative to NIASPAN at the end of the treatment period. In addition, a lower percentage of patients had maximum GFSS reported as moderate, severe, or extreme at week 5 in the ER niacin/laropiprant group versus the group treated with NIASPAN (21.2% vs. 43.2%, respectively). The percentage of patients who had maximum GFSS reported as moderate, severe, or extreme at week 16 was 7.7% for the ER niacin/laropiprant group versus 21.3% for the group treated with NIASPAN.

These results indicate that laropiprant can reduce the intrinsic flushing signal of a 1 g ER niacin dose to less than that of a 0.5 g dose of NIASPAN. The tolerability differences not only persisted for the duration of the study but actually grew larger during the ensuing weeks of the study. Whereas the patients who continued to titrate up on NIA-SPAN experienced a high level of flushing and spikes in the flushing signal with each dose titration step, patients in the ER niacin/laropiprant group who reached the 2 g dose by week 5 experienced a progressive decrease in the frequency of flushing symptoms. By week 8, patients in ER niacin/laropiprant group were receiving near-maximal lipid-altering benefits at the 2 g dose, with fewer than 10% of these patients experiencing moderate, severe, or extreme (GFSS greater than 4) flushing symptoms.

Importantly, superiority of the 1 g → 2 g ER niacin/laropiprant dosing regimen was observed in the setting of patients having the option of taking aspirin or NSAIDs to help alleviate flushing symptoms. Whereas aspirin modestly reduces flushing symptoms with niacin monotherapy, it does not provide additional benefit beyond that of laropiprant in patients receiving ER niacin/laropiprant.[53] Not only did more patients in the group treated with NIA-SPAN use aspirin/NSAIDs to mitigate flushing symptoms (21.6% vs. 11.3%), but only the patients treated with NIASPAN would have seen any decrease in flushing scores as a result of its use.

These data show that the improvement in flushing symptoms that the laropiprant component provides is sufficiently robust to yield a superior tolerability profile for ER niacin/laropiprant, even with an accelerated 1 g → 2 g dose advancement regimen. The improved tolerability of ER niacin/laropiprant persists, even when compared with the recommended gradual titration schedule of NIA-SPAN, with the discretionary use of aspirin and/or other NSAIDS.

DISCONTINUATION BECAUSE OF FLUSHING

The clinical significance of the reduction in flushing provided by laropiprant is underscored by the finding that consistently fewer patients discontinued from ER niacin/laropiprant therapy because of flushing symptoms than comparator niacin formulations. The percentage of patients discontinuing because of flushing was a key secondary endpoint in the placebo-controlled study (Study 020) and an exploratory endpoint in the head-to-head study (Study 054). In Study 020, 10% in the ER niacin/laropiprant and 22% in the ER niacin groups discontinued because of flushing over the 6-month study (*P* < .001). Corresponding rates for groups treated with ER niacin/laropiprant or NIASPAN in Study 054 were 7% and 12% over 16 weeks of treatment, demonstrating superiority with ER niacin/laropiprant, even though patients in the ER niacin/laropiprant group were at a higher dose of niacin for all but the last 4 weeks of the study. This is noteworthy given the short duration of the clinical trials and the inherent encouragement for patients not to discontinue (patients were encouraged strongly to stay in the trials and endure their flushing symptoms rather than discontinue, if possible). Although it is difficult to predict real-world discontinuation rates from clinical trials, one reasonably could presume that the discontinuation rates might have been even higher had these patients not been as highly motivated and encouraged to remain in the studies, as is the case within the unique environment of a controlled clinical trial. Observational studies have shown that approximately 85% of patients discontinue niacin over 12 months, and most cite flushing as the reason.

SAFETY

Data were pooled from three active- or placebo-controlled phase III studies and three, phase II, 1-year safety extensions. The results indicate that ER niacin/laropiprant generally was tolerated well. Apart from the clear advantage of ER niacin/laropiprant on flushing-related adverse events and discontinuations, the tolerability profile of ER niacin/laropiprant was similar to that of ER niacin alone (**Table 4**).

The overall population was comprised of 4747 patients exposed to ER niacin/laropiprant (n = 2548), ER niacin/NIASPAN (n = 1268), or simvastatin/placebo (n = 931). The studies ranged from 12 to 52 weeks in duration. The incidence of consecutive greater than or equal to three times the upper limit of normal (ULN) increases in alanine aminotransaminase (ALT) and/or aspartate aminotransferase (AST) was low and similar across the groups. Elevations were reversible with therapy discontinuation and not associated with clinical hepatotoxicity. There was no evidence that ER niacin/laropiprant had an adverse effect on muscle. There were two cases of myopathy, defined as creatine kinase greater than or equal to 10 times ULN with muscle symptoms and considered

Table 4
Extended-release niacin/laropiprant safety summary

Safety Parameter	Simvastatin/Placebo	Extended-Release Niacin	Extended-Release Niacin/Laropiprant
Drug-related[a] adverse events, n/N (%)	156/931 (16.8)	501/1268 (39.5)	901/2548 (35.4)[d,e]
Drug-related[a] serious adverse events, n/N (%)	1/931 (0.1)	1/1268 (0.1)	8/2548 (0.3)[f,g]
Discontinuations due to drug–related[a] adverse events, n/N (%)	28/931 (3.0)	204/1268 (16.1)	328/2548 (12.9)[d,e]
Confirmed adjudicated cardiovascular events, n/N (%)	3/931 (0.3)	5/1268 (0.4)	8/2548 (0.3)[h,i]
Consecutive ALT/AST elevations ≥3× ULN, n/N (%)	8/920 (0.9)	6/1221 (0.5)	25/2465 (1.0)[h,i]
Drug-related hepatitis, n/N (%)	0/920 (0.0)	0/1221 (0.0)	0/2465 (0.0)
Myopathy,[b] n/N (%)	0/920 (0.0)	1/1221 (0.08)	1/2465 (0.04)[h,i]
CK elevations ≥10 × ULN, n/N (%)	2/920 (0.2)	2/1221 (0.2)	7/2465 (0.3)[h,i]
New-onset diabetes,[c] n/N (%)	1/888 (0.1)	3/1094 (0.3)	12/2276 (0.5)[h,i]

Abbreviations: ALT/AST, alanine aminotransferase and/or aspartate aminotransferase; CK, creatine kinase; ER, extended release; n, number of patients with given event; N, total patients in treatment group; ULN, upper limit of normal.
  [a] Determined to be possibly, probably, or definitely drug-related by the investigator.
  [b] CK ≥ 10 × ULN with muscle symptoms and considered drug-related by the investigator.
  [c] Based on clinical adverse events and change in medication.
  [d] 95% CI for difference with ER niacin does not include 0.
  [e] 95% CI for difference with simvastatin/placebo does not include 0.
  [f] 95% CI for difference with ER niacin includes 0.
  [g] 95% CI for difference with simvastatin/placebo includes 0.
  [h] Not significantly different from ER niacin.
  [i] Not significantly different from simvastatin/placebo.

drug-related by the investigator: one each in the ER niacin (0.08%) and ER niacin/laropiprant (0.04%) groups. Both were associated with unusually high levels of physical activity. ER niacin/laropiprant and ER niacin produced small increases in fasting blood glucose levels (approximately 4 mg/dL median change from baseline), consistent with the known effects of niacin. Very few patients in the pooled population met a prespecified criterion for new-onset diabetes (a clinical adverse event of diabetes mellitus or initiation of antidiabetic medication), and there were no significant differences between the treatment groups receiving ER niacin versus placebo. Overall, there was no difference between the treatment arms with respect to the incidence of confirmed cardiovascular events, although no study to date has been sufficient in power or duration to establish any potential cardiovascular differences. The magnitude of potential benefits of ER niacin/laropiprant on cardiovascular outcomes and atherosclerosis is being assessed in the ongoing 4-year, 20,000-patient clinical outcome study, the Heart Protection Study–Treatment of HDL to Reduce the Incidence of Vascular Events (HPS2-THRIVE). The favorable safety and tolerability profile of ER niacin/laropiprant for up to 12 months supports the use of laropiprant to achieve the optimal therapeutic dosing of niacin, an agent shown to reduce cardiovascular risk.

SUMMARY

ER niacin/laropiprant produces superior lipid-altering efficacy relative to placebo, whether administered as monotherapy or coadministered with concomitant statin. Coadministration of ER niacin/laropiprant with simvastatin was highly efficacious at producing beneficial changes across the lipid profile. The lipid effects of ER niacin/laropiprant 2 g/40 mg were maintained over 52 weeks of treatment.

Laropiprant consistently mitigates niacin-induced flushing, as measured by objective, validated measures of flushing. Given that difficulties with flushing tolerability and the necessary 12-week gradual dose titration regimen remain critical impediments to achieving the target 2 g dose with currently available ER niacin formulations, combining an inhibitor of the flushing pathway with ER niacin supports a fundamental change in the niacin dosing paradigm. Replacing the standard gradual, multistep ER niacin titration regimen with a more streamlined and better-tolerated regimen may allow patients to successfully initiate treatment at the 1 g dose and more rapidly advance to the 2 g target dose, with accompanying improvement in compliance and adherence. Treatment with ER niacin/laropiprant generally was tolerated well, and with the exception of flushing-related adverse events, which occurred more frequently with ER niacin, had a safety profile similar to that of ER niacin. In July 2008, ER niacin/laropiprant was approved for marketing in the European Union, Iceland and Norway.

In conclusion, ER niacin/laropiprant offers the opportunity for a major therapeutic advance. The improvements in the tolerability of niacin observed with ER niacin/laropiprant will allow niacin dosing to initiate therapy at a therapeutic 1 g dose and rapidly advance to the maximum efficacious 2 g dose in a simplified dosing regimen. ER niacin/laropiprant is a generally well-tolerated and easy-to-use, long-term treatment for dyslipidemia that offers the potential for more patients to realize the demonstrated lipid-altering and cardiovascular benefits of niacin, a therapy proven to reduce cardiovascular risk.

REFERENCES

1. Expert Panel on Detection Evaluation and Treatment of High Blood Cholesterol in Adults. Executive summary of the third report of the National Cholesterol Education Program (NCEP) expert panel on detection, evaluation, and treatment of high blood cholesterol in adults (adult treatment panel III). J Am Med Assoc 2001;285(19):2486–97.

2. Wilson PW, D'Agostino RB, Levy D, et al. Prediction of coronary heart disease using risk factor categories. Circulation 1998;97:1837–47.

3. Stamler J, Daviglus ML, Garside DB, et al. Relationship of baseline serum cholesterol levels in 3 large cohorts of younger men to long-term coronary, cardiovascular, and all-cause mortality, and to longevity. J Am Med Assoc 2000;284(3):311–8.

4. DeBacker G, Amronsione E, Borch-Johnsen K, et al. European guidelines on cardiovascular disease prevention in clinical practice. Eur J Cardiovasc Prev Rehabil 2003;10:S1–78.

5. Gotto AM. High-density lipoprotein cholesterol and triglycerides as therapeutic targets for preventing and treating coronary artery disease. Am Heart J 2002;144:S33–42.

6. Shah PK, Kaul S, Nilsson J, et al. Exploiting the vascular protective effects of high-density lipoprotein and its apolipoproteins—an idea whose time for testing is coming, part I. Circulation 2001;104:2376–83.

7. Gordon DJ, Probstfield JL, Garrison RJ, et al. High-density lipoprotein cholesterol and cardiovascular disease. Four prospective American studies. Circulation 1989;79(1):8–15.

8. Assmann G, Nofer JR. Atheroprotective effects of high-density lipoproteins. Annu Rev Med 2003;54:321–41.

9. Durrington PN. Triglycerides are more important in atherosclerosis than epidemiology has suggested. Atherosclerosis 1998;141(Suppl 1):S57–62.

10. Jeppesen J, Hein HO, Suadicani P, et al. Triglyceride concentration and ischemic heart disease: an eight-year follow-up in the Copenhagen Male Study. Circulation 1998;97(11):1029–36.

11. Austin MA, Hokanson JE, Edwards KL. Hypertriglyceridemia as a cardiovascular risk factor. Am J Cardiol 1998;81(4a):7b–12.

12. Assmann G, Schulte H, Funke H, et al. The emergence of triglycerides as a significant independent risk factor in coronary artery disease. Eur Heart J 1998;19(Suppl M):8–14.

13. Brunzell JD. ADA/ACC consensus statement. Diabetes Care 2008;31:811–22.

14. Offermanns S. The nicotinic acid receptor GPR109A (HM74A or PUMA-G) as a new therapeutic target. Trends Pharmacol Sci 2006;27(7):384–90.

15. Altschul R, Hoffer A, Stephen JD. Influence of nicotinic acid on serum cholesterol in man. Arch Biochem 1955;54:558–9.

16. Carlson LA. Nicotinic acid: the broad-spectrum lipid drug. A 50th anniversary review. J Intern Med 2005; 258:94–114.

17. Mahley RW, Bersot TP. Drug therapy for hypercholesterolemia and dyslipidemia. In: Hardman JG, Limblrd LE, Gilman AG, editors. The pharmacological basis of therapeutics. 10th edition. New York: Goodman and Gillman's; 2001. p. 971–1002.

18. National Institutes of Health. National Cholesterol Education Program (NCEP) Expert Panel. Third report of the National Cholesterol Education Program (NCEP) Expert panel on detection, evaluation, and treatment of high blood cholesterol in adults (Adult Treatment Panel III) final report. Circulation 2002; 106:3143–421.

19. Kamanna VS, Kashyap ML. Mechanism of action of niacin on lipoprotein metabolism. Curr Atheroscler Rep 2000;2:36–46.

20. The Coronary Drug Project Research Group. Clofibrate and niacin in coronary heart disease. J Am Med Assoc 1975;231(4):360–81.

21. Brown BG, Zhao X-Q, Chait A, et al. Simvastatinstatin and niacin, antioxidant vitamins, or the combination for the prevention of coronary disease. N Engl J Med 2001;345(22):1583–92.

22. Taylor AJ, Sullenberger LE, Lee HJ, et al. Arterial biology for the investigation of the treatment effects of reducing cholesterol (ARBITER) 2. A double-blind, placebo-controlled study of extended-release niacin on atherosclerosis progression in secondary prevention patients treated with statins. Circulation 2004;110:3512–7.

23. Canner PL, Berge KG, Wenger NK, et al. Fifteen-year mortality in coronary drug project patients long-term benefit with niacin. J Am Coll Cardiol 1986;8(6):1245–55.

24. Blankenhorn DH, Nessim SA, Johnson RL, et al. Beneficial effects of combined colestipol–niacin therapy on coronary atherosclerosis and coronary venous bypass grafts. J Am Med Assoc 1987;257: 3233–40.

25. Brown G, Albers JJ, Fisher LD, et al. Regression of coronary artery disease as a result of intensive lipid-lowering therapy in men with high levels of apolipoprotein B. N Engl J Med 1990;323(19):1289–98.

26. Birjmohun RS, Hutten BA, Kastelein JJ, et al. Increasing HDL cholesterol with extended-release nicotinic acid: from promise to practice. Neth J Med 2004;62:229–34.

27. Morgan JM, Capuzzi DM, Guyton JR. A new extended-release niacin (NIASPAN): efficacy, tolerability, and safety in hypercholesterolemic patients. Am J Cardiol 1998;82:29U–34.

28. Guyton JR, Bays HE. Safety considerations with niacin therapy. Am J Cardiol 2008;99(6A):32C–34.

29. Abbott Pharmaceuticals. NIASPAN (niacin extended-release tablets) US prescribing information. Copyright. Available at: http://www.rxabbott.com/pdf/niaspantablet.pdf. 2005. Accessed August 8, 2008.

30. Knopp RH, Alagona P, Davidson M, et al. Equivalent efficacy of a time-release form of niacin (Niaspan) given once-a-night versus plain niacin in the management of hyperlipidemia. Metabolism 1998; 47(9):1097–104.

31. Kamal-Bahl, Burke T, Watson D. Dosage, titration, and gaps in treatment with extended- release niacin in clinical practice. Curr Med Res Opin 2008;24(6): 1817–21.

32. Kamal-Bahl S, Burke T, Watson D, et al. Discontinuation of lipid-modifying drugs among commercially insured United States patients in recent clinical practice. Am J Cardiol 2007;99:530–4.

33. Kamal-Bahl S, Watson DJ, Kramer B, et al. Flushing experience and discontinuation with niacin in clinical practice. J Am Coll Cardiol 2007;49(9 Suppl A):273A.

34. Trovato AT, Norquist JM, Rhodes T, et al. The impact of niacin-induced flushing during the first week of therapy in a real-world setting. J Am Coll Cardiol 2008;51(Suppl 1):A255.

35. Morrow JD, Roberts LJ. Lipid-derived autacoids, eicosanoids, and platelet-activating factor. In: Hardman JG, Limbird LE, Gilman AG, editors. The pharmacological basis of therapeutics. 10th edition. New York: Goodman and Gillman's; 2001. p. 669–85.

36. Jungnickel PW, Maloley PA, Vander Tuin EL, et al. Effect of two aspirin pretreatment regimens on niacin-induced cutaneous reactions. J Gen Intern Med 1997;12:591–6.

37. Morrow JD, Parsons WG, Roberts LJ. Release of markedly increased quantities of prostaglandin D2 in vivo in humans following the administration of nicotinic acid. Prostaglandins 1989;38(2):263–74.

38. Wilkin JK, Wilkin O, Kapp R, et al. Aspirin blocks nicotinic acid-induced flushing. Clin Pharmacol Ther 1982;31(4):478–82.

39. Whelan AM, Price SO, Fowler SF, et al. The effect of aspirin on niacin-induced cutaneous reactions. J Fam Pract 1992;34(2):165–8.

40. Svedmyr N, Heggelund A, Aberg G. Influence of indomethacin on flush induced by nicotinic acid in man. Acta Pharmacol Toxicol 1977;41:397–400.

41. Phillips WS, Lightman SL. Is cutaneous flushing prostaglandin-mediated? Lancet 1981;1:754–6.

42. Wilkin JK, Fortner G, Reinhardt LA, et al. Prostaglandins and nicotinate-provoked increase in cutaneous blood flow. Clin Pharmacol Ther 1985;38:273–7.

43. Nozaki S, Kihara S, Kubo M. Increased compliance of niceritrol treatment by addition of aspirin: relationship between changes in prostaglandins and skin flushing. Int J Clin Pharmacol Ther Toxicol 1987;25(12):643–7.

44. Eklund B, Kaijser L, Nowak J, et al. Prostaglandins contribute to the vasodilation induced by nicotinic acid. Prostaglandins 1979;17(6):821–30.

45. Heavy DJ, Lumley P, Barrow SE, et al. Effects of intravenous infusions of prostaglandin D2 in man. Prostaglandins 1984;28:755–67.

46. Cheng K, Wu TJ, Wu KK, et al. Antagonism of the prostaglandin D2 receptor 1 suppresses nicotinic acid-induced vasodilation in mice and humans. Proc Natl Acad Sci U S A 2006;103(17):6682–7.

47. Lai E, De Lepeleire I, Crumley TM, et al. Suppression of niacin-induced vasodilation with an antagonist to prostaglandin D2 receptor subtype 1. Clin Pharmacol Ther 2007;81:849–57.

48. Norquist JM, Watson DJ, Yu Q, et al. Validation of a questionnaire to assess niacin-induced cutaneous flushing. Curr Med Res Opin 2007;23(7):1549–60.

49. Sheehan KH, Sheehan DV. Assessing treatment effects in clinical trials with the discan metric of the Sheehan disability scale. Int Clin Psychopharmacol 2008;23(2):70–83.

50. Paolini JP, Mitchel YB, Reyes R, et al. Effects of laropiprant on nicotinic acid-induced flushing in dyslipidemic patients. Am J Cardiol 2008;101:625–30.

51. Maccubbin D, Bays HE, Olsson AG, et al. Lipid-modifying efficacy and tolerability of extended-release niacin/laropiprant in patients with primary hypercholesterolemia or mixed dyslipidemia. Int J Clin Pract 2008; In press.

52. Gleim G, Liu N, Thompson-Bell S, et al. Lipid-altering efficacy and safety profile of coadministered extended-release niacin/laropiprant and simvastatin in patients with dyslipidemia. Circulation 2007;116:II 127 [abstract 683].

53. Merck & Co., Inc., Study memo; data on file.

Management of Heart Failure: a Brief Review and Selected Update

Samuel Unzek, MD[a], Gary S. Francis, MD[a,b],*

KEYWORDS

- Heart failure • Treatment

Clinical trials in heart failure (HF) are designed to identify effective and safe therapies that reduce mortality and improve symptoms. In the past few decades, many novel mechanistic targets have been proposed, and physicians now have an abundance of proven therapies. The early drug development experience from the late 1970s through the 1990s was highly successful, but more recently it has become increasingly difficult to demonstrate efficacy and safety in the development of new drugs for HF.[1]

As pharmacologic targets become more complex, so also do clinical trials. The vasodilator strategy described years ago is still appropriate today, and neurohormonal blockade has proven remarkably durable over time. It is becoming more challenging, however, to investigate new therapeutic targets, design drugs that affect the target, and move on to a clinical trial. Regulatory agencies require one or two large mortality trials, and they do not accept surrogate endpoints such as left ventricular (LV) remodeling or reduced B-type natriuretic peptide (BNP) as primary endpoints. Clinical trials today tend to be multicentered, randomized, placebo-controlled, double-blinded, and require large sample sizes to demonstrate meaningful difference between therapies, all of which makes them very expensive. Control groups are treated with effective drugs, making it more difficult to show survival benefit.

"One size does not fit all" is a frequent claim of clinicians. In this era in medicine, therapy is likely to be increasingly tailored to the individual patient. It is now widely recognized that a medication that benefits one patient may be ineffective in another. Trialists, however, still tend to homogenize their patient samples to reduce the variance of response. In doing so, the sample size of patients can be made smaller (ie, less expensive), but the homogenized sample of patients may ultimately not be very representative of "real world" patients. The elderly and those with serious comorbid conditions, such as renal insufficiency and lung disease, are frequently excluded from clinical trials. This has created problems.

This article first reviews what the authors consider to be the landmark trials that have brought us to where we are today (**Table 1**, a–d). The authors describe and analyze some more novel targets and therapeutic agents, as well as their respective performance in clinical trials. Further, the authors speculate about the future.

LANDMARK CLINICAL TRIALS

Table 1 highlights studies that have created the modern framework on which today's conventional therapy for chronic HF rests. In the 1980s, the Pfeffers and many others developed the concept that the core lesion of chronic HF is progressive left ventricular remodeling.[2] In response to myocardial injury, perverse loading conditions, cardiac inflammation, altered myocardial gene expression, or infiltrative processes within the myocardium, the heart tends to progressively hypertrophy, dilate, and eventually manifests reduced LV systolic function.[3] Some, but not all of these changes in LV geometry and performance are driven by

[a] Department of Cardiovascular Medicine, Cleveland Clinic, 9500 Euclid Avenue, Desk F15, Cleveland, OH 44195, USA
[b] Department of Clinical Cardiology, Cleveland Clinic, 9500 Euclid Avenue, Desk F15, Cleveland, OH 44195, USA
* Corresponding author. Cleveland Clinic, 9500 Euclid Avenue, Desk F15, Cleveland, OH 44195.
E-mail address: francig@ccf.org (G.S. Francis).

Cardiol Clin 26 (2008) 561–571
doi:10.1016/j.ccl.2008.06.001

Table 1
Review of trials

Trial	Study Drug	Patients	Primary Endpoint	Difference Between Treatments
a. ACE Inhibitors				
CONSENSUS[4] NYHA IV	Enalapril versus placebo	253	-All cause mortality	$P = .003$ in favor of enalapril
SOLVD[5] Reduced EF and HF	Enalapril versus placebo	2569	-All cause mortality	$P = .0036$ in favor of enalapril
SAVE[6] Post-MI Study	Captopril versus placebo	2231	-All cause mortality -Mortality from CV causes -CV morbidity -CV morbidity and mortality -HF -Hospitalization to treat HF	Favors captopril ($P = .019$)
AIRE[7] Post-MI Study	Ramipril versus placebo	1986	-All cause mortality	$P = .002$ in favor of ramipril
ATLAS[8] Chronic HF	Lisinopril low versus high dose	3164	-All cause mortality	$P = .128$ in favor of high dose treatment
HOPE[9] High risk patients	Ramipril versus placebo	9541	-MI -Stroke -Death from CV causes	Favors ramipril p = <0.001
EUROPA[10] Stable CAD	Perindopril versus placebo	12,218	-CV mortality -Non-fatal MI -Resuscitated cardiac arrest	Trend in favor of perindopril $P = .10$
PEACE[11] Stable CAD	Trandolapril versus placebo	8290	-Death from CV causes -Non fatal MI -Revascularization	Trend in favor of trandolapril $P = .43$
PEP-CHF[12] Elderly	Perindopril versus placebo	852	-Total mortality -Unplanned heart failure hospitalization	Trend in favor of perindopril $P = .545$
b. β-blockers				
MDC[13] Idiopathic dilated cardiomyopathy	Metoprolol versus placebo	383	-All cause mortality -Clinical deterioration requiring cardiac transplantation.	Trend in favor of metoprolol $P = .058$

Study	Comparison	N	Endpoints	Result
ANZ Carvedilol[14] Chronic HF	Carvedilol versus placebo	415	-Changes in LV ejection fraction. -Changes in treadmill exercise duration.	$P \le .0005$, (LV ejection fraction) and $P \ge 0.5$ (treadmill exercise duration). In favor of carvedilol
US Carvedilol[15] Chronic HF	Carvedilol versus placebo	1094	-All cause mortality	$P < .001$ in favor of carvedilol
CIBIS-II[16] NYHA III-IV.	Bisoprolol versus placebo	2647	-All cause mortality	$P \le .0001$ in favor of bisoprolol
MERIT-HF[17] Chronic HF	Metoprolol CR/XL versus placebo	3980	-Vital status -CV death -Death from HF -Sudden death	$P = .0062$ in favor of the beta-blocker
BEST[18] NYHA III-IV.	Bucindolol versus placebo	2708	-All cause mortality	Trend in favor of bucindolol ($P = .16$)
COPERNICUS[19] NYHA III-IV.	Carvedilol versus placebo	2289	-All cause mortality	$P = .0014$ in favor of carvedilol
COMET[20] Chronic HF	Carvedilol versus Metoprolol	3029	-All cause mortality or admission to hospital	$P = .0017$ in favor of carvedilol
CIBIS-III[21] Chronic HF	Bisoprolol versus Enalapril in drug naive patients	1010	-Combined all cause mortality or hospitalization	Bisoprolol and enalapril similar
SENIORS[22] Elderly	Nebivolol versus placebo	2128	-Death or cardiovascular hospital admission	Trend in favor of nebivolol $P = .039$
c. ARBs				
ELITE II[23] Symptomatic HF-elderly	Losartan versus Captoril	3152	-All cause mortality	Trend in favor of losartan $P = .16$
Val-HeFT[24] Chronic HF	Valsartan versus placebo (most patients already on ACE inhibitor)	5010	-Mortality -Mortality and morbidity	Valsartan similar to ACE inhibitor
OPTIMAAL[25] Post-MI study	Losartan versus Captopril	5477	-All cause mortality	$P = .07$ in favor of losartan
CHARM-Alternative[26] HF patients intolerant to ACE inhibitors	Candesartan versus placebo	2028	-All cause mortality or -Hospital admission for CHF	$P \le .0001$ in favor of candesartan
CHARM-Added[27] HF patients on ACE inhibitors	Candesartan versus placebo	2548	-All cause mortality or -Hospital admission for CHF	$P = .105$ trend in favor of adding candesartan to ACE inhibitors
CHARM-Preserved[28] HF with preserved EF	Candesartan versus placebo	3023	-All-cause mortality or -Hospital admission for CHF	$P = .051$ trend in favor of adding candesartan

(continued on next page)

Table 1
(continued)

Trial	Study Drug	Patients	Primary Endpoint	Difference Between Treatments
VALIANT[29] Post-MI study	Valsartan versus Captopril versus combination of both.	14,703	-All cause mortality	All groups have similar effects
d. Vasodilators				
V-HeFT-I[30] Chronic HF	Prazosin versus hydralazine and isosorbide dinitrate versus placebo	642	-Mortality	$P = .046$ in the hydralazine and isosorbide dinitrate treatment grouptable_head
V-HeFT-II[31] Chronic HF	Hydralazine and isosorbide dinitrate versus Enalapril	804	-Mortality -Peak VO2 -LVEF -Plasma norepinephrine levels	favors enalapril ($P \leq .05$) at 2 years
PRAISE II[32] NYHA III-IV	Amlodipine versus placebo	1652	-All cause mortality	Amlodipine and placebo similar; no harm from amlodipine
VMAC[33] Acute HF	Nesiritide versus nitroglycerine versus placebo	489	-Self-evaluation of dyspnea -Changes in PCWP	$P = .03$ for dyspnea in favor of nesiritide
A-HeFT[34] African-American with HF	Bidil versus placebo. Bidil = combination of isosrbide dinitrate and hydralazine.	1050	-All-cause mortality -Hospitalization for HF -Change of quality of life	Favors Bidil ($P = .01$)
e. Others				
DIG[35] Chronic HF	Digoxin versus placebo	3397	-All cause mortality	$P = .80$, digoxin and placebo similar
RALES[36] NYHA III-IV	Spironolactone versus placebo	1663	-All cause mortality	$P \leq .001$, favors spironolactone
EARTH[37] Chronic HF	Darusentan versus placebo. Darusentan= endothelin receptor blocker	642	-Change in LVESV -6-min walk test -Quality of life	No significant difference between placebo and darusentan

Trial	Intervention	N	Endpoints	Result
ENABLE-1 & 2[38] NYHA IIIb-IV	Bosentan versus placebo Bosentan = endothelin receptor blocker	1613	-Death and -Hospitalization for heart failure	$P = .8976$ (not published)
EPHESUS[39] Post-MI study	Eplerenone versus placebo	6632	-Time to death from any cause and -Time to death from cardiovascular causes or first hospitalization for a cardiovascular event, including heart failure, recurrent acute myocardial infarction, stroke, or ventricular arrhythmia	favors eplerenone ($P = .008$)
MOXCON[40] Chronic HF	Moxonidine versus placebo Moxonidine = sympatholytic agent.	1934	-All cause mortality	Stopped early by DSMB due to excess fatalities from monoxidine group
RENAISSANCE/RECOVER)[41] Chronic HF	Etanercept versus placebo Etanercept = TNFα blocker	925/1123	-Clinical status at 24 weeks	No significant difference
VERITAS[42] Acute HF	Tezosentan versus placebo Tezosentan = endothelin receptor blocker	1435	-All cause mortality -Worsening HF	Stopped early by DSMB due to low probability of achieving a significant treatment effect

Abbreviations: EF, ejection fraction; LVEF, left ventricular ejection fraction; LVESV, left ventricular end-systolic volume; PCWP, pulmonary capillary wedge pressure; Peak VO2, peak oxygen uptake.

neurohormonal activation, including excessive sympathetic activity and heightened activity of the renin-angiotensin-aldosterone system (RAAS). Chronic blockade of these systems with β-adrenergic blocking drugs and agents that inhibit the RAAS such as angiotensin converting enzyme (ACE) inhibitors, aldosterone receptor blockers, and angiotensin receptor blockers (ARBs) reduces progressive LV remodeling and improves patient survival. These agents, along with diuretics, constitute the core treatment for chronic HF today.

Despite many successful clinical trials, the annual mortality for HF remains about 8%–10% per year (down from about 20% per year 30 years ago), and there is an ongoing quest to find newer, safer, and more efficacious drugs. This has been a difficult road because new treatment strategies must be now tested on top of effective therapy.[1] Demonstrating a meaningful incremental improvement in survival by adding additional drugs has been challenging in the face of treatment with baseline β-blockers, ACE inhibitors, ARBs, and aldosterone receptor blockers. Recently, new devices such as cardiac resynchronization therapy (CRT) and implantable cardioverter-defibrillators (ICDs) have accounted for more success in improving patient survival than new drugs. Moreover, there have been almost no new drugs introduced for the treatment of acute HF, as there is the vexing problem as to which clinical endpoints to measure and how to measure them. Lastly, it has become apparent that diuretic therapy is not uniformly effective in acute HF, and new strategies to reduce salt and water retention are being explored.

NEWER MEDICAL THERAPIES
Levosimendan for Acute HF

Intravenous inotropes are still widely used to improve hemodynamic parameters in patients with acute decompensated HF, but these agents have never demonstrated a survival benefit. In fact, inotropic agents almost uniformly increase mortality.[43] Levosimendan, a calcium sensitizer, is a new class of inotropic drug that has been evaluated and is used primarily in Europe. It has a different mechanism of action than the currently more widely used inotropes such as dobutamine and milrinone. The drug induces positive inotropy by binding to the calcium saturated N-terminal domain of cardiac troponin C, thus stabilizing and prolonging the lifespan of the molecule without impairment in filament relaxation. Levosimendan seemingly does not increase myocardial oxygen consumption despite increasing myocardial contractility. Other benefits of the drug include peripheral and coronary vasodilation and anti-ischemic effects mediated by opening of ATP-dependent potassium channels. Levosimendan is highly bound to plasma protein and is metabolized by the liver, rendering the half-life to be quite long (80 hours). The active moiety is likely not the levosimendan molecule but a degradation product. One of the drawbacks of levosimendan is prolonged hypotension, which can be prevented by keeping LV filling pressures adequate. Levosimendan is used in Europe but is not approved in the United States.[44]

Several clinical studies evaluating the efficacy and safety of levosimendan have been performed. They have demonstrated improvement in acute hemodynamic parameters and symptoms, with a trend toward prolonging short-term survival (Randomized Study on Safety and Effectiveness of Levosimendan in Patients with Left Ventricular Failure due to an Acute Myocardial Infarct [RUSSLAN], Levosimendan Infusion versus Dobutamine [LIDO] and Calcium Sensitizer or Inotrope or None in Low-Output Heart Failure [CASINO] trials). However, these trials were relatively small trials performed in Europe and they were generally of short duration.

Survival of Patients with Acute Heart Failure in Need of Intravenous Inotropic Support (SURVIVE) was a large randomized, double-blind study conducted in Europe that compared levosimendan to dobutamine. The study included 1327 patients with acute decompensated HF and a left ventricular ejection fraction (LVEF) <30% who were followed for 180 days after randomization. The primary endpoint of this study was all-cause mortality. At 30 and 180 days, there was no difference between the two groups ($P = .29$ and $.40$ respectively). After 5 days, BNP was lower in the levosimendan group compared with dobutamine (46% reduction versus 13% reduction respectively). The study showed evidence of regional heterogeneity in results, suggesting that differences in clinical practice may have influenced outcome.[45] Traditionally, comparator studies such as SURVIVE have a difficult time demonstrating a robust and clear "winner," and this may be particularly the case in acute HF where there is ambiguity about which clinical outcome to measure and when to measure it, making interpretation even more difficult.

The Second Randomized Multicenter Evaluation of Intravenous Levosimendan Efficacy (REVIVE-2) compared levosimendan versus placebo in 600 patients with acute decompensated HF unresponsive to conventional therapy who were followed up for 90 days after randomization. The primary endpoint of this study was a composite outcome including changes in symptoms, death or worsening HF over 5 days. There was no significant reduction in mortality between the two groups (15.1% versus 11.6% [P = .210]). In the levosimendan group, there was 33% improvement in patient symptoms, and 30% fewer patients worsened compared with placebo (P = .015). The length of stay was 2 days shorter (P = .001) and BNP levels were lower in the levosimendan group. There were 10 more deaths at 90 days in the levosimendan arm, but this difference was not statistically significant because of the small sample size. Another observation was that the levosimendan group had more hypotension and atrial fibrillation than the control group. The lack of positive survival data is disappointing,[46] and, to date, the levosimendan portfolio has not been forwarded to the Food and Drug Administration for approval in the United States.

Nesiritide for Acute Heart Failure

Nesiritide is an approved form of human B-type natriuretic peptide synthesized by using recombinant DNA techniques. It is prescribed for patients who have acute HF. Nesiritide has modest natriuretic properties and is a systemic vasodilator. It has been widely used in the United States but not in the rest of the world. Its high-tech production makes the drug relatively expensive. Nesiritide was quickly adopted in the United States soon after its approval, but its use has waned over time, in part due to concerns raised about its efficacy and safety.[47] It produces its pharmacologic effects by binding to the guanylate cyclase receptor on endothelial and smooth muscle cells in the arteries and veins. Like all vasodilators, nesiritide can increase cardiac output and reduce LV filling pressure. It has a long half-life (18 minutes) relative to nitrates and nitroprusside, and has no positive inotropic action. However, it can produce prolonged hypotension, especially if the patient is volume depleted. Nesiritide tends to inhibit neurohormonal activity and blocks proliferative/fibrotic response to injury in the heart in vitro, but the importance of these effects is understudied in patients. The pivotal clinical study leading to approval of nesiritide was done in the United States (Vasodilation in the Management of Acute CHF-VMAC).[33] This study demonstrated improvement in dyspnea in a large, randomized, controlled setting and on this basis nesiritide was approved for use in acute HF. It was rapidly adopted by clinicians, indicating a perceived need for such therapy. Eventually, pooled analysis of several studies suggested a possible increased risk of worsening renal function (RR 1.54, 95% CI, 1.20-1.99; P = .001).

A recent large study of serial infusions of nesiritide for chronic severe HF (ie, The Second Follow-up Serial Infusions of Nesiritide- FUSION II) has not replicated this risk.[48] The FUSION II study used intermittent infusions of nesiritide versus placebo in a prospective, randomized, parallel, multicenter, double-blind, placebo-controlled trial in patients with advanced HF (NYHA class III-IV) and a LVEF <40%. The trial was performed on an outpatient basis. Treatment with nesiritide and placebo was allocated using a 2:1 ratio and the treatments were administered once or twice weekly. A total of 911 patients were randomized (306 patients in the placebo group and 605 patients in the nesiritide group). The primary endpoint was time to all-cause mortality or first occurrence of hospitalization for cardiovascular and/or renal causes through week 12. All cause mortality and cardiorenal hospitalization were similar in both groups (P = .98 and 0.95 respectively).[49,50] There were no apparent safety concerns.

A large mortality study with nesiritide, ASCEND-HF (Acute Study of Clinical Effectiveness of Nesiritide in Decompensated Heart Failure) is now underway and its results are awaited.

Vasopressin Antagonists for Chronic Heart Failure

Inappropriately excessive circulating plasma vasopressin levels occur in patients with chronic HF.[51] These levels might contribute to increased vascular resistance and to positive water balance observed in patients with HF. There are at least two vasopressin receptors types in the body. The V1 (V_{1a}, V_{1b}) receptors are located in vasculature and subserve intense vasoconstriction. V2b receptors are located in the distal nephron segments of the kidneys and mediate water re-absorption. Because the goal of most HF drugs is to alleviate symptoms of fluid congestion, removal of excessive water (but not salt) via aquaresis could lead to improvement in hyponatemia and reduce pulmonary and tissue congestion. This was the basis of development of vasopressin antagonists.

Tolvaptan, is an oral, selective vasopressin V2-receptor antagonist that facilitates an aquaresis of mainly electrolyte-free water. There is an associated improvement in hyponatremia, as observed in the very large Efficacy of Vasopressin Antagonism in Heart Failure Outcome Study with Tolvaptan (EVEREST) trial.[52,53] This placebo-controlled study evaluated the short- and long-term effects of tolvaptan versus placebo in optimally treated patients hospitalized with acute HF. The primary endpoints for the EVEREST program were all-cause mortality and cardiovascular death or hospitalization for HF. Candidates for this trial were patients with an LVEF of 40% or less hospitalized for HF. Additional endpoints were a composite score of changes from baseline in patient-assessed global clinical status and body weight at day 7 or discharge. A total of 4133 patients were randomized. Tolvaptan improved serum sodium levels at hospital discharge in patients who were hyponatremic at baseline. At discharge, mean reduction from baseline was grater in the tolvaptan group than placebo (55.6 mg per day versus 42.9 mg per day; p=0.002). Despite the improvements in signs and symptoms of HF, there was no benefit in global clinical status at day 7 or at hospital discharge. Moreover, long-term tolvaptan treatment had no effect on all-cause mortality (P = .68) or the combined endpoints of cardiovascular mortality or subsequent hospitalization for worsening HF (P = .55). It also failed to show any favorable effect on cardiac remodeling, a surrogate endpoint usually associated with improvement in survival.[54] There is no question that these new aquaretic agents, including tolvaptan, conivaptan and other novel arginine vasopressin antagonists provide short-term improvement in hyponatremia and promote water loss. Whether they are useful in improving the long-term natural history of HF is open to question. More clinical investigation will be necessary.

MECHANICAL INTERVENTIONS AND DEVICES
Ultrafiltration

Diuretics have been used to treat HF since the 1950s. However, diuretic refractoriness can occur in patients with acute HF, despite large doses of loop diuretics and metolazone. The Ultrafiltration versus Intravenous Diuretics for Patients Hospitalized for Acute Decompensated Congestive Heart Failure (UNLOAD) trial[55] is the first randomized comparison of intravenous loop diuretic therapy versus ultrafiltration in hypervolemic patients hospitalized with acute HF. It was designed as a prospective, randomized, multicenter trial. There was no ejection fraction inclusion criterion. All patients received conventional HF therapy. The duration and rate of acute fluid removal was at the discretion of the treating physician. The primary endpoint was weight loss and patient's dyspnea assessment 48 hours after randomization to ultrafiltration or medical therapy. The trial also included several secondary endpoints. One hundred patients were enrolled in each arm and followed for 90 days or until death. At 48 hours following randomization, ultrafiltration produced more weight loss than conventional medical therapy (5.0 $\pm$ 3.1 Kg versus 3.1 $\pm$ 3.5 Kg; P = .001), but dyspnea assessment

indicated similar scores in both groups. Fewer patients required vasoactive medications for hypotension in the ultrafiltration group than the conventional group (P = .015). Somewhat surprisingly, there was no correlation between the 48-hour dyspnea score and the 48-hour weight or fluid loss. Changes in serum creatinine were similar in both groups at the end of the trial and changes were not reflected by the amount of fluid that was removed. However, serum creatinine did increase more during ultrafiltration more than with loop diuretics, but it returned to baseline by the end of the ultrafiltration treatment, and thus was not an adverse event. The rise in creatinine during ultrafiltration may be related to how aggressively fluid is removed, which varied from center to center. The patients in the ultrafiltration group required less diuretic, were rehospitalized fewer times (P = .037), and had fewer emergency department visits due to symptoms of congestion after release from the hospital. There were nine deaths in the ultrafiltration group compared with eleven in the diuretic arm. There was a very small number of adverse events secondary to the technical aspects of ultrafiltration (bleeding, clotted filters, infection). Ultrafiltration was associated with a 44% reduction in the percentage of patients rehospitalized for HF, and more than 50% reduction in the number and length of HF rehospitalizations and in the occurrence of unscheduled medical visits for HF. Length of index hospitalization stay was comparable (6.3 $\pm$ 4.9 days versus 5.8 $\pm$ 3.8 days; P = .979). These results clearly demonstrate the potential of an alternative therapeutic modality for patients admitted to the hospital with acute decompensated HF. However, the filters are expensive and personnel must be trained to use the technique. It is not entirely clear if bedside ultrafiltration can be easily used outside the setting of an intensive care unit, which would possibly offset the cost of the filters. The additional costs will have to be offset by reduced hospitalization stay and re-admissions to hospital. More experience will be useful in determining how and when to use this new strategy.

Cardiac Resynchronization Therapy

Another example of device innovation is biventricular pacing. Dyssynchrony in myocardial contraction commonly occurs in patients with HF and left bundle branch block, leading to impaired LV function and worsening mitral regurgitation. CRT restores more normal contraction to the LV wall while improving overall heart function. Longitudinal follow-up data suggest that CRT induces reverse remodeling as early as 3 months after implantation. Experimental data show that restoration of more normal contraction is accompanied by improvement in local loading conditions leading to changes in myocyte protein synthesis.[56] CRT should be considered only after conventional pharmacologic treatment has been optimized. Published data suggest that about 70% of patients receiving a biventricular pacemaker improve clinically.[57] Proper patient selection is perhaps the most important issue key to success with this therapeutic modality, and is a subject of ongoing discussion, but is still under intense study.[58]

Indications for CRT include: EF <35%, NYHA class III; QRS-interval of more than 130 msec; medically refractory, LV end diastolic diameter of 55 mm or more; and dyssynchrony on echocardiogram. Studies performed the last few years have demonstrated that CRT in addition to an ICD can lower the composite endpoint of death and hospitalization (Comparison of Medical Therapy, Pacing, and Defibrillation in Heart Failure [COMPANION] trial[59]). The European Cardiac Resynchronization — Heart Failure (CARE-HF) trial was a multicenter, randomized, controlled mortality trial that compared a population of patients who had systolic dysfunction (LVEF <35%), HF symptoms (NYHA class III-IV), and dyssynchrony by echocardiography with two different treatment strategies: 1) conventional drug therapy and 2) conventional drug therapy plus cardiac resynchronization. Patients were required to have a QRS-duration of more than 120 msec on the electrocardiogram. Those randomized to a device received a Medtronic InSync or InSync III device (Bi-ventricular pacemaker). Patients were followed for a mean of 29.4 months. The primary endpoint was a composite of all-cause mortality or an unplanned hospitalization for a major cardiovascular event. All patients received optimal medical therapy and 409 were additionally randomized to receive a biventricular pacer. Nearly 85% of the study population was on β-blockers. By the end of the study, 224 medically treated patients reached the primary endpoint compared with 159 in the resynchronization group (P < .001). Mortality was strikingly reduced. Unplanned hospitalization was also less in the device group than in the medically treated group (P < .002). CRT significantly reduced death, hospitalization for worsening HF, and symptoms/NYHA classification, while improving quality of life and echocardiographic parameters. The data suggest that for every nine devices implanted, one can prevent one death and three hospitalizations for major cardiovascular events. Biventricular pacing has proved to be a powerful tool in the management of HF. In the United States, it is usually performed in conjunction with implantation of an ICD, but in Europe this is not the case. Patients with class IV HF make up a small subset of these CRT studies, and to date, CRT cannot be considered a form of "rescue" therapy for the critically ill class IV patient. However, more stable class IV patients may occasionally benefit from CRT.

SUMMARY

Patients with HF are clearly receiving better treatment today than was the case 20 years ago. However, the mortality, morbidity, and costs of caring for patients with HF remain substantial. Four new trends are emerging in the development of new therapies: (1) pharmacogenomics is beginning to identify more clearly who the responders and nonresponders might be; (2) designer drugs, including new natriuretic peptides, that include the most effective moieties of several molecules are being hybridized to create highly creative new drugs that may favorably alter specific pathophysiologic components of HF; (3) in the future, small interference ribonucleotides (si RNAs) may be used to silence or activate specific genes that regulate the synthesis of proteins known to alter the clinical course of HF; and (4) stem cell therapy may emerge to stabilize or even reverse the failing heart and some of its associated signs and symptoms. Clinicians may look back some day at how primitive our current armamentarium of drugs and devices, such as intra-aortic balloon pumps, LV assist devices, defibrillators and CRT, might appear. Many challenges remain, but as long as HF is a major public health problem, medical practitioners can expect even more highly creative and innovative therapeutic approaches to the problem.

REFERENCES

1. Packer M. The impossible task of developing a new treatment for heart failure. J Card Fail 2002;8:193–6.
2. Cohn JN, Ferrari R, Sharpe N, et al. Cardiac remodeling—concepts and clinical implications: a consensus paper from an international forum on cardiac remodeling. J Am Coll Cardiol 2000;35:569–82.
3. Hill JA, Olson EN. Mechanisms of disease: cardiac plasticity. N Eng J Med 2008;358:1370–80.
4. The CONSENSUS trial study group. Effects of enalapril on mortality in severe congestive heart failure. Results of the cooperative north scandinavian enalapril survival study (CONSENSUS). N Eng J Med 1987;316:1429–35.
5. The SOLVD investigators. Effect of enalapril on survival in patients with reduced left ventricular ejection fractions and congestive heart failure. N Eng J Med 1991;325:293–302.

6. Pfeffer MA, Braunwald E, Moye LA, et al. Effect of captopril on mortality and morbidity in patients with left ventricular dysfunction after myocardial infarction. Results of the survival and ventricular enlargement trial. The SAVE investigators. N Eng J Med 1992;327:669–77.

7. AIRE study investigators. Effect of ramipril on mortality and morbidity of survivors of acute myocardial infarction with clinical evidence of heart failure. Lancet 1993;342:821–8.

8. Packer M, Poole-Wilson PA, Armstrong PW, et al. Comparative effects of low and high doses of the angiotensin-converting enzyme inhibitor, lisinopril, on morbidity and mortality in chronic heart failure. Circulation 1999;100:2312–8.

9. The heart outcomes prevention evaluation study investigators. Affects of angiotensin-converting-enzyme inhibitor, ramipril, on cardiovascular events in high-risk patients. N Eng J Med 2000;342: 145–53.

10. The European trial on reduction of cardiac events with perindopril in stable coronary artery disease investigators. Efficacy of perindopril in reduction of cardiovascular events among patients with stable coronary artery disease: randomised, double-blind, placebo-controlled, multicenter trial (the EUROPA study). Lancet 2003;362:782–8.

11. The PEACE trial investigators. Angiotensin-converting-enzyme inhibition in stable coronary artery disease. N Engl J Med 2004;351:2058–68.

12. Cleland JG, Tendera M, Adamus J, et al. The perindopril in elderly people with chronic heart failure (PEP-CHF) study. Eur Heart J 2006;27:2338–45.

13. Waagstein F, Bristow MR, Swedberg K, et al. Beneficial effects of metoprolol in idiopathic dilated cardiomyopathy. Lancet 1993;342:1441–6.

14. Australia-New Zeland heart failure research collaborative group. Effects of carvedilol, a vasodilator-beta-blocker, in patients with congestive heart failure due to ischemic heart disease. Circulation 1995;92:212–8.

15. Packer M, Bristow MR, Cohn JN, et al. The effect of carvedilol on morbidity and mortality in patients with chronic heart failure. N Eng J Med 1996;334: 1349–55.

16. CIBIS-II investigators. The cardiac insufficiency bisoprolol study II (CIBIS-II): a randomised trial. Lancet 1999;353:9–13.

17. MERIT-HF study group. Effect of metoprolol CR/XL in chronic heart failure: metoprolol CR/XL randomised intervention trial in congestive heart failure (MERIT-HF). Lancet 1999;353:2001–7.

18. Packer M, Coats AJ, Fowler MB, et al. Effect of carvedilol on survival in severe chronic heart failure. N Eng J Med 2001;344:1651–8.

19. Beta-blocker evaluation of survival trial investigators. A trial of the beta-blocker bucindolol in patients with advanced chronic heart failure. N Eng J Med 2001; 344:1659–67.

20. Poole-Wilson PA, Swedberg K, Cleland JG, et al. Comparison of carvedilol and metoprolol on clinical outcomes in patients with chronic heart failure in the carvedilol or metoprolol european trial (COMET): randomised controlled trial. Lancet 2003;362:7–13.

21. Willenheimer R, van Veldhuisen DJ, Silke B, et al. Effect on survival and hospitalization of initiating treatment for chronic heart failure with bisoprolol followed by enalapril, as compared with the opposite sequence. Results of the randomized cardiac insufficiency bisoprolol study (CIBIS) III. Circulation 2005;112:2426–35.

22. Flather MD, Shibata MC, Coats AJS, et al. Randomized trial to determine the effect of nebivolol on mortality and cardiovascular hospital admission in elderly patients with heart failure (SENIORS). Eur Heart J 2005;26:215–25.

23. Pitt B, Poole-Wilson PA, Segal R, et al. Effect of losartan compared with captopril on mortality in patients with symptomatic heart failure: randomized trial- the losartan heart failure survival study ELITE II. Lancet 2000;355:1582–7.

24. Cohn JN, Tognoni G. A randomized trial of the angiotensin-receptor blocker valsartan in chronic heart failure. N Eng J Med 2001;345:1667–75.

25. Dickstein K, Kjekshus J. Effects of losartan and captopril on mortality and morbidity in high-risk patients after acute myocardial infarction: the OPTIMAAL randomised trial. Lancet 2002;360:752–60.

26. Granger CB, McMurray JJ, Yusuf S, et al. Effects of candesartan in patients with chronic heart failure and reduced left-ventricular systolic function intolerant to angiotensin-converting-enzyme inhibitors: the CHARM-Alternative trial. Lancet 2003;362:772–6.

27. Yusuf S, Pfeffer MA, Swedberg K, et al. Effects of candesartan in patients with chronic heart failure and preserved left ventricular ejection fraction: the CHARM-Preserved trial. Lancet 2003;362:777–81.

28. McMurray JJV, Östergren J, Swedberg K, et al. Effects of candesartan in patients with chronic heart failure and reduced left-ventricular systolic function taking angiotensin-converting-enzyme inhibitors: the CHARM-Added trial. Lancet 2003;362:767–71.

29. White HD, Aylward PE, Huang Z, et al. Mortality and morbidity remain high despite captopril and/or valsartan therapy in elderly patients with left ventricular systolic dysfunction, heart failure, or both after acute myocardial infarction. Results from the valsartan in acute myocardial infarction trial (VALIANT). Circulation 2005;112:3391–9.

30. Cohn JN, Archibald DG, Ziesche S, et al. Effect of vasodilator therapy on mortality in chronic congestive heart failure. Results of a veterans administration cooperative study. N Eng J Med 1986;314: 1547–52.

31. Cohn JN, Johnson G, Ziesche S, et al. A comparison of enalapril with hydralazine-isosrbide dinitrate in the treatment of congestive heart failure. N Eng J Med 1991;325:303–10.

32. Thackray S, Witte K, Clark AL, et al. Clinical trials update: OPTIME-CHF, PRAISE-2, ALL-HAT. Eur J Heart Fail 2000;2:209–12.

33. VMAC Investigators. Intravenous nesiritide vs nitroglycerine for treatment of decomependated congestive heart failure. A randomized controlled trial. JAMA 2002;287:1531–40.

34. Taylor AL, Ziesche S, Yancy C, et al. Combination of isosorbide dinitrate and hydralazine in blacks with heart failure. N Eng J Med 2004;351:2049–57.

35. The Digitalis Investigation Group. The effect of digoxin on mortality and morbidity in patients with heart failure. N Eng J Med 1997;336:525–33.

36. Pitt B, Zannad F, Remme WJ, et al. The effect of spironolactone on morbidity and mortality in patients with severe heart failure. N Eng J Med 1999;341:709–17.

37. Coletta AP, Clark AL, Nikitin N, et al. Clinical trials update from the European Society of Cardiology: CARMEN, EARTH, OPTIMAAL, ACE, TEN-HMS, MAGIC, SOLVD-X and PATH-CHF II. Eur J Heart Fail 2002;4:661–6.

38. Teerlink JR. Recent heart failure trials of neurohormonal modulation (OVERTURE and ENABLE): approaching the asymptote of efficacy? J Card Fail 2002;8:124–7.

39. Pitt B, Remme W, Zannad F, et al. Eplerenone, a Selective aldosterone blocker, in patients with left ventricular dysfunction after myocardial infarction. N Engl J Med 2003;348:1309–21.

40. Cohn JN, Pfeffer MA, Rouleau J, et al. Adverse mortality effect of central sympathetic inhibition with sustained-release oxonidine in patients with heart failure (MOXCON). Eur J Heart Fail 2003;5:659–67.

41. Mann DL, McMurray JJV, Packer M, et al. Targeted anticytokine therapy in patients with chronic heart failure. Results of the randomized etanercept worldwide evaluation (RENEWAL). Circulation 2004;109:1594–602.

42. McMurray JJV, Teerlink JR, Cotter G, et al. Effects of tezosentan on symptoms and clinical outcomes in patients with acute heart failure. JAMA 2007;298:2009–19.

43. Cuffe MS, Califf RM, Adams KF Jr, et al. Short-term intravenous milrinone for acute exacerbations of chronic heart failure. A randomized controlled trial. JAMA 2002;287:1541–7.

44. Lehtonen L, Poder P. The ultility of levosimendan in the treatment of heart failure. Ann Med 2007;39:2–17.

45. Mebazaa A, Nieminen MS, Packer M, et al. Levosimendan vs dobutamine for patients with acute decompensated heart failure. JAMA 2007;297:1883–91.

46. Cleland JGF, Freemantle N, Coletta AP, et al. Clinical trials update from the american heart association: REPAIR-AMI, ASTAMI, JELIS, MEGA, REVIVE-II, SURVIVE and PROACTIVE. Eur J Heart Fail 2006;8:105–10.

47. Sackner-Bernstein JD, Skopicki HA, Aaronson KD. Risk of worsening renal function with nesiritide in patients with acutely decompensated heart failure. Circulation 2005;111(12):1487–91.

48. Circulation CHF, in press.

49. Yancy CW, Krum H, Massie BM, et al. The second follow-up serial infusions of nesiritide (FUSION II) trial for advanced heart failure: Study rationale and design. Am Heart J 2007;153:478–84.

50. Cleland JGF, Coletta AP, Clark AL. Clinical trials update from the American College of Cardiology 2007: ALPHA, EVFREST, FUSION II, VALIDD, PARR-2, REMODEL, SPICE, COURAGE, COACH, REMADHE, pro-BNP for the evaluation of dyspnoea and THIS-diet. Eur J Heart Fail 2007;9:740–5.

51. Goldsmith SR, Gheorghiade M. Vasopressin antagonism in heart failure. J Am Coll Cardiol 2005;46:1785–91.

52. Konstam MA, Gheorghiade M, Burnet JC Jr, et al. Effects of oral tolvaptan in patients hospitalized for worsening heart failure. The EVEREST outcome trial. JAMA 2007;297:1319–31.

53. Gheorghiade M, Konstam MA, Burnett JC Jr, et al. Short-term clinical effects of Tolvaptan, an oral vasopressin antagonist, in patients hospitalized for heart failure. JAMA 2007;297:1332–43.

54. Udelson JE, McGrew FA, Flores E, et al. Multicenter, randomized, double-blind, placebo-controlled study on the effect of oral tolvaptan on left ventricular dilation and function in patients with heart failure and systolic dysfunction. J Am Coll Cardiol 2007;49:2151–9.

55. Costanzo MR, Guglin ME, Saltzberg MT, et al. Ultrafiltration versus intravenous diuretics for patients hospitalized for acute decompensated heart failure. J Am Coll Cardiol 2007;49:675–83.

56. Kass DA. An epidemic of dyssynchrony: but what does it mean? J Am Coll Cardiol 2008;51:12–7.

57. Cleland JGF, Daubert JC, Erdmann E, et al. The effect of cardiac resynchronization on morbidity and mortality in heart failure. N Engl J Med 2005;352:1539–49.

58. Beshai JF, Grimm RA, Nagueh SF, et al. Cardiac-resynchronization therapy in heart failure with narrow QRS complexes. N Engl J Med 2007;357:2461–71.

59. Bristow MR, Saxon LA, Boehmer J, et al. Cardiac-resynchronization therapy with or without an implantable defibrillator in advanced chronic heart failure. N Engl J Med 2004;350:2140–50.

Statins in Heart Failure

Prakash C. Deedwania, MD, FACC, FACP, FCCP, FAHA*,
Usman Javed, MD

KEYWORDS

- Statin • Heart failure

Heart failure (HF) is a complex syndrome that is comprised of hemodynamic, metabolic, and neurohormonal abnormalities. It is the leading cause of hospital admissions in the United States. Over the past decade, the mortality and number of hospitalizations caused by HF are surging despite rapid advancements in clinical management. At the organ level, the structural remodeling of the left ventricle leads to progression of HF. At the cellular level, patients who have HF exhibit endothelial dysfunction, increased inflammation and oxidative stress, cellular migration and apoptosis.[1,2] In patients who have New York Heart Association class II through III HF, it has been demonstrated that short-term treatment with atorvastatin improves forearm vasodilatory response to reactive hyperemia and decreases serum levels of cytokines like endothelin-I and coenzyme 10.[3] These findings indicate that statins may be useful in patients who have HF and normal cholesterol levels, by affecting forearm vasodilatory response to reactive hyperemia and inflammatory process.

Coronary artery disease (CAD) is the most common underlying cause of HF. HF occurs in patients who have CAD primarily after they have had a coronary event such as myocardial infarction (MI).[4,5] The structural changes that occur after MI lead to left ventricular (LV) remodeling, which, unless interrupted by neurohormonal modulation, progresses to increasing LV dimensions and geometric changes.[6] Obviously, a therapy effective at preventing the coronary event will be effective in preventing development of HF in most patients who have CAD.

The benefits of statins (3-hydroxy 3-methyl glutaryl coenzyme A reductase inhibitors) in ischemic heart disease have been established to extend beyond their lipid-lowering effects. Pleiotropic effects of statins include inhibition of cellular proliferation and migration, plaque stabilization, and improved endothelial function.[7]

Based on the fact that CAD is the predominant etiology of HF, most patients who have HF would appear to be candidates for statin therapy. Landmark clinical trials of statins, however, largely have excluded patients who have advanced/decompensated HF. Based on limited data from various different clinical trials, several recent reports have shown beneficial effects of statins in patients who have HF. It is important to note that these results are based primarily upon limited data available from small numbers of patients who have stable/mild HF. Therefore, safety and efficacy of statins in HF remain elusive.

This article reviews the results from several recent reports describing the safety and efficacy of statin therapy in the setting of HF. It additionally discusses the ongoing controversy regarding the lipid paradox and possible mechanisms responsible for potential benefit of statin therapy in HF.

THE PLEIOTROPIC EFFECTS OF STATINS

The hallmark of chronic HF (CHF) is the adverse remodeling of the left ventricle associated with progressive LV dilatation and LV dysfunction.[2] It now is recognized increasingly that HF also is associated with systematic and vascular inflammation as denoted by increased levels of inflammatory biomarkers and cell adhesion molecules. This remains an issue despite advancements in medical management and successful employment of Renin Angiotensin Aldosterone System and β-blockers. Statins have been used widely in chronic ischemic heart disease and have been shown to improve vascular endothelial function by amplification of

Division of Cardiology, Veterans Affairs Central California Health Care System, University of California, San Francisco Program at Fresno, 2615 E Clinton Avenue (111), Fresno, CA 93703, USA
* Corresponding author.
E-mail address: deed@fresno.ucsf.edu (P.C. Deedwania).

Cardiol Clin 26 (2008) 573–587
doi:10.1016/j.ccl.2008.06.006
0733-8651/08/$ – see front matter. Published by Elsevier Inc.

endogenous nitric oxide (NO) production[8] and mitigation of inflammatory biomarkers such as C-reactive protein (CRP), oxidized low-density lipoprotein (LDL), and cytokines like tumor necrosis factor α (TNF-α) and interleukin (IL)-6.[9,10] The end result is reduction in hypertrophy and prevention of cardiac remodeling through effects of statins on matrix secretion.[11] A significant reduction in cardiac remodeling also might occur because of a decrease in oxidative stress at the molecular level by statins. This potentially is achieved by local control of the renin angiotensin system, local inflammation, and modulation of cytokine activation.[12] This effect appears to be exclusive to statins and not related to other lipid- lowering agents. In one HF study, simvastatin but not ezetimibe improved endothelial function, despite a similar degree of cholesterol lowering in both groups.[13]

Neurohormonal and Cytokine Effects of Statins in Heart Failure

Progression of HF leads to an activation of the neurohormonal system promoting an overexpression of cytokine as described previously. Monocyte adherence to endothelium in HF is overexpressed and leads to further production of cytokines by endothelium. Reduction of these inflammatory mediators by statin therapy in patients who have HF has been validated in small pilot studies, but this had not been confirmed in randomized clinical trials.[14,15] The effects of statins on anti-inflammatory markers appear to be independent of their effects on cholesterol levels. Tousoulis and colleagues[9,10] have demonstrated reduction in antithrombin III, protein C, IL-6, factor V, tPA, vascular cell adhesion molecule, P-selectin, and TNF-α involving patients who have NYHA class II through IV HF in two different trials. Whether the anti-inflammatory activities of statins directly translate to clinical benefits has yet to be shown in randomized clinical trials.

Myocardial Effects

In several studies of patients with acute MI ST segment Elevation Myocardial Infarction (STEMI) or Non ST segment Elevation Myocardial Infarction (NSTEMI), new or continued use of statins within the first 24 hours of the acute event has been shown to reduce 24-hour morbidity and mortality. In animal models of experimental MI, statins also have been shown to improve endothelial function, increase endogenous production of NO, inhibit platelet activation, and attenuate ventricular remodeling during the postinfarction period. This is postulated to be linked to the effects of statin on protein kinase called Akt, which has been

shown to prevent apoptosis.[16,17] In a rat model of cardiomyopathy, Lovastatin reduced LV hypertrophy and fibrosis;[18] however in human studies, the results are conflicting. Observational data from the The Hypertension High Risk Management (HYRIM) trial study showed reduction in LV mass. In this study, patients were followed for up to 4 years on fluvastatin.[19]

Reduced Oxidative Stress with Statins

It is known that there is evidence of increased oxidative stress after MI. In experimental models, use of antioxidants has been shown to impede the adverse remodeling process. Reduced oxidative stress potentially can improve LV dysfunction and reduce ventricular dilatation by virtue of deactivation of matrix metalloproteinases, which drive matrix turnover and advance the left ventricle remodeling that subsequently can lead to progressive LV dysfunction.[20]

Statins have antioxidant properties and inhibit reactive oxygen species (ROS) generation through modulation of nicotinamide adenine dinucleotide phosphate (NADPH) pathway, hence blunting the injurious effects of ROS, including effects on antioxidant enzymes, lipid peroxidation, LDL cholesterol oxidation, and NO synthase.

In HF, an increase in ROS may be driven by various mechanisms, including the activation of the renin angiotensin system, cytokine activation, local inflammation, and mechanical stimuli.[12] Upregulation of angiotensin 2 type 1 (AT1) in HF leads to vasoconstriction, fluid and sodium retention, increased sympathetic activity, and myocyte hypertrophy.[17] Angiotensin-converting enzyme (ACE) inhibitors and angiotensin receptor blockers are highly effective inhibitors of angiotensin 2-dependent NADPH oxidase activation. Statins appear to inhibit the NADPH pathway through small GTPases such as Rac.[21] Several experimental studies have indicated favorable effects of statins on cardiac hypertrophy and remodeling after MI.[17]

DOES LIPID PARADOX EXIST IN HEART FAILURE?

There are limited clinical data supporting the fact that statins may harm patients who have HF. Small observational studies have shown that lower cholesterol concentrations are associated with a poor prognosis and increased mortality in HF. This phenomenon is postulated to be multifactorial and may reflect the onset of cardiac cachexia, liver dysfunction, and impaired nutrition. In theory, statin use in HF remains controversial. This essentially has been based upon the so- called endotoxin hypothesis, which requires the presence of lipoproteins to eliminate bacterial lipopolysaccharides and inhibit cytokine release.[22] On the contrary, lowering of lipoproteins by statins would increase the lipopolysaccharides and promote infection in patients who have HF.[23]

Statins are known to cause a decrease in coenzyme Q10, thus worsening oxidative stress and decreasing mitochondrial and myocardial function.[24] In patients who have HF, cholesterol modulates inflammatory immune activity, in particular endotoxin levels. Therefore, it is conceivable that lowering cholesterol levels with the use of statins may prove detrimental in some patients who have HF.[25] Further studies are needed to elucidate on these aspects of statin therapy in patients who have HF.

CURRENT LEVEL OF EVIDENCE ABOUT ROLE OF STATINS IN HEART FAILURE

Although some experimental evidence from small studies suggest that statins are beneficial in HF, one should exercise caution in interpreting clinical outcome data that largely are obtained from various statin trials and studies done in patients who have HF. In most of the recent reports, the evidence comes primarily from observation made by retrospective analyses. These results are limited further by small and relatively poorly defined cohorts of HF patients in the study. Also, the endpoints are not prespecified pertaining to the impact of statin therapy on HF. Hence, the available information is weak and incomplete regarding the long-term efficacy of statins in HF (**Box 1**).

RETROSPECTIVE ANALYSIS OF STATIN AND HEART FAILURE TRIALS
The Statin Trials

First indirect information about the beneficial effects of statins in HF came from the posthoc analyses of two landmark clinical trials of statin therapy (**Table 1**). In the 4S study,[28] patients who had known CAD and hypercholesterolemia were included. Patients who had symptomatic HF were excluded. Of the 4444 patients on statin therapy, 412 developed symptomatic HF during follow-up. A lower incidence of symptomatic HF was observed in the simvastatin group, compared with the placebo group (184 vs. 228). Also, there was a 19% relative risk reduction (RRR) in 5-year mortality with statin therapy in patients who had HF (25.5% vs. 31.9%, CI not reported).

The Cholesterol and Recurrent Events study[26] was a randomized trial of pravastatin for secondary prevention of cardiovascular events after MI. This study excluded symptomatic patients who

Box 1
Beneficial and adverse effects of statins in heart failure
Beneficial effects
Reduced in coronary events
Improved endothelial function
Anti-inflammatory effects
Decreased endothelial adhesion markers
Reduced oxidative stress
Increased angiogenesis
Prevention of cardiac remodeling
Reduced platelet activation and thrombosis
Reduction in apoptosis
Reduced myocardial hypertrophy
Improved neurohormonal balance
Improved renal function
Adverse effects
Reduced synthesis of ubiquinone (coenzyme Q10)
Decreased binding of lipopolysaccharides
Probable impairment of cellular function

had HF or those who had LV ejection fraction (LVEF) less than 25%. Of 4159 patients, 706 had LVEF between 25% and 40%, while the rest had LVEF greater than 40%. A posthoc analysis compared the outcome in two subgroups regarding the rate of cardiovascular death or nonfatal MI, and showed 28% versus 23% RRR, respectively, in patients who had LVEF greater or less than 40%.

The Treat to New Targets (TNT) study evaluated efficacy of atorvastatin in 10,001 patients who had stable CAD and LDL less than 130.[37] A subgroup analysis of 781 patients who had HF demonstrated that 80 mg of atorvastatin reduced HF hospitalizations to a greater extent than 10 mg. This study suggested an incremental benefit of high-dose statin therapy in preventing HF hospitalizations, with an RRR of 26% (hazard ratio [HR] 0.74, CI 0.59 to 0.94, $P = .01$) with high-dose statin. For each 1 mg/dL reduction in LDL cholesterol on treatment, the risk of hospitalization for HF was reduced by 0.6% ($P < .007$). This study was limited by the fact that no information on systolic or diastolic function was available. Also, patients who had advanced HF (NYHA classes III to IV) were excluded.

Subgroup analysis from the Incremental Decrease in Events through Aggressive Lipid

Table 1
Subgroup analysis of heart failure patients in major randomized trails of statin therapy

Study	Population	Major Characteristic	Patients with Heart Failure	Outcomes in Heart Failure Subgroup	Outcomes Result	Statin	Follow-up (Years)
CARE[26]	4159	Myocardial infarction (MI) and high cholesterol	706	Death from coronary artery disease (CAD), ejection fraction >40 versus <40	Reduction	Pravastatin	5
LIPID (1998)[38]	9014	MI and unstable angina	None at baseline	Death	Reduction	Pravastatin	6.1
4S (1999)[28]	4444	CAD and high cholesterol	412	Mortality	Positive effect	Simvastatin	5.4
MIRACL[29]	3086	Unstable angina, NSTEMI	253	Onset of heart failure (HF), rehospitalization	No difference	Atorvastatin	4 wks
PROSPER[27]	5814	Peripheral vascular disease or related risk factors	HF NYHA class III–IV excluded	hospitalization for HF	No difference	Pravastatin	3.2
GREACE[30]	1600	CAD	118	Death, nonfatal MI, unstable angina	Reduction in primary endpoints	Atorvastatin	3
A-Z[31]	4497	Acute coronary syndrome	221	New onset heart failure	Reduction in new onset HF	Simvastatin	0.5-2
GRACE[32]	19,537	ACS	N/A	HF during hospitalization	Reduction	Atorvastatin	3.5
ALLIANCE[33]	2442	CAD	162 HF patients	Hospitalization	Reduction (p = not significant)	Atorvastatin	4.3
IDEAL[34]	8888	Acute MI	537	Risk of hospitalization	No effect	Atorvastatin versus simvastatin	4.8
HYRIM[19]	568	Hypertension	None at baseline	LV mass	Reduction	Fluvastatin	4
PROVE IT (2006)[35]	4162	ACS	N/A	Hospitalization	Reduction	Atorvastatin versus pravastatin	2
HPS (2007)[36]	20,536	Diabetes mellitus, vascular disease	Severe HF excluded	Hospitalization or death	Reduction	Simvastatin	5
TNT (2007)[37]	10,001	Stable CAD and LDL <130	781	Hospitalization	Positive effect	Atorvastatin 10 mg versus 80 mg	4.9

Lowering study[34] also exhibited a 19% nonsignificant reduction (HR 0.81, CI 0.62 to 1.05 P = .11) in risk of hospitalization in patients receiving atorvastatin 80 mg/d compared with simvastatin 40 mg/d. In the Aggressive Lipid Lowering to Alleviate New Cardiovascular Endpoints (ALLIANCE) study,[33] treatment with atorvastatin was associated with a 27% reduction in hospitalization because of HF (CI 0.49 to 1.09, P = not significant [NS]), while Pravastatin or Atorvastatin Evaluation and Infection Therapy - Thrombolysis in Myocardial Infarction 22 (PROVE IT-TIMI 22) reported a 45% reduction in HF hospitalization[35] with 80 mg of atorvastatin (CI 0.35 to 0.85, P = .008).

The Long-Term Intervention with Pravastatin in Ischemic Disease (LIPID)[38] trial observed mortality benefit of pravastatin in HF (P < .05), while the Heart Protection Study (HPS) showed a marginal reduction in mortality (3.4% in simvastatin vs. 3.9% in placebo group) and hospitalization.[36] The A to Z trial[31] showed reduction of new-onset heart failure by 18%. In retrospective analysis of the HYRIM study,[19] a reduction of LV mass was observed over 2 years of follow-up during treatment with fluvastatin (P = .014).

Contrary to the previously mentioned reports of benefit with statin therapy, the Prospective Study of Pravastatin in the Elderly at Risk (PROSPER)[27] trial included elderly patients (70 to 82 years) with history or risk factors for vascular disease and found no difference in hospitalization for HF between pravastatin and usual care groups. Also, the Myocardial Ischemia Reduction with Acute Cholesterol Lowering (MIRACL)[29] trial showed no difference in onset or hospitalization for HF in patients treated with statins. The MIRACL trial, however, was a short-term study lasting only 16 weeks, and this period might not be sufficiently long enough to have significant impact on HF outcome.

Observation from the Heart Failure Trials

Retrospective reviews of statin use in patients enrolled in HF trials have evaluated the role of statins on the mortality and hospitalization for HF extensively (**Table 2**). First compelling evidence came from the Prospective Randomized Amlodipine Survival Evaluation (PRAISE) trial, in which data from the subset of 134 HF patients on statin (out of a total of 1153 patients) were evaluated.[45] Ninety-three patients were on statin at enrollment, while others were started on during follow-up. Compared with those not on statin therapy, there was a 62% RRR (HR 0.44, CI 0.26 to 0.75) for total mortality.

Horwich and colleagues[45] also studied effect of statin therapy in patients with systolic HF. In a population of 551 patients, statin therapy improved survival in ischemic and nonischemic cardiomyopathy (P = .001 for both). Krum and colleagues[43] reported similar effect in (CIBIS)-II and Valsartan Heart Failure Trial (Val-HeFT) trials.[44] In the Cardiac Insufficiency Bisoprolol (CIBIS)-II trial, survival was compared in patients who had HF on statin/bisoprolol, statin/placebo, placebo/bisoprolol, and placebo-only groups. Overall, statin use was associated with better survival compared with no statin use (P < .05), with greatest survival benefit in statin/bisoprolol group. A posthoc analysis of data from the Val-HeFT study examined the effect of statin use at baseline on outcomes in 5010 patients who had NYHA class II to III CHF. Statin use significantly reduced the risk of mortality with 19% RRR (HR 0.81, 95% CI 0.70-0.94). Patients with an ischemic etiology appeared to derive more survival benefit from statin therapy than those with a nonischemic etiology.[44]

In the OPTIMAAL[41] trial, the outcomes were evaluated in patients receiving statin and beta blockers alone, versus both of them or none. In 2467 patients, statin use was associated with reduced hospitalization (RR of 9%, P < .05), cardiovascular death as well as all cause mortality and recurrent infarction.

The COMPANION[48] trial enrolled 1520 patients with advanced HF randomized to cardiac resynchronization therapy with or without automatic implantable cardioverter defibrillator compared with medical therapy alone. Of the total 608 patients, 40% were on statin. The patients on statin therapy had a 28% RRR (HR 0.72, CI 0.56 to 0.92) in mortality.

Evaluation of Statin Therapy in Observational Studies of HF Cohorts

Several systematic reviews of HF cohorts also suggest that statins may be beneficial in this patient population (**Table 3**). Ray and colleagues[52] studied the impact of statin therapy in patients hospitalized for newly diagnosed CHF. Of 28,828 patients, only 1146 were on various statins. In the observation period of 1.3 years for statin users and 2 years in nonusers, mortality, nonfatal MI, and stroke were studied as primary outcomes. A 38% RRR (CI 0.63 to 0.83) in combined outcomes and a 33% RRR (CI 0.57 to 0.78) in mortality were observed in patients on statin therapy.

In a recent large retrospective observational study of Medicare beneficiaries hospitalized for HF, Foody and colleagues[54] evaluated the association between statin use and survival using the

Table 2
Statin use from major heart failure trials

Study	N	Major Characteristics	Patients on Statin	Outcomes in Statin Subgroup	Outcome Results	Statin	Follow-up (Years)
ELITE II[39]	3152	NYHA II–IV, losartan versus captopril	359	Mortality	Positive	Any	1.5
PRAISE[40]	1153	NYHA III–IV, amlodipine versus placebo	134	Mortality, sudden cardiac death	Positive	Lovastatin, pravastatin, simvastatin	1.3
OPTIMAAL[41]	5477	Acute myocardial infarction (MI) associated with heart failure (HF)	2467	All-cause mortality, hospitalization, reinfarction	Positive	Not specified	3.1
Val-HeFT[42]	5010	NYHA II–IV, EF <40	1602	Mortality	Positive	Any	1.9
CIBIS-II[43]	2647	NYHA III–IV, bisoprolol	226	Mortality	Positive	Any	1.3
Val-HeFT[44]	5010	NYHA II–IV, EF <40	1602	Mortality (ischemic vs. nonischemic)	Improved only in ischemic	Any	1.3
Horwich et al[45]	551	HF, EF <40	248	Mortality/cardiac transplantation	Positive	Atorvastatin, simvastatin, pravastatin	2
Ezekowitz et al[46]	6427	Ischemic cardiomyopathy	2545	Mortality	Positive	Any	1
Sola et al[47]	446	NYHA II–III, EF <35	NA	Mortality, hospitalization	Positive	Any	2
COMPANION[48]	1520	NYHA III–IV, cardiac resynchronization therapy versus AICD versus medical therapy alone	608	Mortality	Positive	Any	1.3
ELITE II[49]	3132	NYHA II–IV, losartan versus captopril	398	Mortality	Positive	Any	1
Anker et al[49]	2068	HF	705	Mortality	Positive	Any	1
Dikinson[50]	2521	HF	965	Mortality	Positive	Any	3.8

Table 3
Observational studies of statin therapy in heart failure cohorts

Study	Population	Major Characteristics	Patients on Statin	Outcomes in Statin Subgroup	Results	Statin	Follow-up (Years)
Howlett et al[51]	4888	Heart failure (HF) admission or discharge diagnosis	714	Mortality	Positive	Any	2
Ray et al[52]	23,328	Newly diagnosed HF	1146	Mortality/ myocardial infarction (MI)/ cerebrovascular accident	Positive	Any	2
Jaganmohan et al[53]	32,463	Veterans with HF	19,838	Mortality	Positive	Any	NA
Nul et al[55]	2331	Ambulatory HF	2331	Mortality, admission	Positive	Any	206
Foody et al[54]	54,940	Medicare patients discharged diagnosis HF	9175	Mortality	Positive	Any	3
Go et al[56]	24,598	HF patients eligible for statin therapy	24,598	Mortality	Positive	Any	2.4
Folkeringa et al[57]	840	HF admissions	524	Mortality	Positive	Any	2.5

Cox proportional hazard model. Of the 54,940 patients hospitalized with a primary discharge diagnosis of HF, 16.7% were discharged on statin therapy. Treatment of with a statin at the time of discharge was associated with significant improvements in mortality at 1 and 3 years (HR 0.80, 95% CI 0.76 to 0.84 and HR 0.82, 95% CI 0.79 to 0.85, respectively, **Fig. 1**). This benefit was noted independent of demographics, treatments, physician specialty, and hospital characteristics.

Another study by Go and colleagues[56] evaluated a large (n = 24,589) Kaiser Permanente CHF cohort to confer an association between

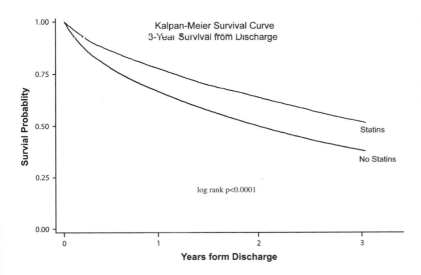

Kalpan-Meier Survival Curve
3-Year Survival from Discharge

Survial Probability

Statins

No Statins

log rank p<0.0001

Years form Discharge

Fig. 1. Association of statin use with survival in patients discharged with diagnosis of heart failure. (*From* Foody JM, Shah R, Galusha D, et al. Statins and mortality among elderly patients hospitalized with heart failure. Circulation 2006;113:1090; with permission.)

initiating statin therapy and the risk of death and hospitalization among adults who had HF after a median follow-up of 2.4 years. Statin therapy was associated with a 24% (HR 0.74 CI 0.72 to 0.80) lower risk for death and a 21% (HR 0.79 CI 0.74 to 0.85) lower risk of hospitalization for heart HF. Difference in mortality was independent of total cholesterol level or coronary disease status. It is important to note that statins were more likely to be prescribed in younger patients and those known to have CAD, diabetes, or hypertension.

Jaganmohan and colleagues[53] retrospectively studied 32,463 veterans who had a diagnosis of HF. Of the total, 31% of the patients had an underlying CAD, and 61% (n = 19,838) were on statins. When adjusted for demographics and CAD therapy including aspirin, ACEI, and β-blockers, statin therapy was associated

with 10% RRR (HR 0.9, CI 0.88 to 0.92) in mortality.

Overall, most observational data (see **Table 3**) from these large cohorts of patients with HF have shown that treatment with statins was associated with improvement in survival. It is, however, difficult to assess whether the benefit of statin therapy is related to reduction in coronary events or other direct effect on HF-related processes.

Prospective Trials Evaluating Mechanistic Effects of Statins in Heart Failure

Table 4 summarizes results of several small pilot studies that have evaluated the effects of statin therapy on various parameters related to HF. In general, these are small studies that have evaluated different parameters or biomarkers, and

Table 4
Observational studies of statins therapy in heart failure cohorts

Study	Population	Major Characteristics	Outcomes	Results	Statin	Follow-up (Years)
Node et al[58]	51	NYHA II–III, EF <35, dilated cardiomyopathy	EF, functional class, biomarkers	Positive	Simvastatin	0.25
Hong et al[59]	202	Left ventricular ejection fraction (LVEF) <40, ischemic	Left ventricular (LV), Cardiovascular death, restenosis, CVA	Positive	Simvastatin	0.2
Laufs et al[60]	15	NYHA II–-III, DCM	Functional capacity, quality of life, biomarkers	Positive	Cerivastatin	0.4
Landmesser et al[13]	20	NYHA IV, simvastatin versus ezetimibe	Endothelial function	Positive	Simvastatin	10 wks
Tousoulis et al[9]	35	NYHA II–IV	Angiotensin III, protein C and factory V, tPA and PAI-1	Reduced	Atorvastatin	4 wks
Tousoulis et al[10]	38	NYHA II–IV	Interleukin (IL)-6, tumor necrosis factor (TNF), VCAM-1	Reduced	Atorvastatin	4 wks
Strey et al[3]	24	NYHA II–III, EF <40	Flow mediated vasodilatation, coenzyme Q, ET-1	Positive	Atorvastatin	6 wks
UNIVERSE[61]	87	NYHA II–III, EF <40	LV remodeling	No effect	Rosuvastatin	0.5
Sola et al[62]	108	Non Ischemic cardiomyopathy	LVEF	Positive	Atorvastatin	1

most of them fail to relate changes in these parameters to clinical benefits.

The Rosuvastatin Impact on Ventricular Remodelling Lipids and Cytokines (UNIVERSE) trial[61] was a prospective and randomized trial that analyzed effect of statin therapy in HF. In this trial, 87 patients who had ischemic and nonischemic cardiomyopathy, NYHA class II to III HF, and LVEF less than 40% were randomized to take rosuvastatin 40 mg or placebo in addition to standard HF therapy for 6 months. This study failed to demonstrate an improvement in LVEFor end diastolic volume or reduction in neurohormonal or inflammatory markers.

In contrast, Sola and colleagues[62] evaluated the effects of 20 mg of atorvastatin in a prospective cohort of 108 patients who had nonischemic cardiomyopathy. They demonstrated an improvement in LVEF (0.004), Left Ventricular end systolic dimension ($P = .01$) and Left Ventricular end diastolic dimension ($P = .01$) and statistically significant reduction in inflammatory markers including TNF-α, CRP, IL-6, and erythrocyte superoxide dismutase. Mean NYHA functional class was 2.9 and 2.2, respectively, in treatment and placebo arms. However, there was no difference in hospitalizations or total mortality between the two groups.

In two separate studies, Tousoulis and colleagues[9,10] observed the effect of atorvastatin on flow-mediated vasodilatation in patients who had HF. In a subset of 38 patients who had NYHA class II to IV and LVEF less than 35%, 10 mg of atorvastatin were used, and efficacy was determined by measuring various biomarkers and flow-mediated vasodilatation at baseline and 4 weeks.[9] Reactive hyperemia caused by flow-mediated vasodilatation increased significantly ($P < .01$) and so was reduction in inflammatory markers including IL-6 ($P < .05$), CVAM-1 ($P < .01$) and TNF-α ($P < .01$). In another study of 35 patients who had NYHA class II to IV HF, flow-mediated reactive hyperemia and inflammatory biomarkers were evaluated after 4 weeks of treatment with 10 mg of atorvastatin.[10] Compared with placebo, atorvastatin had no effect on reactive hyperemia. Antithrombin III, protein C and factor V ($P < .01$ for all), and PAI-1 and tPA ($P < .05$ for both) were reduced significantly, however.

Laufs and colleagues[60,63] confirmed beneficial effect of cerivastatin with improved brachial artery flow mediated dilation, quality-of-life score, functional ability, and reduced levels of PAI-1, CRP, and TNF-α. This study refutes the notion that the differences between UNIVERSE and other trials that reported positive results may have been related to the inclusion of ischemic and nonischemic patients in the UNIVERSE trial.

Prospective Randomized Clinical Trials

The inconsistent findings of available studies emphasize the need for large, randomized, double-blind placebo-controlled clinical trials to elucidate the role of statins for treating HF (**Table 5**). The results from the Controlled Rosuvastatin in Multinational Trial in Heart Failure CORONA[64] and the Gruppo Italiano per lo Studio della Sopravvivenza nell'Insufficienza Cardica Gruppo Italiano per lo Studio della Sopravvivenza nell'Infarto Miocardico (GISSI-HF)[65] trials have been awaited. Results of the CORONA trial were reported recently, and the GISSI-HF trial is anticipated to provide important information concerning the use of rosuvastatin in HF by 2009.

In the CORONA trial, 5011 elderly patients (age greater than 60), with ischemic cardiomyopathy and NYHA class II to IV HF were enrolled and had a median follow-up of 32.8 months.[64] They randomly were assigned to receive 10 mg/d of rosuvastatin or placebo. The primary composite outcome was cardiovascular death, nonfatal MI, or nonfatal stroke, analyzed as time to the first event. Secondary outcomes included death from any cause, any coronary event, death from cardiovascular causes, and the number of hospitalizations. In the rosuvastatin group, there was a significant reduction in LDL cholesterol (136 vs. 76 mg/dL, 45%, $P < .001$) and also a reduction in high-sensitivity CRP (difference between groups, 37.1%; $P < .001$). The primary events (**Fig. 2**) occurred in 692 patients in the rosuvastatin group and 732 in the placebo group (HR, 0.92; 95% CI, 0.83 to 1.02; $P = .12$). Deaths from cardiovascular causes (**Fig. 3**) were in 593 patients in drug group and 581 in control group (HR, 0.97; 95% CI, 0.87 to 1.09; $P = .6$). There was no effect on the cardiovascular outcome, NYHA class or quality of life. Fewer hospitalizations for cardiovascular causes, however, were reported in the rosuvastatin group (2193) compared with the placebo group ($n = 2564$) ($P < .001$).

This trial is limited by the fact that it enrolled elderly patients (mean age 73) in whom the burden of comorbidities may be high, and this may have blunted the benefits in an ailing population. Also raised is potential interaction of the drug with a complex medical regimen in an elderly population. Although the molecular configuration of rosuvastatin helps lower LDL significantly, it might not have a favorable clinical effect in patients who have HF. Further evaluation in prospectively designed clinical trials is needed to compare the effects of rosuvastatin with other statins that have shown beneficial effects in observational studies.

Table 5
Randomized controlled trial of statin use in heart failure

Study	Population	Major Characteristics	Outcomes in Statin Subgroup	Results	Statin	Follow-up (Years)
CORONA[64]	692	NYHA II–IV	Nonfatal myocardial infarction (MI), death, stroke, hospitalization	Improved hospitalization	Rosuvastatin	2.6
GISSI-HF[65]	~7000	NYHA II–IV	Nonfatal MI, all-cause death	Not applicable	Rosuvastatin versus omega-3 fish oil	1.5

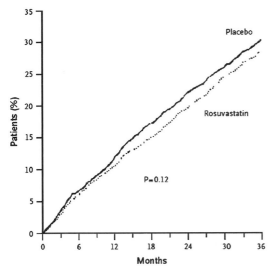

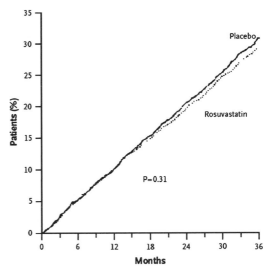

Fig. 2. Controlled Rosuvastatin in Multinational Trial in Heart Failure (CORONA) showed no significant risk reduction in primary outcome (death from cardiovascular causes, nonfatal myocardial infarction, and nonfatal stroke) with use of rosuvastatin in HF. (*From* Kjekshus J, Apetrei E, Barrios V, et al. the CORONA Group. Rosuvastatin in older patients with systolic heart failure. N Engl J Med 2007;357:2252; with permission. Copyright © 2007, Massachusetts Medical Society.)

Fig. 3. Controlled Rosuvastatin in Multinational Trial in Heart Failure (CORONA) showed no risk reduction in cardiovascular deaths from use of rosuvastatin in HF. (*From* Kjekshus J, Apetrei E, Barrios V, et al. the CORONA Group. Rosuvastatin in older patients with systolic heart failure. N Engl J Med 2007;357:2252; with permission. Copyright © 2007, Massachusetts Medical Society.)

Another ongoing study[65] is the GISSI-HF trial. This trial will randomize around 7000 patients with NYHA functional class II to IV HF regardless of etiology and with ejection fractions less than or equal to 40% to receive either omega-3 polyunsaturated fatty acids or placebo. Patients who have no indication to statin therapy will be randomized to receive rosuvastatin 10 mg or placebo with a follow-up for 18 months. The study endpoints include all-cause mortality or cardiovascular hospitalization. This trial may give a better insight based upon etiology, as patients with nonischemic cardiomyopathy and diastolic HF also will be enrolled. It is expected to be reported in 2009.

Meta-analysis of Statin Use in Heart Failure

A recent meta-analysis of thirteen HF trials[66] estimated survival benefit of statin use in patients who had HF of ischemic and nonischemic etiologies. All trials included in this meta-analysis had evaluated mortality as primary outcome and reported results as HRs. Eleven of the trials included were retrospective, while two were prospective studies. This meta-analysis suggested that statin use among patients who had HF was associated with 26% RRR in mortality (HR, 0.74; 95% CI, 0.68 to 0.8) (**Fig. 4**). A stratified analysis of 8 out of these 13 studies also suggested that statin use was associated with an improved

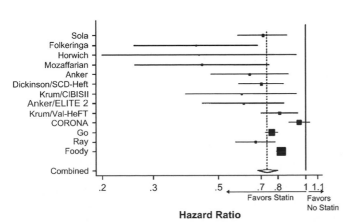

Fig. 4. Meta-analysis of mortality among patients with heart failure (HF). HF patients using statins (n = 30,107); HF patients not using statins (n = 101,323). (*From* Ramasubbu K, Estep J, White DL, et al. Experimental and clinical basis for the use of statins in patients with ischemic and nonischemic cardiomyopathy. J Am Coll Cardiol 2008;51:422; with permission.)

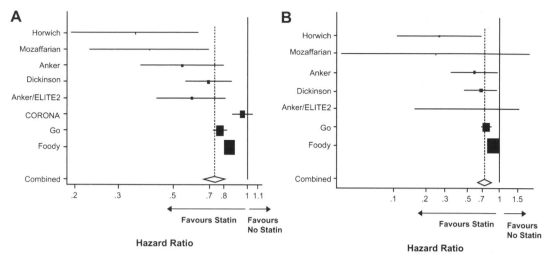

Fig. 5. Mortality among patients with heart failure (HF): ischemic and nonischemic etiology. (*A*) Adjusted mortality among patients with ischemic etiology (n = 62,273) using statins, compared with those not using statins (*B*). Mortality among patients with HF of nonischemic etiology (n = 31,551) using statins compared with those not using statins. (*From* Ramasubbu K, Estep J, White DL, et al. Experimental and clinical basis for the use of statins in patients with ischemic and nonischemic cardiomyopathy. J Am Coll Cardiol 2008;51:423; with permission.)

survival among patients who had HF when added to currently recommended therapy for HF (**Fig. 5**). This effect was noted to be independent of the etiology for HF (for ischemic etiology, HR 0.73; 95% CI 0.65 to 0.82, while for nonischemic etiology, HR, 0.73; 95% CI 0.61 to 0.87).

SUMMARY

As described in the review of clinical data, mostly from the observational studies and posthoc evaluations from the large randomized clinical trials (conducted for various reasons), it seems reasonable to conclude that statin therapy is beneficial in patients who have HV. The third Adult Treatment Panel of the National Cholesterol Education Program recommends the use of statins in HF patients who have underlying CAD.[67] There is no official endorsement for the use of statins in other patients who have HF, as the available data are based upon observational or retrospective, nonrandomized (for statin use) studies. The results of the CORONA trial fail to show any significant benefit, and one must await the results of the GISSI-HF to give further insight regarding the use of statins in all patients who have HF. In summary, patients who have HF should be treated based upon underling cardiac risk factors and etiology of HF. Patients who have ischemic cardiomyopathy and/or diabetes should be treated aggressively with a statin to lower LDL cholesterol levels to at least less than 100 mg/dL and preferably to less than 70 mg/dL. The role of statin therapy in the remaining patients

who have HF remains controversial, and one must wait for the results of the ongoing GISSI-HF trial before making any further recommendations.

REFERENCES

1. Braunwald E, Bristow MR. Congestive heart failure: fifty years of progress. Circulation 2000;102:14–23.
2. Anker SD, von Haehling S. Inflammatory mediators in chronic heart failure: an overview. Heart 2004; 90:464–70.
3. Strey CH I, Young JM, Molyneux SL, et al. Endothelium-ameliorating effects of statin therapy and coenzyme Q10 reductions in chronic heart failure. Atherosclerosis 2005;179:201–6.
4. Aronow WS, Ahn C. Frequency of congestive heart failure in older persons with prior myocardial infarction and serum low-density lipoprotein cholesterol <125 mg/dL treated with statins versus no lipid-lowering drug. Am J Cardiol 2002;90:147–9.
5. Kjekshus J, Pedersen TR, Olsson AG, et al. The effects of simvastatin on the incidence of heart failure in patients with coronary heart disease. J Card Fail 1997;3:249–54.
6. Mann DL. Mechanisms and models in heart failure: a combinatorial approach. Circulation 1999;100: 999–1008.
7. Seta Y, Shan K, Bozkurt B, et al. Basic mechanisms in heart failure: the cytokine hypothesis. J Card Fail 1996;2:243–9.
8. Maack C, Kartes T, Kilter H, et al. Oxygen-free radical release in human failing myocardium is associated with increased activity of rac1-GTPase and

represents a target for statin treatment. Circulation 2003;108:1567–74.

9. Tousoulis D, Antoniades C, Bosinakou E, et al. Effects of atorvastatin on reactive hyperemia and inflammatory process in patients with congestive heart failure. Atherosclerosis 2005;178:359–63.

10. Tousoulis D, Antoniades C, Bosinakou E, et al. Effects of atorvastatin on reactive hyperaemia and the thrombosis–fibrinolysis system in patients with heart failure. Heart 2005;91:27–31.

11. Ichiki T, Takeda K, Tokunou T, et al. Down regulation of angiotensin II type 1 receptor by hydrophobic 3-hydroxy-3-methylglutaryl coenzyme A reductase inhibitors in vascular smooth muscle cells. Arterioscler Thromb Vasc Biol 2001;21:1896–901.

12. Landmesser U, Spiekermann S, Dikalov S, et al. Vascular oxidative stress and endothelial dysfunction in patients with chronic heart failure: role of xanthine–oxidase and extracellular superoxide dismutase. Circulation 2002;106:3073–8.

13. Landmesser U, Bahlmann F, Mueller M, et al. Simvastatin versus ezetimibe: pleiotropic and lipid-lowering effects on endothelial function in humans. Circulation 2005;111:2356–63.

14. Levine B, Kalman J, Mayer L, et al. Elevated circulating levels of tumor necrosis factor in severe chronic heart failure. N Engl J Med 1990;323:236–41.

15. Bleske BE, Nicklas JM, Bard RL, et al. Neutral effect on markers of heart failure, inflammation, endothelial activation and function, and vagal tone after high-dose HMG-CoA reductase inhibition in nondiabetic patients with nonischemic cardiomyopathy and average low-density lipoprotein level. J Am Coll Cardiol 2006;47:338–41.

16. Dimmeler S, Aicher A, Vasa M, et al. HMG-CoA reductase inhibitors (statins) increase endothelial progenitor cells via the PI 3-kinase/Akt pathway. J Clin Invest 2001;108:391–7.

17. Nickenig G, Baumer AT, Temur Y, et al. Statin-sensitive dysregulated AT1 receptor function and density in hypercholesterolemic men. Circulation 1999;100:2131–4.

18. Oi S, Haneda T, Osaki J, et al. Lovastatin prevents angiotensin II-induced cardiac hypertrophy in cultured neonatal rat heart cells. Eur J Pharmacol 1999;376:139–48.

19. Anderssen SA, Hjelstuena AK, Hjermanna I, et al. Fluvastatin and lifestyle modification for reduction of carotid intima–media thickness and left ventricular mass progression in drug-treated hypertensives. Atherosclerosis 2005;178:387–97.

20. Bellosta S, Via D, Canavesi M, et al. HMG-CoA reductase inhibitors reduce MMP-9 secretion by macrophages. Arterioscler Thromb Vasc Biol 1998;18:1671–8.

21. Habibi J, Whaley-Connell A, Qazi MA, et al. Rosuvastatin, a 3-hydroxy-3-methylglutaryl coenzyme A reductase inhibitor, decreases cardiac oxidative stress and remodeling in Ren2 transgenic rats. Endocrinology 2007;148:2181–8.

22. Horwich TB, Hamilton MA, Maclellan WR, et al. Low serum total cholesterol is associated with marked increase in mortality in advanced heart failure. J Card Fail 2002;8:216–24.

23. Rauchhaus M, Coats AJ, Anker SD. The endotoxin–lipoprotein hypothesis. Lancet 2000;356:930–3.

24. Rundek T, Naini A, Sacco R, et al. Atorvastatin decreases the coenzyme Q10 level in the blood of patients at risk for cardiovascular disease and stroke. Arch Neurol 2004;61:889–92.

25. Rauchhaus M, Clark AL, Doehner W, et al. The relationship between cholesterol and survival in patients with chronic heart failure. J Am Coll Cardiol 2003;42:1933–40.

26. Sacks FM, Pfeffer MA, Moye LA, et al. The effect of pravastatin on coronary events after myocardial infarction in patients with average cholesterol levels. Cholesterol and Recurrent Events Trial investigators. N Engl J Med 1996;335:1001–9.

27. Shepherd J, Blauw GJ, Murphy MB, et al. PROspective Study of Pravastatin in the Elderly at Risk pravastatin in elderly individuals at risk of vascular disease (PROSPER): a randomized–controlled trial. Lancet 2002;360:1623–30.

28. Randomised trial of cholesterol lowering in 4444 patients with coronary heart disease: the Scandinavian Simvastatin Survival Study (4S). Lancet 1994;344:1383–9.

29. Schwartz GG, Olsson AG, Ezekowitz MD, et al. Effects of atorvastatin on early recurrent ischemic events in acute coronary syndromes: the MIRACL study: a randomized–controlled trial. JAMA 2001;285:1711–8.

30. Athyros VG, Papageorgiou AA, Mercouris BR, et al. Treatment with atorvastatin to the National Cholesterol Educational Program goal versus usual care in secondary coronary heart disease prevention. The GREek Atorvastatin and Coronary-heart-disease Evaluation (GREACE) study. Curr Med Res Opin 2002;18:220–8.

31. de Lemos JA, Blazing MA, Wiviott SD, et al. Early Intensive vs a Delayed Conservative Simvastatin Strategy in Patients With Acute Coronary Syndromes: Phase Z of the A to Z Trial. JAMA 2004;292:1307–16.

32. Spencer FA, Allegrone J, Goldberg R, et al. Association of statin therapy with outcomes of acute coronary syndromes: the GRACE study. Ann Intern Med 2004;140:857–66.

33. Koren MJ, Hunninghake DB, ALLIANCE Investigators. Clinical outcomes in managed care patients

with coronary heart disease treated aggressively in lipid-lowering disease management clinics: the alliance study. J Am Coll Cardiol 2004;44:1772–9.

34. Pedersen TR, Faergeman O, Kastelein JJ, et al. High-dose atorvastatin vs. usual-dose simvastatin for secondary prevention after myocardial infarction: the IDEAL study: a randomized–controlled trial. JAMA 2005;294:2437–45.

35. Scirica BM, Morrow DA, Cannon CP, et al. Intensive statin therapy and the risk of hospitalization for heart failure after an acute coronary syndrome in the PROVE IT-TIMI 22 study. J Am Coll Cardiol 2006; 47:2326–31.

36. Heart Protection Study Collaborative Group. The effects of cholesterol lowering with simvastatin on cause-specific mortality and on cancer incidence in 20,536 high-risk people: a randomised placebo-controlled trial. BMC Med 2005;3:6.

37. Khush KK, Waters DD, Bittner V, et al. Effect of high-dose atorvastatin on hospitalizations for heart failure subgroup analysis of the Treating to New Targets (TNT) study. Circulation 2007;115:576–83.

38. The Long-Term Intervention with Pravastatin in Ischaemic Disease (LIPID) study group. Prevention of cardiovascular events and death with pravastatin in patients with coronary heart disease and a broad range of initial cholesterol levels. N Engl J Med 1998;339:1349–57.

39. Segal R, Pitt P, Poole-Wilson P, et al. Effects of HMG-COA reductase inhibitors (statins) in patients with heart failure. Eur J Heart Fail 2000;2(Suppl 1):96.

40. Mozaffarian D, Nye R, Levy WC. Statin therapy is associated with lower mortality among patients with severe heart failure. Am J Cardiol 2004;93: 1124–9.

41. Hognestad A, Dickstein K, Myhre E, et al. Effect of combined statin and beta-blocker treatment on one-year morbidity and mortality after acute myocardial infarction associated with heart failure. Am J Cardiol 2004;93:603–6.

42. Anand I, Florea V, Kuskowski M, et al. Total cholesterol, statin therapy, and survival in ischemic and nonischemic heart failure results from the Val-HeFT. Circulation 2004;110(2590 Suppl):556.

43. Krum H, Bailey M, Meyer W, et al. Impact of statin therapy on mortality in CHF patients according to h-blocker use: results of CIBIS II. Circulation 2004; 110(2031 Suppl):431.

44. Krum H, Caretta E, Latini R, et al. Are statins of clinical benefit in patients with established systolic chronic heart failure? A retrospective analysis of 5010 patients enrolled in Val-HeFT. Circulation 2004;110(3150 Suppl):680.

45. Horwich TB, MacLellan WR, Fonarow GC. Statin therapy is associated with improved survival in ischemic and nonischemic heart failure. J Am Coll Cardiol 2004;43:642–8.

46. Ezekowitz J, McAlister FA, Humphries KH, et al. The association among renal insufficiency, pharmacotherapy, and outcomes in 6427 patients with heart failure and coronary artery disease. J Am Coll Cardiol 2004;44:1587–92.

47. Sola S, Mir MQ, Lerakis S, et al. Atorvastatin improves left ventricular systolic function and serum markers of inflammation in nonischemic heart failure. J Am Coll Cardiol 2006;47:332–7.

48. Sumner A, Boehmer J, Saxon L, et al. Statin use is associated with a marked improvement in survival in an advanced heart failure population from the COMPANION trial. J Am Coll Cardiol 2005;45(Suppl A): 183A.

49. Anker SD, Clark AL, Winkler R, et al. Statin use and survival in patients with chronic heart failure: results from two observational studies with 5200 patients. Int J Cardiol 2006;112:234–42.

50. Dickinson MG, Ip JH, Olshansky B, et al. Statin use was associated with reduced mortality in both ischemic and nonischemic cardiomyopathy and in patients with implantable defibrillators: mortality data and mechanistic insights from the Sudden Cardiac Death in Heart Failure Trial (SCDHeFT). Am Heart J 2007;153:573–8.

51. Howlett J, Johnstone D, Cox J. Statins are associated with improved survival in advanced heart failure irrespective of total cholesterol levels. J Card Fail 2004;10(4 Suppl):S101 [309 Suppl].

52. Ray JG, Gong Y, Sykora K, et al. Statin use and survival outcomes in elderly patients with heart failure. Arch Intern Med 2005;165:62–7.

53. Jaganmohan S, Khurana V. Statins improve survival in congestive heart failure: a study of 32,000 US veterans. J Am Coll Cardiol 2005;45(Suppl A):183A [abstract].

54. Foody JM, Shah R, Galusha D, et al. Statins and mortality among elderly patients hospitalized with heart failure. Circulation 2006;113:1086–92.

55. Nul D, Fernandez A, Zambrano C, et al. Statins and mortality in congestive heart failure: benefit beyond cholesterol reduction? J Am Coll Cardiol 2005; 45(Suppl A):182A [abstract].

56. Go AS, Lee WY, Yang J, et al. Statin therapy and risks for death and hospitalization in chronic heart failure. JAMA 2006;296:2105–11.

57. Folkeringa RJ, Van Kraaij DJ, Tieleman RG, et al. Statins associated with reduced mortality in patients admitted for congestive heart failure. J Card Fail 2006;12:134–8. 92.

58. Node K, Fujita M, Kitakaze M, et al. Short-term statin therapy improves cardiac function and symptoms in patients with idiopathic dilated cardiomyopathy. Circulation 2003;108:839–43.

59. Hong YJ, Jeong MH, Hyun DW, et al. Prognostic significance of simvastatin therapy in patients with ischemic heart failure who underwent percutaneous

coronary intervention for acute myocardial infarction. Am J Cardiol 2005;95:619–22.

60. Laufs U, Wassmann S, Schackmann S, et al. Beneficial effects of statins in patients with nonischemic heart failure. Z Kardiol 2004;93:103–8.

61. Krum H, Tonkin A. The Rosuvastatin Impact on Ventricular Remodeling, Cytokines, and Neurohormones (UNIVERSE) Study. J Am Coll Cardiol 2006;47: 61A–2A [abstract].

62. Sola S, Mir M, Rajagopalan S, et al. Statin therapy improves mortality, cardiovascular outcomes, and levels of inflammatory markers in patients with heart failure. Circulation 2004;110(2591 Suppl):556.

63. Laufs U, La Fata V, Plutzky J, et al. Up-regulation of endothelial nitric oxide synthase by HMG CoA reductase inhibitors. Circulation 1998;97:1129–35.

64. Kjekshus J, Apetrei E, Barrios V, et al. The CORONA group. Rosuvastatin in older patients with systolic heart failure. N Engl J Med 2007;357:2248–61.

65. Tavazzi L, Tognoni G, Franzosi MG, et al. Rationale and design of the GISSI heart failure trial: a large trial to assess the effects of n-3 polyunsaturated fatty acids and rosuvastatin in symptomatic congestive heart failure. Eur J Heart Fail 2004;6:635–41.

66. Ramasubbu K, Estep J, White DL, et al. Experimental and clinical basis for the use of statins in patients with ischemic and nonischemic cardiomyopathy. J Am Coll Cardiol 2004;51:415–28.

67. Grundy SM, Cleeman JI, Bairey CN, et al. Implications of recent clinical trials for the National Cholesterol Education Program Adult Treatment Panel III guidelines. Circulation 2004;110:227–9.

Cyclooxygenase-2 Inhibitors, Nonsteroidal Anti-inflammatory Drugs, and Cardiovascular Risk

Orly Vardeny, PharmD[a], Scott D. Solomon, MD[b],*

KEYWORDS

- Cyclooxygenase-2 inhibitors • Cardiovascular disease
- Thrombosis

Cyclooxygenase-2 (cox-2) inhibitors, also known as coxibs, were introduced with the promise that they would provide pain relief similar to that of traditional nonsteroidal anti-inflammatory drugs (NSAIDs) but would be better tolerated with lower risk for gastrointestinal (GI) side effects. Although coxibs were associated with lower GI risk, experimental and observational data raised the specter of increased cardiovascular risk associated with this class of drugs. When a randomized controlled trial of rofecoxib for colonic polyp prevention was stopped in September 2004 because of a twofold risk for cardiovascular events, the entire class of agents became the subject of intense scrutiny, culminating in withdrawal of two coxibs from the market and a US Food and Drug Administration (FDA)–mandated black-box warning on the remaining agent. Nevertheless, coxibs remain an important part of the pain-management armamentarium for patients who have osteoarthritis, rheumatoid arthritis, and various other conditions. This article describes the pharmacologic and biologic basis of cardiovascular risk associated with coxibs, summarizes the evidence for cardiovascular risk associated with cox-2 inhibitors, and weighs the risks and potential benefits of pain management with these agents.

Analgesics are among the most commonly used medications in the United States and among the most frequently prescribed medications to patients older than 65 years of age. It has been estimated that more than 70 million NSAID prescriptions are written per year in the United States. Moreover, NSAIDs have been potentially implicated in thousands of deaths and an even greater number of hospitalizations, primarily because of an excess risk for GI bleeds or renal impairment. Treatment of nonsteroidal-related GI side effects has been estimated to account for up to one third of the cost of arthritis therapy. Cyclooxygenase-2 inhibitors were designed and introduced in an attempt to reduce the potential GI risk of traditional NSAIDs. Their adoption was driven by the enormous profit potential in safer analgesics, and a medical community and consumers eager to reduce the GI risks with similar pain relief.

PHARMACOLOGY OF CYCLOOXYGENASE-2 INHIBITORS

Cyclooxygenase-2 inhibitors and traditional NSAIDS inhibit enzymes that convert prostaglandins to tissue-specific isomerases (**Fig. 1**). The prostaglandin cascade begins with the release of arachidonic acid from membrane phospholipids through actions of lipases (primarily phospholipase A2 type).[1,2] Thereafter, four distinct pathways contribute to oxidizing arachidonic acid to

[a] School of Pharmacy, University of Wisconsin, 777 Highland Avenue, Madison, WI 53705-2222, USA
[b] Cardiovascular Division, Brigham and Women's Hospital, Harvard Medical School, 75 Francis Street, Boston, MA 02115, USA
* Corresponding author.
E-mail address: ssolomon@rics.bwh.harvard.edu (S.D. Solomon).

Cardiol Clin 26 (2008) 589–601
doi:10.1016/j.ccl.2008.06.004
0733-8651/08/$ – see front matter © 2008 Elsevier Inc. All rights reserved.

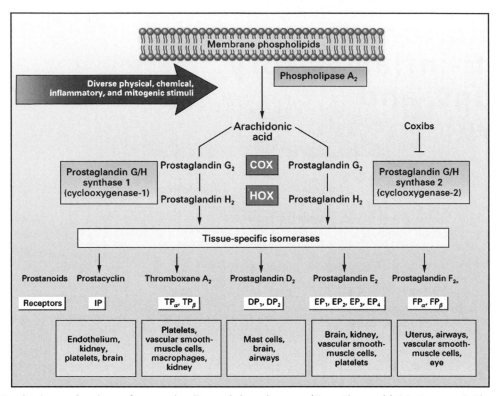

Fig. 1. Production and actions of prostaglandins and thromboxane. (*From* Fitzgerald GA, Patrono C. The coxibs, selective inhibitors of cyclooxygenase-2. N Engl J Med 2001;345:433–42; with permission. Copyright © 2001, Massachusetts Medical Society.)

form eicosanoids, which serve numerous roles in biologic systems and disease, including cardiovascular, GI, blood coagulation, nervous, and reproductive systems. One of the four eicosanoid-forming pathways is that of prostaglandin G/H synthase, otherwise known as the cyclooxygenase (COX) enzyme. The enzyme converts arachidonic acid into prostaglandin G2 and subsequently to prostaglandin H2. Specific eicosanoids formed subsequent to this reaction are termed prostanoids, referring to various prostaglandins and thromboxane compounds. The distribution of prostanoid types is determined by the cell category in which the prostanoids are produced and tissue-specific isomerases contained within.[3] For example, endothelial cells express PGI synthase and produce the antithrombotic vasodilator prostanoid PGI2, or prostacyclin. Platelets express PGE synthase, and are capable of forming the inflammatory, prothrombotic PGE2 prostanoid.

The cyclooxygenase enzyme exists as two distinct isoenzymes, the COX-1 and COX-2 isoenzymes, with differential expression in various tissues.[4] It was originally believed that the COX-1 isoenzyme functioned primarily as a housekeeping enzyme in the cytoprotection of gastric mucosa, regulation of renal blood flow, and platelet

aggregation. This enzyme is constitutively expressed, detectable in the bloodstream, and is the only isoenzyme expressed in platelets. In contrast, COX-2 levels and activities are normally undetectable in blood vessels, but are rapidly upregulated on exposure to cytokines, endotoxins, tumor promoters, and mitogens, giving rise to the notion that this enzyme mediates production of inflammatory response prostanoids.[5] The mechanistic distinction between COX-1 and COX-2 isoenzymes is not that clear-cut. Although COX-1 is the predominant isoenzyme in normal gastric mucosa, there are increasing data to support that COX-2 mRNA and protein are either constitutive or inducible during acute stages of gastric erosion and ulceration in areas of the GI tract.[6,7] Similarly, it is not just the COX-2 isoenzyme that is inducible during inflammation; COX-1 induction occurs in arthritic synovia or in atherosclerotic plaques.[8,9]

COX-1 products, which include PGI2 and PGE2, maintain GI system integrity by decreasing gastric acid secretion, increasing the thickness of the gastric mucus layer, enhancing blood flow to mucosal tissues, and stimulating bicarbonate secretion.[10,11] PGE2 in particular is responsible for gastric mucosal secretion through activation of cAMP in gastric epithelial cells.[12] Blockade of

COX-1 prevents formation of the cytoprotective prostaglandin PGE2, and in addition to reduced production of thromboxane A2 (TxA2) in platelets, increases the risk for gastric mucosal damage and bleeding.[13] Aspirin and traditional NSAIDs, which inhibit COX-1 and COX-2 enzymes, thus increase the risk for gastric mucosal injury.

The development of numerous NSAIDS that block both COX isoenzymes flourished in the 1980s, resulting in various compounds differing in their relative affinity for and blockade of COX-1 versus COX-2 and their anti-inflammatory actions. Concerns of hemorrhagic risk of therapeutic agents that nonselectively block COX-1 and COX-2, with subsequent adverse GI outcomes,[14] led to the idea that selective blockade of the COX-2 enzyme would mitigate negative GI effects[15] and thus lead to drugs with the promise of fewer adverse GI effects while still decreasing inflammation and pain.

The coxibs were approved based on their reduced rates of endoscopically visualized gastroduodenal ulcerations in comparison to equivalent doses of traditional NSAIDS. These approvals were based on three year-long and one short-term outcome study examining incidence of serious GI complications in larger populations.[16–18]

Tertiary structure differences of COX isoenzymes account for pharmacologic disparities between COX-1/COX-2 nonselective and COX-2 selective agents. A hydrophobic pocket in the binding channel of COX-2 is absent in COX-1.[4,19] Selective inhibitors of COX-2 have side chains that fit within the hydrophobic pocket but are too large to block COX-1 with equally high affinity. The interaction of all NSAIDS and coxibs with COX-1 and COX-2 is therefore conditioned by their molecular structure. There is no absolute selectivity for one isoform versus another, and the relative affinities to the two isoforms are just as variable within the NSAID and coxib classes as between them. COX-2 selectivity is best described as a continuous scale on which the agents can be ranked. The concentration of drug required to inhibit the activities of COX-1 and COX-2 enzymes by 50% is termed the IC_{50}. The COX-1 IC_{50} value:COX-2 IC_{50} value ratio can be used to determine a selectivity index.[20] A value less than 1 indicates the drug is more COX-1 selective, whereas a value greater than 1 indicates the drug is more COX-2 selective.[21] First-generation coxibs include celecoxib and rofecoxib, which are the least COX-2 selective of the coxibs. The second-generation coxibs, such as etoricoxib and lumiracoxib, are more selective for COX-2 than rofecoxib, an agent possessing higher relative COX-2 affinity than celecoxib (**Table 1**).[22] Evaluation of traditional NSAIDS has

Table 1
Pharmacologic differences among COX-2 inhibitors

Compound	COX-1:COX-2 IC_{50} Ratio[a]	Half-Life (h)
First generation		
Celecoxib	6	6–12
Rofecoxib	38	15–18
Second generation		
Valdecoxib	28	6–10
Etoricoxib	105	20–26
Lumiracoxib	515	2–6

[a] Measured with human whole blood assay; the concentration required to inhibit COX activity by 50%.
Data from Coruzzi G, Venturi N, Spaggiari S. Gastrointestinal safety of novel nonsteroidal antiinflammatory drugs: selective COX-2 inhibitors and beyond. Acta Biomed. Aug 2007;78(2):96–110.

shown that some compounds, including diclofenac, nimesulide, and nabumetone, display similar selectivity as that of celecoxib.[23] Similarly, coxibs vary widely in their duration of action (half-life), such that etoricoxib possesses the longest half-life and celecoxib and lumiracoxib have shorter half-lives. Selectivity ratio of various coxibs is highly variable, depending on the assay and experimental conditions used. Additionally, differences in selectivity may not correlate with therapeutic efficacy after dosing.

GASTROINTESTINAL EFFECTS OF COXIBS

Because coxibs were developed with the promise of a lower risk for GI side effects, much of the initial clinical research on coxibs sought to document the beneficial GI profile of these agents compared with traditional NSAIDS. In the VIGOR trial,[16] rofecoxib was associated with approximately a 50% reduction in the risk for serious lower GI events. Similarly, in the CLASS trial[17] celecoxib was associated with fewer upper GI tract complications compared with patients treated with NSAIDs. This benefit was completely absent in the patients who were taking low-dose aspirin for cardiovascular reasons, however, which suggests that concomitant use of aspirin—even low-dose aspirin—simultaneously with coxibs may actually attenuate their potential GI benefits. Although celecoxib was associated with less upper GI bleeding in the CLASS study after 6 months, further follow-up out to 1 year (which was reported to the FDA but not published in the initial manuscript) failed to show a clear-cut benefit of celecoxib use.

Although the GI benefits of coxibs in comparison to traditional NSAIDs have been supported by several studies and with several agents, the GI safety of coxibs over placebo has not been as clear. In the APPROVe trial,[24] rofecoxib was associated with an increased risk for GI ulcers and bleeding compared with placebo, suggesting that although coxibs may reduce the risk for GI side effects compared with traditional NSAIDs, the risk is not nullified when compared with placebo. Interestingly, hospital admissions for GI hemorrhage increased around the time of the introduction of celecoxib and rofecoxib, and it has been postulated that this increased observed incidence may be directly related to the introduction of the coxib medications with resultant overprescribing, preferential prescription to high-risk subjects, and concomitant use of low-dose aspirin.[25]

Other potential GI benefits, supported by experimental literature and early clinical trials, have also been attributed to coxibs. COX-2 is expressed at all stages of human colon carcinogenesis, has been shown to be a promoter of intestinal tumorigenesis, and may be an important promoter of tumorigenesis in various epithelial carcinomas.[26] Overexpression of COX-2 in experimental models results in tumor production of angiogenic factors and proteolytic enzymes and prostaglandin-mediated resistance to apoptosis. These experimental findings led to enormous interest in the therapeutic potential for coxibs to prevent cancer and provided a rationale for numerous chemoprevention trials, particularly in the arena of colon cancer. In the Familial Adenomatous Polyposis (FAP) trial, celecoxib in doses of 400 mg twice daily resulted in a 28% reduction in the number of colorectal polyps in patients at high risk for development of colon cancer.[27] This trial was the basis of additional trials testing coxibs more broadly for colon cancer prevention—trials that ultimately led to a greater understanding of the cardiovascular risk associated with coxibs.

PHARMACOLOGIC BASIS OF CARDIOVASCULAR RISK

Before the existence of compelling clinical data suggesting increased cardiovascular risk associated with coxibs, experimental data had raised concerns of increased risk, especially that of thrombosis. The mechanistic support for this risk came from experimental data, which suggested that coxibs might lead to an imbalance between two downstream prostanoids, thromboxane and prostacyclin.

Thromboxane A2 (TxA2) is formed in the platelet by the action of thromboxane synthase. It possesses potent vasoconstrictor activity, facilitates cholesterol uptake, induces proliferation of vascular smooth muscle cells, and stimulates platelet aggregation. TxA2 binds to a G-protein–coupled receptor on platelet plasma membranes. Ultimately, TxA2 induces a conformational change of the integrin α2β3, which mediates the finals steps in platelet activation, resulting in platelet binding to fibrinogen and fibronectin.

Conversely, prostaglandin I2 (PGI2, or prostacyclin) causes vasodilation, decreases platelet aggregation, reduces cholesterol uptake, inhibits vascular smooth muscle cell proliferation,[22] and may have a cardioprotective role in the vasculature in the context of ischemia-reperfusion injury.[28]

Recent studies have demonstrated that genomic or pharmacologic removal of prostacyclin led to platelet-dependent and platelet-independent induction of thrombosis, plaque destabilization, or atherogenesis.[29–32] In murine models, deficiency of PGI2 signaling did not result in spontaneous thrombosis, but once the thrombotic process was induced by endothelial damage, it proceeded more vigorously than in mice with intact PGI2 function.[33]

The notion that coxibs might be associated with increased risk for thrombosis in humans originated from a series of experiments by Fitzgerald and colleagues [34,35] showing that administration of coxibs to normal volunteers was associated with a reduction in prostacyclin production in a dose-dependent fashion without changes in thromboxane. By selectively blocking production of the vasodilatory and platelet-inhibitory properties of prostacyclin, coxibs may create a prothrombotic environment dominated by TxA2.[2,5,36] This alteration in the balance between these two prostanoids allows TxA2 to function unopposed, and has been proposed to lead to a more thrombogenic state, which under the correct clinical circumstances might result in pathologic thrombosis (**Fig. 2**).

Opponents to the prothrombotic hypothesis argue that murine models do not adequately translate to human models when it comes to inhibition of prostacyclin production, as its synthesis is not completely blocked in humans as it is in mice. COX-2 inhibitors depress PGI2 by 50% to 70% in humans.[35,37] Nonetheless, data suggest that a mere 50% reduction in prostacyclin production is sufficient to increase susceptibility to thrombotic stimuli.[38] This finding does raise the question, however, whether incomplete blockade of prostacyclin production in humans leads to varying risk profiles between coxibs with differing duration of activity. Another argument opposing the prothrombotic hypothesis involves the source of

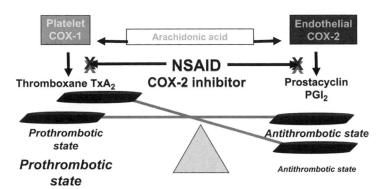

Fig. 2. Mechanism-based Fitzgerald hypothesis of cardiovascular risk for coxibs. (*Data from* Fitzgerald GA, Patrono C. The coxibs, selective inhibitors of cyclooxygenase-2. N Engl J Med 2001;345:433–42; and García Rodríguez LA. The effect of NSAIDs on the risk of coronary heart disease: fusion of clinical pharmacology and pharmacoepidemiologic data. Clin Exp Rheumatol. 2001;19(6 Suppl 25):S41–4.)

PGI2. Biosynthesis of PGI2 is quantified by the measurement of its urinary metabolite, 2,3 dinor 6-keto PGF1a.[34] Rofecoxib and celecoxib were shown to suppress 2,3 dinor 6-keto PGF1a to a significant degree.[39,40] Although a good measure of whole-body PGI2 biosynthesis, measuring urinary metabolites does not allow for quantification of PGI2 in the vessel wall, and may therefore not reflect COX-2–dependent inhibition of vasculature PGI2 production. MacAdam and colleagues[35] measured urinary prostacyclin levels in healthy volunteers 6 to 12 hours after a dose of celecoxib or ibuprofen and found that prostacyclin levels were reduced by approximately 80% in patients receiving 400 or 800 mg of celecoxib. Prostacyclin levels were also reduced, but to a somewhat lesser extent, in patients receiving ibuprofen.

Regardless of the controversies surrounding the prothrombotic hypothesis and the strength of its association with cardiovascular risk, it is recognized that other mechanisms may also contribute to adverse cardiac events with coxibs, including disrupted blood pressure homeostasis. Although the COX-1 isoenzyme is predominant in the kidneys, COX-2 serves to regulate renal blood flow. PGE2 and PGI2 increase renal medullary blood flow, which drives diuresis and reduces blood pressure.[41] Inhibition of COX-2 production of PGE2 induces a reduction in daily urinary sodium excretion by approximately 30%. The retention of sodium and water clinically manifests as increased systemic blood pressure.[42] In patients who have normal renal function, the kidneys increase sodium excretion to compensate for the antinatriuretic effects of the COX inhibitor.[41] This process occurs without significant increases in blood pressure or plasma volume. In patients who have chronic kidney disease, this compensatory mechanism is impaired, leading to increases in blood pressure and edema, in some cases causing heart failure.[43]

In a randomized controlled trial of patients who had osteoarthritis and type II diabetes who were on stable antihypertensive medication, celecoxib,

naproxen, and rofecoxib were associated with 16%, 19%, and 30% incidence of development of hypertension (systolic blood pressure [SBP] >135), respectively, in patients who were previously normotensive.[44] In a case-control analysis of a Medicare population, new-onset hypertension developed in 21%, 23%, and 27% of those prescribed celecoxib, NSAIDS, or rofecoxib, respectively.[45] The increased rates of hypertension induced by rofecoxib were thus significantly higher than with celecoxib or nonselective NSAIDS. The risk was higher in those who had renal or hepatic disease, as well as heart failure. Another study evaluated effects of rofecoxib and celecoxib on clinic SBP in 1094 patients on stable doses of antihypertensives. Rofecoxib induced significant increases in SBP in individuals taking angiotensin-converting enzyme inhibitors and β-blockers, but not in those taking calcium antagonists.[43]

OBSERVATIONAL AND CLINICAL TRIALS DATA ON CARDIOVASCULAR RISK ASSOCIATED WITH CYCLOOXYGENASE-2 INHIBITORS

Several early observational studies suggested that rofecoxib might be associated with increased cardiovascular risk. These data came from prescription databases and case-control studies in which rofecoxib has been associated with as high as a fourfold increased risk for cardiovascular events. In the FDA-sponsored Kaiser Permanente study[46] looking at the risk for acute myocardial infarction and sudden cardiac death associated with current use of cox-2 selective and nonselective NSAIDs, similar hazard ratios were observed with virtually all NSAIDs with the exception of rofecoxib in doses greater than 25 mg daily (**Fig. 3**). Although the hazard ratios associated with indomethacin and diclofenac were greater than 1 and, in the case of indomethacin, statistically significant, rofecoxib use at higher than 25 mg was associated with a threefold increased risk for events. In contrast, much of the observational data associated with

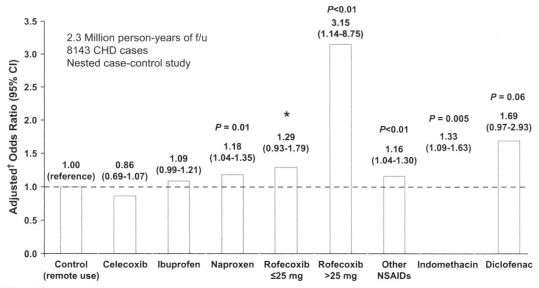

AMI = acute myocardial infarction; SCD = sudden coronary death.

*P = 0.04 compared with celecoxib.

†Adjusted for age, sex, health plan region, medical history, smoking, and medication use.

Fig. 3. FDA-Sponsored Kaiser Permanente Study: risk for acute myocardial infarction and sudden coronary death with current use of COX-2 selective and nonselective NSAIDs. (*Data from* Graham DJ, Campen D, Hui R, et al. Risk of acute myocardial infarction and sudden cardiac death in patients treated with cyclo-oxygenase 2 selective and non-selective non-steroidal anti-inflammatory drugs: nested case-control study. Lancet 2005;365(9458):475–81.)

celecoxib was not so unfavorable, with hazard ratios that were almost uniformly less than 1, albeit with wide confidence intervals, when comparing celecoxib use to nonusers of NSAIDs (**Fig. 4**).

Some important caveats always need to be considered when interpreting the results of observational data. It is difficult or impossible to account for all confounders in observational studies, and especially difficult to address intrinsic biases, including recall bias. Fortunately, the most compelling data for cardiovascular risk associated with coxibs came not from observational studies, but from randomized controlled trials (RCTs). The first such trial to raise concern was VIGOR, which randomized patients who had rheumatoid arthritis to rofecoxib 50 mg a day compared with naproxen 500 mg twice a day. The primary endpoint of the study was GI side effects, which were indeed reduced in patients receiving rofecoxib. The trial demonstrated a higher rate of cardiovascular adverse events in patients receiving rofecoxib compared with those receiving naproxen. Although these data were reported in the initial manuscript, the interpretation was that naproxen was associated with a reduction in risk, and not that rofecoxib was associated with increased risk, and the authors remarked that "…our results are consistent with the theory that naproxen has a coronary protective effect…."[16] This interpretation was only minimally challenged until more definitive data became available years later.

On September 30, 2004, Merck halted the ongoing APPROVe trial and withdrew rofecoxib from the market, citing evidence of increased cardiovascular risk in that study. APPROVe, a colonic polyp prevention study, compared rofecoxib 25 mg to placebo, and followed patients for approximately 3 years. The study was stopped because of a nearly twofold increased risk for cardiovascular death, myocardial infarction, or stroke (**Fig. 5**). Importantly, APPROVe was testing a relatively common dose of rofecoxib, 25 mg daily, which was the dose being prescribed to most patients who had arthritis. APPROVe was the first direct placebo-controlled evidence of risk associated with rofecoxib that could not be attributed to a benefit associated with an active comparator. The stopping of this trial, and the subsequent withdrawal of rofecoxib from the market, led to an immediate reassessment of all agents in this class.

Several aspects of the APPROVe trial proved subsequently controversial. Safety data in APPROVe were censored 14 days after discontinuation of study drug, with the result that any adverse cardiovascular events occurring after 14 days after study drug would not have been attributed to the drug. This approach has raised several concerns. First, although risk associated with a drug might be expected to dissipate after discontinuation, the timing of that dissipation is unclear, and the most conservative approach

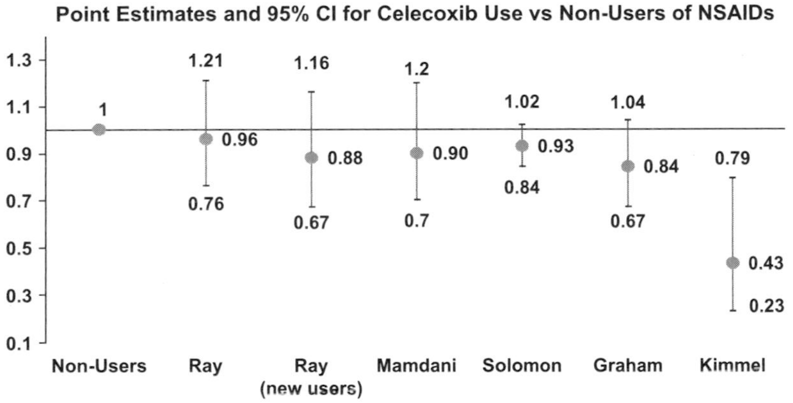

Point Estimates and 95% CI for Celecoxib Use vs Non-Users of NSAIDs

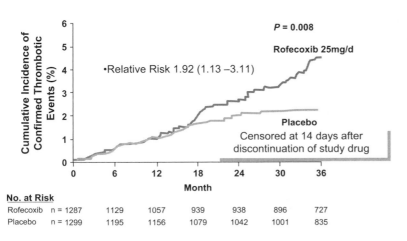

Ray and Graham end points = MI + SCD; Others MI only.
MI = myocardial infarction; SCD = sudden coronary death.

Fig. 4. Summary of observational studies of celecoxib and cardiovascular disease. (*Data from* Ref[46]. and Kimmel SE, Berlin JA, Reilly M, et al. Patients exposed to rofecoxib and celecoxib have different odds of nonfatal myocardial infarction. Ann Intern Med 2005;142(3):157–64; Mamdani M, Rochon P, Juurlink DN, et al. Effect of selective cyclooxygenase 2 inhibitors and naproxen on short-term risk of acute myocardial infarction in the elderly. Arch Intern Med 2003;163(4):481–6; Ray WA, Stein CM, Daugherty JR, et al. COX-2 selective non-steroidal anti-inflammatory drugs and risk of serious coronary heart disease. Lancet 2002;360(9339):1071–3; Solomon DH, Schneeweiss S, Glynn RJ, et al. Relationship between selective cyclooxygenase-2 inhibitors and acute myocardial infarction in older adults. Circulation. 2004;109(17):2068–73.)

generally is to perform an intention-to-treat analysis, wherein adverse event data are counted throughout the duration of follow-up. The APPROVe data have also been used to argue that the risk associated with rofecoxib only began after approximately 18 months of therapy (see **Fig. 5**). A reanalysis of the APPROVe data based on publicly available data using an intention-to-treat approach has refuted this claim, because it shows curves diverging earlier.[47]

CELECOXIB CLINICAL TRIALS DATA

Following termination of the APPROVe study, the data safety monitoring boards of two similar ongoing colon polyp prevention trials, the Adenoma

Prevention with Celecoxib (APC) trial and the PreSAP trial, commissioned an independent review of the cardiovascular data from those trials. Review of the APC data demonstrated a dose-dependent increased risk for a combined endpoint of cardiovascular death, myocardial infarction, stroke, or heart failure associated with celecoxib, with 200 mg twice a day demonstrating a greater than twofold risk and 400 mg twice a day demonstrating a greater than threefold risk (**Fig. 6**).[48] On December 17, 2004, these data were made public and the APC and PreSAP trials—and several other trials—were halted. Unlike rofecoxib, celecoxib was not withdrawn from the market. In contrast to APC, the PreSAP trial, which was a similarly designed trial but used a different dose regimen of celecoxib

Fig. 5. Cardiovascular data APPROVe APTC events. (*From* Bresalier RS, Sandler RS, Quan H, et al. Cardiovascular events associated with rofecoxib in a colorectal adenoma chemoprevention trial. N Engl J Med 2005;352(11):1092–102; with permission. Copyright © 2005, Massachusetts Medical Society.)

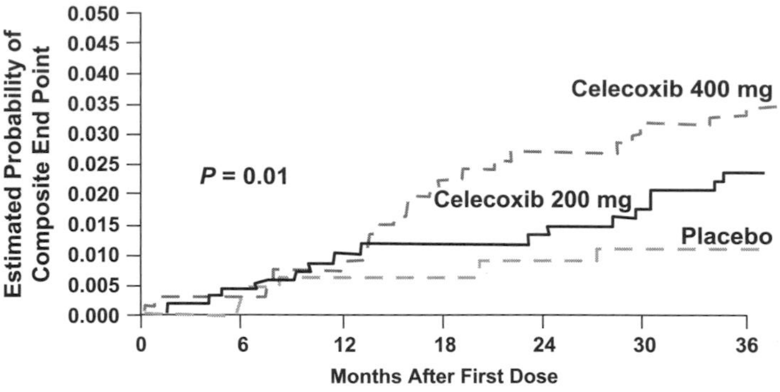

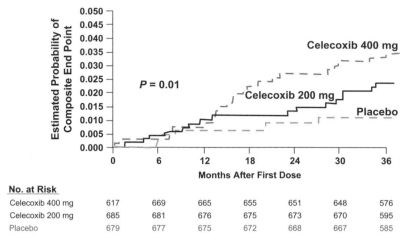

No. at Risk							
Celecoxib 400 mg	617	669	665	655	651	648	576
Celecoxib 200 mg	685	681	676	675	673	670	595
Placebo	679	677	675	672	668	667	585

Fig. 6. Cardiovascular risk in the APC study. (*From* Solomon SD, McMurray JJV, Pfeffer MA, et al for the Adenoma Prevention with Celecoxib (APC) Study Investigators. Cardiovascular risk associated with celecoxib in a clinical trial for colorectal adenoma prevention. N Engl J Med 2005;352:1071–80; with permission. Copyright © 2005, Massachusetts Medical Society.)

(400 mg once daily), did not demonstrate clear evidence of cardiovascular risk. For the same combined endpoint, PreSAP showed a hazard ratio of 1.3 with 95% confidence interval that ranged from 0.6 to 2.6.[49] Although elevated risk was not observed in PreSAP, these wide confidence intervals suggest that celecoxib may have been associated with as much as a 2.6-fold increased risk or a 40% reduction in risk. Although several potential differences between these two trials, including study population and baseline cardiovascular risk, might account for the differences in the results, dosing interval was the major difference, with PreSAP using a once-daily dose of celecoxib and APC using twice-daily doses.

Review of the APC and PreSAP blood pressure data demonstrated a pattern of blood pressure elevation that paralleled the outcomes data.[49] In APC, 200 mg twice a day and 400 mg twice a day of celecoxib were associated with a significant 2.9 and 5.2 mmHg increase in blood pressure, respectively. In PreSAP, however, no blood pressure elevation was observed. The primary efficacy measures in all three of the colon polyp prevention trials, APC, PreSAP, and APPROVe, were very positive, with between a 25% and 60% reduction in the risk for colonic polyps in patients receiving coxibs.[50–52]

Nearly simultaneous to the reports from the colon cancer prevention trials was the report of an additional study using valdecoxib (Bextra) in patients after bypass surgery.[53] These findings—also demonstrating increased cardiovascular events in the patients receiving coxibs—together with the reports from the colonic polyp prevention trials, were the subject of a special FDA hearing in February 2005. Subsequent to this hearing, valdecoxib was voluntarily withdrawn from the market, and celecoxib, which remains the only COX-2 inhibitor available in the United States, was given a black-box warning.

The National Institutes of Health–commissioned Cross-Trials Safety Analysis (CTSA) with celecoxib pooled the data from the APC and PreSAP trials with similarly adjudicated data from four other randomized placebo-controlled clinical trials studying the three dose regimens that were studied in APC and PreSAP.[54] These data showed a similar pattern in which the risk increased with dose regimen and was lowest for the 400-mg daily dose (hazard ratio, 1.1; 95% CI, 0.6 to 2.0), intermediate for the 200-mg twice-daily dose (hazard ratio, 1.8; 95% CI, 1.1 to 3.1), and highest for the 400-mg twice-daily dose (hazard ratio, 3.1; 95% CI, 1.5 to 6.1) (**Fig. 7**A). Moreover, these data demonstrated an interaction with baseline cardiovascular risk, so that patients who had the lowest baseline risk had not only lower absolute risk but also lower relative risk for a celecoxib-related event (see **Fig. 7**B).

The results of CTSA confirmed the dose-regimen response observed in APC and PreSAP, with another 400-mg once-daily dose trial showing a hazard ratio near 1.0. The importance of dosing interval in celecoxib-related risk is supported by experimental data showing that within about 12 hours of a celecoxib dose, prostacyclin levels, originally diminished, begin to return to normal.[35] It is conceivable, thus, that once-daily dosing might allow enough prostacyclin recovery to attenuate the thrombotic effect of the celecoxib dose, and thus might explain why divided doses might be potentially more toxic than a single dose of the same overall daily amount.

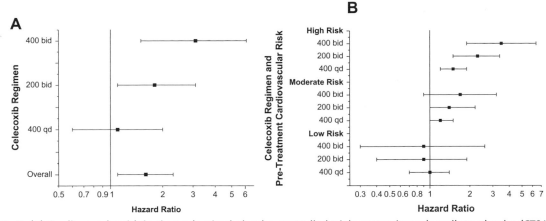

Fig. 7. (*A*) Cardiovascular risk in six randomized placebo-controlled trials comparing celecoxib to placebo (CTSA). (*B*) Relationship between baseline risk, dose, and celecoxib risk. (*From* Solomon SD, Wittes J, Finn PV, et al. Cardiovascular risk of celecoxib in 6 randomized placebo-controlled trials: the cross trial safety analysis. Circulation 2008;117(16):2104–13; with permission.)

That baseline risk was an important determinant of celecoxib-related risk suggests that preexisting atherosclerotic disease might be a prerequisite for coxib-related risk, and argues that patients at very low risk for cardiovascular disease in general are probably at very low risk for coxib-related risk. These findings argue for even more caution in using coxibs in patients at increased risk for cardiovascular events.

The CTSA results also need to be considered in light of the high doses of celecoxib tested in these trials, all of which were for conditions other than arthritis. The average daily dose of celecoxib taken by patients who had osteoarthritis was 200 mg daily, much lower than even the lowest 400-mg daily doses in the CTSA trials. The results of these trials thus cannot be extrapolated easily to the lower doses, for which few long-term placebo-controlled data exist.

Since the introduction of rofecoxib, celecoxib, and valdecoxib, other so-called "second-generation" coxibs have emerged. Lumiracoxib, currently approved for use in Canada but not in the United States, was compared with ibuprofen and naproxen in separate randomizations and showed similar rates of cardiovascular outcomes.[18] Similarly, the MEDAL trial,[55] comparing etoricoxib with diclofenac, showed similar rates of adverse cardiovascular events, although the choice of an active comparator in this trial has been criticized because diclofenac, considered a traditional NSAID, has similar COX1:COX2 selectivity as a coxib.

Despite all the available data that have emerged regarding the cardiovascular risk of coxibs over the last several years, the potential cardiovascular

risk associated with traditional NSAIDs remains a major gap in our knowledge. There have been few placebo-controlled trials of NSAIDs in which cardiovascular risk was reported, and most head-to-head comparisons with coxibs have shown similar overall risk. Non-adjudicated data from the ADAPT trial, a study comparing celecoxib or naproxen with placebo in patients at risk for Alzheimer disease, showed clear increased risk associated with naproxen use.[56] Other observational studies have similarly suggested that traditional NSAIDs, which can elevate blood pressure and result in prostacyclin/thromboxane imbalances, can also be associated with increased cardiovascular risk.[57] The ongoing PRECISION trial will prospectively assess the risk of celecoxib compared with ibuprofen and naproxen on cardiovascular risk in patients who have osteoarthritis and rheumatoid arthritis. Still, the lack of a non-NSAID arm will not allow us to interpret the real risks associated with each of these drugs.

CURRENT RECOMMENDATIONS

Recently the American Heart Association (AHA) put forth a treatment approach for patients who have concomitant arthritis and heart disease.[58] A "stepped care" strategy promotes the short-term use of aspirin, acetaminophen, nonacetylated salicylates, tramadol, and opioid analgesics as first-line therapies. These specific recommendations are controversial because of the paucity of evidence comparing COX-2 inhibitors and opioids with respect to efficacy or adverse effects, lack of long-term studies with opioids, and limited efficacy data and potential side effects with tramadol. Nonetheless, the AHA recommendations advocate use of agents with the lowest risk for cardiovascular events. Thereafter, progression to other agents, such as NSAIDS and COX-2 inhibitors, should coincide with a risk–benefit consideration at each step. COX-2 inhibitors are reserved as last choice given their cardiovascular hazard. The AHA recommends using the lowest dose of NSAIDS required to control symptoms and adding aspirin 81 mg daily and a proton pump inhibitor (PPI) to COX-2 selective agents in patients at an increased risk for thrombotic events.

The most recent guidelines on management of osteoarthritis of the hip and knee by the American College of Rheumatology (ACR) were published in 2000,[59] just before release of information about cardiovascular risk with coxibs. As such, pharmacologic recommendations following acetaminophen as first line include use of low-dose NSAIDS or coxibs. Patients who have risk factors for GI events should only receive NSAIDS in combination with a PPI or misoprostol. Nonacetylated salicylates were recommended for high-risk patients as an alternative, recognizing risks for ototoxicity and central nervous system toxicity.

In 2002, the American Pain Society (APS) issued guidelines for management of pain in osteoarthritis, rheumatoid arthritis, and juvenile chronic arthritis. These guidelines recommended use of coxibs following acetaminophen before choosing NSAIDS. Again, the most compelling data about cardiovascular risks of coxibs had yet to surface; therefore the ACR and APS guidelines will likely be updated.

CLINICAL CONSIDERATIONS

A treatment regimen for pain relief takes into account the type of pain, available therapeutic modalities (nonpharmacologic and pharmacologic choices), and patient-specific risk factors for GI and cardiovascular events. Based on the current available evidence, it seems prudent that to minimize cardiovascular risk from coxibs, patients who have active atherosclerotic processes or recent cardiovascular events (such as bypass surgery, unstable angina, or acute myocardial infarction) or ischemic cerebrovascular events should avoid coxib use if possible.[58] If coxibs are indicated, the smallest effective dose for the shortest duration should be used. Traditional NSAIDS also carry cardiovascular risk, however, and similar to coxibs, these vary with individual agents. Although most guidelines suggest that naproxen may carry the least risk for major thrombotic events, the data to support these recommendations are scarce. Moreover, for patients taking an aspirin for cardiovascular protection, data suggest that ibuprofen may interfere with aspirin's antiplatelet actions, theoretically undermining its protective effects, although this has not been proved.[60] Additionally, the use of aspirin likely negates the GI protective effects of a coxib. Treatment considerations for analgesics include careful assessment of GI and cardiovascular risk, individual pain relief needs, and use of potential concomitant therapies for GI and cardiovascular protection.

SUMMARY

Coxibs have become an important part of the armamentarium of clinicians treating patients who have arthritis. Although celecoxib remains the only coxib available in the United States currently, other agents are available outside the United States and may undergo FDA review in the near future. Although the data strongly support increased risk associated with multiple cox-2 inhibitors, the risk seems to be dose and possibly dosing interval dependent. Moreover, that risk may vary enough by a patient's individual baseline cardiovascular risk that these factors should be considered when prescribing coxibs to individual patients. Although the current AHA recommendations suggest naproxen as the best NSAID alternative to coxibs, it is not entirely clear that traditional NSAIDS, which are available over-the-counter, such as naproxen or even ibuprofen, are risk-free.

In summary, multiple COX-2 selective inhibitors have been associated with increased cardiovascular risk in randomized, placebo-controlled trials. It is difficult not to consider this a class effect, although there may be real differences in the degree of risk between drugs. The data strongly suggest a dose response and that there may be real differences between dosing regimens and dosing intervals. Prescribers of cox-2 inhibitors should thus use the lowest possible dose, and as with all drugs, potential risks must be weighed against potential benefits.

REFERENCES

1. Smith WL, DeWitt DL, Garavito RM. Cyclooxygenases: structural, cellular, and molecular biology. Annu Rev Biochem 2000;69:145–82.
2. Grosser T, Fries S, FitzGerald GA. Biological basis for the cardiovascular consequences of COX-2 inhibition: therapeutic challenges and opportunities. J Clin Invest 2006;116(1):4–15.
3. Marcus AJ. Transcellular metabolism of eicosanoids. Prog Hemost Thromb 1986;8:127–42.

4. Picot D, Loll PJ, Garavito RM. The X-ray crystal structure of the membrane protein prostaglandin H2 synthase-1. Nature 1994;367(6460):243–9.

5. Grosser T. The pharmacology of selective inhibition of COX-2. Thromb Haemost 2006;96(4):393–400.

6. Kargman S, Charleson S, Cartwright M, et al. Characterization of prostaglandin G/H synthase 1 and 2 in rat, dog, monkey, and human gastrointestinal tracts. Gastroenterology 1996;111(2):445–54.

7. Zimmermann KC, Sarbia M, Schror K, et al. Constitutive cyclooxygenase-2 expression in healthy human and rabbit gastric mucosa. Mol Pharmacol 1998;54(3):536–40.

8. Crofford LJ, Wilder RL, Ristimaki AP, et al. Cyclooxygenase-1 and -2 expression in rheumatoid synovial tissues. Effects of interleukin-1 beta, phorbol ester, and corticosteroids. J Clin Invest 1994;93(3):1095–101.

9. Schonbeck U, Sukhova GK, Graber P, et al. Augmented expression of cyclooxygenase-2 in human atherosclerotic lesions. Am J Pathol 1999;155(4):1281–91.

10. Hawkey CJ. Nonsteroidal anti-inflammatory drug gastropathy. Gastroenterology 2000;119(2):521–35.

11. Khanna IK, Yu Y, Huff RM, et al. Selective cyclooxygenase-2 inhibitors: heteroaryl modified 1,2-diarylimidazoles are potent, orally active antiinflammatory agents. J Med Chem 2000;43(16):3168–85.

12. Tani S, Suzuki T, Kano S, et al. Mechanisms of gastric mucus secretion from cultured rat gastric epithelial cells induced by carbachol, cholecystokinin octapeptide, secretin, and prostaglandin E2. Biol Pharm Bull 2002;25(1):14–8.

13. Warner TD, Giuliano F, Vojnovic I, et al. Nonsteroid drug selectivities for cyclo-oxygenase-1 rather than cyclo-oxygenase-2 are associated with human gastrointestinal toxicity: a full in vitro analysis. Proc Natl Acad Sci U S A 1999;96(13):7563–8.

14. Coruzzi G, Venturi N, Spaggiari S. Gastrointestinal safety of novel nonsteroidal antiinflammatory drugs: selective COX-2 inhibitors and beyond. Acta Biomed 2007;78(2):96–110.

15. Seibert K, Masferrer J, Zhang Y, et al. Mediation of inflammation by cyclooxygenase-2. Agents Actions Suppl 1995;46:41–50.

16. Bombardier C, Laine L, Reicin A, et al. Comparison of upper gastrointestinal toxicity of rofecoxib and naproxen in patients with rheumatoid arthritis. VIGOR Study Group. N Engl J Med 2000;343(21):1520–8, 1522. p. following 1528.

17. Silverstein FE, Faich G, Goldstein JL, et al. Gastrointestinal toxicity with celecoxib vs nonsteroidal anti-inflammatory drugs for osteoarthritis and rheumatoid arthritis: the CLASS study: a randomized controlled trial. Celecoxib Long-term Arthritis Safety Study. JAMA 2000;284(10):1247–55.

18. Schnitzer TJ, Burmester GR, Mysler E, et al. Comparison of lumiracoxib with naproxen and ibuprofen in the Therapeutic Arthritis Research and Gastrointestinal Event Trial (TARGET), reduction in ulcer complications: randomised controlled trial. Lancet 2004;364(9435):665–74.

19. Garavito RM, DeWitt DL. The cyclooxygenase isoforms: structural insights into the conversion of arachidonic acid to prostaglandins. Biochim Biophys Acta 1999;1441(2–3):278–87.

20. Patrono C, Patrignani P, Garcia Rodriguez LA. Cyclooxygenase-selective inhibition of prostanoid formation: transducing biochemical selectivity into clinical read-outs. J Clin Invest 2001;108(1):7–13.

21. Cryer B, Feldman M. Cyclooxygenase-1 and cyclooxygenase-2 selectivity of widely used nonsteroidal anti-inflammatory drugs. Am J Med 1998;104(5):413–21.

22. FitzGerald GA, Patrono C. The coxibs, selective inhibitors of cyclooxygenase-2. N Engl J Med 2001;345(6):433–42.

23. Capone ML, Tacconelli S, Di Francesco L, et al. Pharmacodynamic of cyclooxygenase inhibitors in humans. Prostaglandins Other Lipid Mediat 2007;82(1–4):85–94.

24. Bresalier RS, Sandler RS, Quan H, et al. Cardiovascular events associated with rofecoxib in a colorectal adenoma chemoprevention trial. N Engl J Med 2005;352(11):1092–102.

25. Mamdani M, Juurlink DN, Lee DS, et al. Cyclo-oxygenase-2 inhibitors versus non selective non-steroidal anti-inflammatory drugs and congestive heart failure outcomes in elderly patients: a population-based cohort study. Lancet 2004;363(9423):1751–6.

26. Pai R, Soreghan B, Szabo IL, et al. Prostaglandin E2 transactivates EGF receptor: a novel mechanism for promoting colon cancer growth and gastrointestinal hypertrophy. Nat Med 2002;8(3):289–93.

27. Steinbach G, Lynch PM, Phillips RK, et al. The effect of celecoxib, a cyclooxygenase-2 inhibitor, in familial adenomatous polyposis. N Engl J Med 2000;342(26):1946–52.

28. Bolli R, Shinmura K, Tang XL, et al. Discovery of a new function of cyclooxygenase (COX)-2: COX-2 is a cardioprotective protein that alleviates ischemia/reperfusion injury and mediates the late phase of preconditioning. Cardiovasc Res 2002;55(3):506–19.

29. Rudic RD, Brinster D, Cheng Y, et al. COX-2-derived prostacyclin modulates vascular remodeling. Circ Res 2005;96(12):1240–7.

30. Egan KM, Wang M, Fries S, et al. Cyclooxygenases, thromboxane, and atherosclerosis: plaque destabilization by cyclooxygenase-2 inhibition combined with thromboxane receptor antagonism. Circulation 2005;111(3):334–42.

31. Francois H, Athirakul K, Howell D, et al. Prostacyclin protects against elevated blood pressure and cardiac fibrosis. Cell Metab 2005;2(3):201–7.

32. Rabausch K, Bretschneider E, Sarbia M, et al. Regulation of thrombomodulin expression in human vascular smooth muscle cells by COX-2-derived prostaglandins. Circ Res 2005;96(1):e1–6.

33. Murata T, Ushikubi F, Matsuoka T, et al. Altered pain perception and inflammatory response in mice lacking prostacyclin receptor. Nature 1997;388(6643):678–82.

34. FitzGerald GA, Brash AR, Falardeau P, et al. Estimated rate of prostacyclin secretion into the circulation of normal man. J Clin Invest 1981;68(5):1272–6.

35. McAdam BF, Catella-Lawson F, Mardini IA, et al. Systemic biosynthesis of prostacyclin by cyclooxygenase (COX)-2: the human pharmacology of a selective inhibitor of COX-2. Proc Natl Acad Sci U S A 1999;96(1):272–7.

36. Marwali MR, Mehta JL. COX-2 inhibitors and cardiovascular risk. Inferences based on biology and clinical studies. Thromb Haemost 2006;96(4):401–6.

37. Belton O, Byrne D, Kearney D, et al. Cyclooxygenase-1 and -2-dependent prostacyclin formation in patients with atherosclerosis. Circulation 2000;102(8):840–5.

38. Cheng Y, Wang M, Yu Y, et al. Cyclooxygenases, microsomal prostaglandin E synthase-1, and cardiovascular function. J Clin Invest 2006;116(5):1391–9.

39. Yamagata K, Andreasson KI, Kaufmann WE, et al. Expression of a mitogen-inducible cyclooxygenase in brain neurons: regulation by synaptic activity and glucocorticoids. Neuron 1993;11(2):371–86.

40. Breder CD, Dewitt D, Kraig RP. Characterization of inducible cyclooxygenase in rat brain. J Comp Neurol 1995;355(2):296–315.

41. Whelton A, Schulman G, Wallemark C, et al. Effects of celecoxib and naproxen on renal function in the elderly. Arch Intern Med 2000;160(10):1465–70.

42. Aw TJ, Haas SJ, Liew D, et al. Meta-analysis of cyclooxygenase-2 inhibitors and their effects on blood pressure. Arch Intern Med 2005;165(5):490–6.

43. Whelton A, White WB, Bello AE, et al. Effects of celecoxib and rofecoxib on blood pressure and edema in patients ≥65 years of age with systemic hypertension and osteoarthritis. Am J Cardiol 2002;90(9):959–63.

44. Sowers JR, White WB, Pitt B, et al. The effects of cyclooxygenase-2 inhibitors and nonsteroidal anti-inflammatory therapy on 24-hour blood pressure in patients with hypertension, osteoarthritis, and type 2 diabetes mellitus. Arch Intern Med 2005;165(2):161–8.

45. Solomon DH, Schneeweiss S, Levin R, et al. Relationship between COX-2 specific inhibitors and hypertension. Hypertension 2004;44(2):140–5.

46. Graham DJ, Campen D, Hui R, et al. Risk of acute myocardial infarction and sudden cardiac death in patients treated with cyclo-oxygenase 2 selective and non-selective non-steroidal anti-inflammatory drugs: nested case-control study. Lancet 2005;365(9458):475–81.

47. Nissen SE. Adverse cardiovascular effects of rofecoxib. N Engl J Med 2006;355(2):203–4 author reply 203–05.

48. Solomon SD, McMurray JJ, Pfeffer MA, et al. Cardiovascular risk associated with celecoxib in a clinical trial for colorectal adenoma prevention. N Engl J Med 2005;352(11):1071–80.

49. Solomon SD, Pfeffer MA, McMurray JJ, et al. Effect of celecoxib on cardiovascular events and blood pressure in two trials for the prevention of colorectal adenomas. Circulation 2006;114(10):1028–35.

50. Bertagnolli MM, Eagle CJ, Zauber AG, et al. Celecoxib for the prevention of sporadic colorectal adenomas. N Engl J Med 2006;355(9):873–84.

51. Arber N, Eagle CJ, Spicak J, et al. Celecoxib for the prevention of colorectal adenomatous polyps. N Engl J Med 2006;355(9):885–95.

52. Baron JA, Sandler RS, Bresalier RS, et al. A randomized trial of rofecoxib for the chemoprevention of colorectal adenomas. Gastroenterology 2006;131(6):1674–82.

53. Nussmeier NA, Whelton AA, Brown MT, et al. Complications of the COX-2 inhibitors parecoxib and valdecoxib after cardiac surgery. N Engl J Med 2005;352(11):1081–91.

54. Solomon SD, Wittes J, Finn PV, et al. Cardiovascular risk of celecoxib in 6 randomized placebo-controlled trials: the cross trial safety analysis. Circulation 2008;117(16):2104–13.

55. Cannon CP, Curtis SP, FitzGerald GA, et al. Cardiovascular outcomes with etoricoxib and diclofenac in patients with osteoarthritis and rheumatoid arthritis in the Multinational Etoricoxib and Diclofenac Arthritis Long-term (MEDAL) programme: a randomised comparison. Lancet 2006;368(9549):1771–81.

56. Martin BK, Breitner JCS, Evans D, et al. ADAPT Research Group. Cardiovascular and cerebrovascular events in the randomized, controlled Alzheimer's Disease Anti-Inflammatory Prevention Trial (ADAPT). PLoS Clin Trials 2006;1(7):e33.

57. Fosbol EL, Gislason GH, Jacobsen S, et al. The pattern of use of non-steroidal anti-inflammatory drugs (NSAIDs) from 1997 to 2005: a nationwide study on 4.6 million people. Pharmacoepidemiol Drug Saf Mar 28 2008;17:822–33.

58. Antman EM, Bennett JS, Daugherty A, et al. Use of nonsteroidal antiinflammatory drugs: an update for

clinicians: a scientific statement from the American Heart Association. Circulation 2007;115(12):1634–42.

59. Recommendations for the medical management of osteoarthritis of the hip and knee: 2000 update. American College of Rheumatology Subcommittee on Osteoarthritis Guidelines. Arthritis Rheum 2000; 43(9):1905–15.

60. Catella-Lawson F, Reilly MP, Kapoor SC, et al. Cyclooxygenase inhibitors and the antiplatelet effects of aspirin. N Engl J Med 2001;345(25):1809–17.

Ranolazine: New Paradigm for Management of Myocardial Ischemia, Myocardial Dysfunction, and Arrhythmias

Peter H. Stone, MD

KEYWORDS

- Myocardial ischemia • Angina • Ranolazine • Heart failure
- Diastolic dysfunction

Anti-ischemia medications have traditionally focused on optimizing the determinants of the myocardial O_2 supply: demand balance. Because myocardial oxygen extraction is maximal at rest, the only way to improve the balance pharmacologically has been to reduce myocardial O_2 demand (ie, heart rate, blood pressure or afterload, myocardial contractility, or preload). The approved antianginal medications in the United States are effective by reducing one or more of these O_2 demand determinants (**Table 1**).

There are many patients, however, who have chronic coronary disease in whom this pharmacologic approach is inadequate. Many patients either cannot tolerate these conventional agents or have continuing symptoms of ischemia and angina despite their use.[1] Ranolazine, which was approved by the US Food and Drug Administration in January 2006, provides a mechanism of action to treat ischemia that has not hitherto been available. Ranolazine is effective to reduce manifestations of ischemia and angina, and it also holds potential promise to be effective in the management of left ventricular dysfunction, particularly diastolic dysfunction, and arrhythmias. This article provides an update on the available studies concerning the value of ranolazine across the spectrum of cardiovascular disease.

MECHANISM OF ACTION

Ranolazine was first believed to be effective by inhibiting free fatty acid metabolism,[2] but it was later appreciated that ranolazine exerted this effect only at serum levels that are much higher than those observed in therapeutic usage.[3] The mechanism of action now seems to be related to inhibition of the late inward sodium channel (late I_{Na}),[4] which pathologically remains open in a wide variety of adverse stimuli to the myocardium. Electrical activation of the cardiomyocytes leads to brief opening of the membrane sodium channel, through which sodium ions rapidly enter the cell, generating the rapid depolarization or upstroke of the action potential (**Fig. 1**A).[4] In the normal setting, the inward sodium channels then inactivate rapidly and remain closed during the plateau phase of the action potential. Other ion channels open following electrical activation, including calcium channels, and the calcium ions that enter the cell during the plateau phase of the action potential then trigger the release of the large stores of calcium ions from the sarcoplasmic reticulum. This increased concentration of cytoplasmic calcium initiates the interaction between actin and myosin and enables the contraction process to occur (see **Fig. 1**A). Following the myocardial

Cardiovascular Division, Brigham and Women's Hospital, Harvard Medical School, 75 Francis Street, Boston, MA 02115-6110, USA
E-mail address: pstone@partners.org

Cardiol Clin 26 (2008) 603–614
doi:10.1016/j.ccl.2008.06.002

Table 1
Antianginal pharmacologic management

Determinant of O$_2$ Demand	β-Blocker	Nitrates	Ca^{++} Blocker Dihydropyridine	Ca^{++} Blocker Verap/Dilt
Heart rate	↓↓	0	↑/↑↑	↓↓
Afterload (BP)	↓	↓	↓↓↓↓	↓↓
Preload	0	↓↓↓	0	0
Contractility	↓↓	↑	↑↑	↓↓
Determinant of O$_2$ supply				
Vasomotor tone	↑	↓↓	↓↓↓↓	↓↓↓↓

Abbreviations: BP, blood pressure; verap/dilt, verapamil/diltiazem; 0, no effect.

contraction, calcium ions are actively taken up back into the sarcoplasmic reticulum again and myocardial relaxation occurs.

In the setting of a wide variety of myocardial insults, however, including myocardial ischemia, hypertrophy, and oxidative stress, the late sodium channels either fail to inactivate (ie, fail to close) or reopen, such that sodium ions continue to enter the cell (see **Fig. 1**B).[4,5] This intracellular overload of sodium ions leads to several major contractility, metabolic, and electrophysiologic disturbances.[6] The elevation of intracellular sodium concentration leads to an increased exchange of intracellular sodium for extracellular calcium through the Na$^+$/Ca^{++} exchanger mechanism, such that the initial sodium overload leads to a subsequent intracellular calcium overload. The increased cytosolic calcium from the calcium overload state leads to the continued exposure of the actin and myosin contractile elements to the calcium ions, leading to a tonic contracture (see **Fig. 1**B). In the intact heart, this increased diastolic stiffness

leads to an abnormal elevation in myocardial contractile work, oxygen consumption, and compression of the vascular space during diastole.[4,7] Compression of the vascular space causes a reduction in myocardial blood flow, which further reduces myocardial O$_2$ supply. This deleterious positive feedback system is detrimental in that the presence of ischemia leads to further exacerbation of ischemia (**Fig. 2**).

Ranolazine reduces the late sodium influx in a concentration-, voltage-, and frequency-dependent manner.[4,6,7] By preventing the most upstream deleterious consequence of myocardial cellular dysfunction (ie, the intracellular sodium overload), all of the downstream consequences of the sodium overload, and the subsequent calcium overload, are reduced or prevented. In animal models ranolazine thus facilitates diastolic relaxation, preserves myocardial blood flow during ischemia and reperfusion, reduces myocardial O$_2$ consumption, and restores electrical stability.[4,6–8] In healthy nonischemic, nonfailing myocytes, in

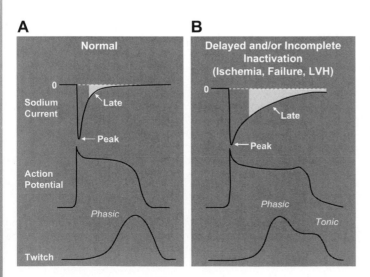

A Normal

B Delayed and/or Incomplete Inactivation (Ischemia, Failure, LVH)

Fig. 1. Relation between late Na$^+$ current and ventricular action potential and contraction. (*A*) Normal conditions. (*B*) Delayed or incomplete inactivation in the setting of ischemia, heart failure, or left ventricular hypertrophy (*From* Belardinelli L, Antzelevitch C, Fraser H. Inhibition of late (sustained/persistent) sodium current: a potential drug target to reduce intracellular sodium-dependent calcium overload and its detrimental effects on cardiomyocyte function. Eur Heart J 2004;6:14; with permission.)

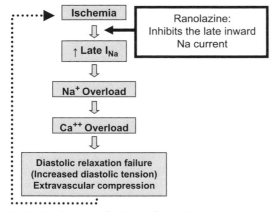

Fig. 2. Mechanism of action of ranolazine.

compounds such as ketoconazole, which inhibit the CYP3A isoenzymes, increase ranolazine levels in the range of 2.5 to 4.5 fold.[9] Clearance of rano-lazine is reduced by renal insufficiency and moderate hepatic impairment.[9]

Drug–drug interactions primarily are related to effects on the CYP3A metabolic pathway.[9] Diltiazem, ketoconazole, verapamil, macrolide antibiotics, HIV protease inhibits, and grapefruit juice inhibit the CYP3A enzyme system, and their concomitant use with ranolazine should be done with caution. Ranolazine also is a substrate and an inhibitor of P-glycoprotein. Verapamil, which inhibits P-glycoprotein, increases the absorption of ranolazine, with a consequent increased in plasma levels. Ranolazine increases digoxin levels.

which the contribution of late I_{Na} is small, the drug does not have a measurable effect on cardiovascular performance at therapeutic plasma concentrations.[9] The effect of ranolazine on late I_{Na} is more pronounced in ischemic or failing myocytes in which the current is amplified.[9] Each of these pharmacologic effects may have important therapeutic application for patients who have cardiovascular disease, as discussed later.

PHARMACOKINETICS AND METABOLISM

Ranolazine is an active piperazine derivative available in oral and intravenous forms and is now manufactured in a sustained-release form.[9] Its maximal plasma concentration is typically 4 to 6 hours after administration, and the average terminal elimination half-life is approximately 7 hours. The peak/trough difference is 1.6-fold with dosing of 500 to100 mg twice a day.[9] Ranolazine plasma concentrations that are therapeutically effective for chronic angina are in the range of 2 to 6 μmol/L.[9] Oral bioavailability is in the range of 30% to 55%. Most of the metabolic biotransformation is through the cytochrome P450 3A4-mediated pathway,[9] which is critical because

THERAPEUTIC USES
Chronic Angina Pectoris

Conventional anti-ischemia medications reduce the development of ischemia primarily by reducing the determinants of myocardial O_2 demand: heart rate, blood pressure, preload, or contractility (**Fig. 3**). As myocardial ischemia develops intracellular calcium overload occurs, which leads to the consequences of ischemia, including systolic and diastolic myocardial dysfunction and electrical instability. Ranolazine has no clinically meaningful effects on the myocardial O_2 demand determinants, but exerts its anti-ischemic effect by preventing the calcium overload state and thereby reducing the subsequent myocardial stiffness that leads to reduced myocardial perfusion (see **Fig. 3**). A recent study demonstrated that the dose-related improvement in myocardial ischemia at submaximal and maximal exercise in patients who had stable coronary artery disease was attributable to an improvement in myocardial blood flow without meaningfully affecting heart rate or blood pressure.[10] One can therefore anticipate that ranolazine would be an ideal complementary agent to

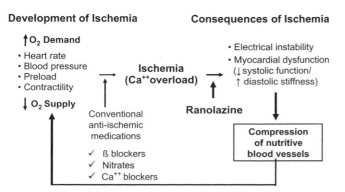

Fig. 3. Sites of action of anti-ischemia medication.

be used with medications that reduce the development of ischemia by reducing O_2 demand.

Monotherapy

The early studies of ranolazine in patients who had stable angina used the immediate-release formulation, whereas the more recent studies have used the sustained-release formulation. In comparison with placebo, ranolazine in the immediate-release formulation significantly reduced anginal episodes and nitroglycerin use, and significantly improved exercise duration and time to exercise-induced myocardial ischemia,[11] and was at least equally as effective as atenolol 100 mg every day (**Fig. 4**). The anti-ischemia effect of atenolol was attributable to its well-known reduction in the rate–pressure product at rest and during exercise, whereas the anti-ischemic effect of ranolazine occurred without any appreciable change in the determinants of myocardial O_2 demand (**Fig. 5**).[11]

The Monotherapy Assessment of Ranolazine in Stable Angina (MARISA) trial investigated the effect of the sustained-release formulation as single agent therapy of 500 mg twice a day, 1000 mg twice a day, or 1500 mg twice a day versus placebo twice a day in 191 patients who had chronic exertional angina with reproducible treadmill-induced myocardial ischemia and angina in a 4-week, double-blind, placebo-controlled crossover trial.[12] All three doses resulted in a significant, dose-dependent increase in exercise duration, exercise time to angina, and exercise time to 1-mm ST segment depression at trough and at peak drug effect compared with placebo

($P < .005$), although the incremental benefit was attenuated at dosages greater than 1000 mg twice a day.[12] The maximal increase in exercise duration compared with placebo was 56 seconds, whereas the maximal increase in time to angina or time to 1-mm ST-segment depression was 69 seconds (**Fig. 6**).

Combination regimens

The Combination Assessment of Ranolazine in Stable Angina (CARISA) trial was designed to evaluate the effect of the addition of ranolazine to a regimen of concomitant antianginal drugs, including atenolol (50 mg every day), diltiazem (180 mg every day), or amlodipine (5 mg every day).[13] A total of 823 patients were studied in a parallel design, and ranolazine 750 mg or 1000 mg or placebo twice a day was administered in addition to the concomitant medications. Exercise tests were performed 2, 6, and 12 weeks after randomization. The addition of ranolazine was associated with a significant reduction in anginal frequency and nitroglycerin consumption, and an increase in exercise duration, time to angina, and time to 1-mm ST-segment depression compared with placebo both at trough and peak drug effect (**Fig. 7**). There was not a major difference between the ranolazine 750 mg and 1000 mg twice a day regimens. The increase in exercise duration of 115.6 seconds above baseline in both ranolazine groups versus 91.7 seconds in the placebo group ($P = .01$) did not depend on changes in blood pressure or heart rate, and this improvement in performance was sustained over the 12 weeks of therapy. The treatment-by-background interaction

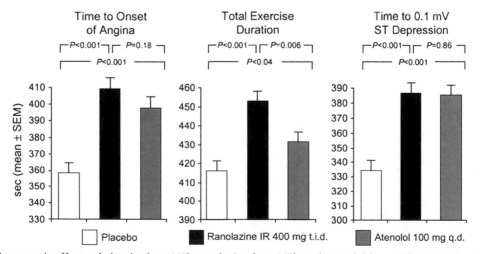

Fig. 4. Therapeutic effects of placebo (n = 142), ranolazine (n = 142), and atenolol (n = 142) on exercise tolerance and ischemic ST-segment depression in patients who have stable coronary disease. (*From* Rousseau MF, Pouleur H, Cocco G, et al. Comparative efficacy of ranolazine versus atenolol for chronic angina pectoris. Am J Cardiol 2005;95:313; with permission.)

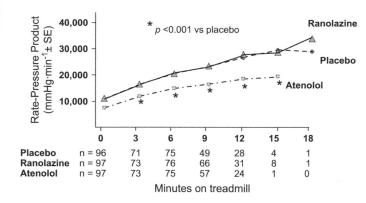

Fig. 5. Anti-ischemic effect of ranolazine without affecting heart rate or blood pressure at rest or during exercise. (*From* Rousseau MF, Pouleur H, Cocco G, et al. Comparative efficacy of ranolazine versus atenolol for chronic angina pectoris. Am J Cardiol 2005;95:314; with permission.)

term indicated no evidence of differential treatment effect according to background therapy received. Adverse events were reported in 26.4% of patients in the placebo group, 31.2% of patients in the ranolazine 750 mg group, and 32.7% of the ranolazine 1000 mg group. The most common dose-related adverse effects were constipation, dizziness, nausea, and asthenia, which occurred in less than 7% of the ranolazine-treated patients and less than 1% of the placebo-treated patients. There was a small, dose-related increase in the QTc interval of 6.1 and 9.2 milliseconds in the 750 mg and 1000 mg ranolazine groups, respectively, but there were no evident arrhythmias. Five patients taking 1000 mg ranolazine twice a day experienced syncope, but all were also taking an angiotensin-converting enzyme inhibitor and 4 of the 5 were also taking diltiazem, which is known to increase ranolazine levels. Although little or no effect of ranolazine was observed on blood pressure on 750 or 1000 mg twice a day dosages, postural hypotension and syncope have occurred in healthy volunteers given higher doses, up to 2000 mg twice a day, and this is believed likely because of α_1-adrenergic receptor blocking activities at higher plasma concentrations.[13] The patients in CARISA treated with

ranolazine who were diabetic experienced a significant reduction in hemoglobin A_{1c} compared with placebo (-0.70%, $P = .002$), although the mechanism of this improvement is not clear.

A more recent study investigated the antianginal effect of ranolazine versus placebo given to 565 patients who had persisting angina symptoms despite maximal dose amlodipine (10 mg every day) (Efficacy of Ranolazine in Chronic Angina [ERICA] trial).[14] Compared with placebo, the addition of ranolazine 1000 mg twice a day was associated with a significant reduction in weekly anginal episodes and nitroglycerin consumption (to 3.31 episodes/wk on placebo versus to 2.88 episodes/wk on ranolazine, $P = .028$).[14] There was a consistent treatment effect of ranolazine across the subgroups analyzed, including those also on long-acting nitrates versus those not on long-acting nitrates, men versus women, and patients aged less than 65 years versus those older than 65 years. An interesting subgroup analysis dividing patients on the basis of being above or below the median of weekly anginal frequency (4.5 episodes) indicated that those patients who had more frequent angina per week had a much more marked beneficial response to the addition of ranolazine, compared with those patients who had less frequent angina,

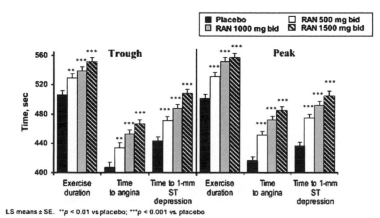

Fig. 6. Monotherapy with ranolazine increases exercise performance at trough and peak pharmacologic effect: the MARISA trial. (*From* Chaitman BR, Skettino SL, Parker JO, et al. Anti-ischemic effects and long-term survival during ranolazine monotherapy in patients with chronic severe angina. *Modified from* J Am Coll Cardiol 2004;43:1378; with permission.)

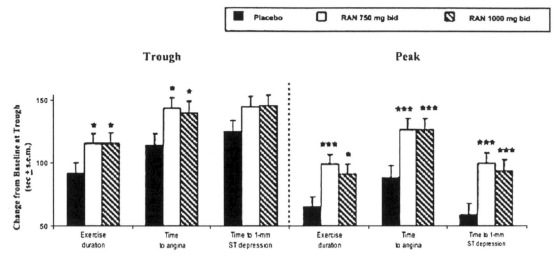

Fig. 7. Effect of ranolazine 1000 mg twice a day on exercise treadmill performance when combined with atenolol 50 mg every day, diltiazem 120 mg every day, or amlodipine 5 mg every day. (*From* Chaitman BR, Pepine CJ, Parker JO, et al. Effects of ranolazine with atenolol, amlodipine, or diltiazem on exercise tolerance and angina frequency in patients with severe chronic angina: a randomized controlled trial. *Data from* JAMA 2004;291:312.)

in reduction in angina, nitroglycerin consumption, and Seattle Angina Questionnaire (**Fig. 8**).[14] These results suggest that those patients who have the most frequent angina may have the most sustained left ventricular dysfunction from their repetitive bouts of ischemia, and that these patients are the ones most likely to experience a substantial benefit from ranolazine's effects on ischemia-associated left ventricular dysfunction.

Unstable Angina/Non–ST Segment Elevation Myocardial Infarction

The recent MERLIN TIMI-36 trial addressed the value of an intravenous infusion of ranolazine, followed by oral ranolazine, in patients who had a non–ST segment elevation acute coronary syndrome (ACS).[15] A total of 6560 patients who had either unstable angina or NSTEMI were enrolled within 48 hours of ischemic symptoms and were

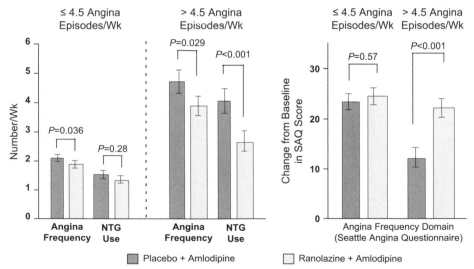

Fig. 8. Effect of ranolazine 1000 mg twice a day in patients who have refractory angina despite maximum amlodipine therapy: the ERICA trial. (*From* Stone PH, Gratsiansky NA, Blokhin A, et al. Antianginal efficacy of ranolazine when added to treatment with amlodipine: the ERICA (Efficacy of Ranolazine in Chronic Angina) trial. J Am Coll Cardiol 2006;48:572; with permission.)

treated with ranolazine (initiated intravenously and followed by oral ranolazine extended release 1000 mg twice a day) or matching placebo. They were followed up for a median of 348 days. The primary efficacy endpoint was a composite of cardiovascular death, myocardial infarction (MI), or recurrent ischemia and occurred in 21.8% of the ranolazine-treated patients and 23.5% of the placebo-treated patients (hazard ratio [HR] 0.92, 95% CI 0.83–1.02, $P = .11$) (**Fig. 9**A). Although there was no difference in the occurrence of the primary composite endpoint between the two treatment groups, or in two of the individual components of the primary composite endpoint (cardiovascular death or MI), there was a significant difference in the endpoint of recurrent ischemia (13.9% in the ranolazine-treated patients versus 16.1% in the placebo-treated group; HR 0.87, 95% CI 0.76–0.99, $P = .03$) (see **Fig. 9**B and **Fig. 10**). A trend toward an early reduction in recurrent ischemic complications with ranolazine was evident with respect to the 30-day endpoint of cardiovascular death, MI, severe recurrent ischemia, or positive Holter for ischemia ($P = .055$). An effect of long-term treatment with ranolazine on angina was evident with respect to several prespecified exploratory endpoints: reduction in worsening angina by at least one Canadian Cardiovascular Society class requiring intensification of medical therapy, less frequent escalation in antianginal medication, and improvement in anginal frequency using the Seattle Angina Questionnaire. There was no significant heterogeneity of the effect of ranolazine on the primary endpoint across the major subgroups examined.

Ranolazine also had a significant effect of preventing ventricular and atrial arrhythmias in these high-risk patients who had a non–ST elevation ACS,[16] as discussed later.

In a substudy analysis stratifying patients on the basis of brain natriuretic peptide (BNP) measurements obtained at the time of randomization, those patients who had an elevated BNP greater than 80 pg/mL, likely reflecting diastolic stiffness resulting from more severe or more prolonged ischemia, experienced a significantly higher incidence of cardiovascular death, MI, or recurrent ischemia compared with patients who had ACS with a BNP value less than 80 pg/mL ($P < .001$).[17] Furthermore, ranolazine was associated with a significant reduction in the composite primary endpoint of cardiovascular death, MI, or recurrent ischemia in those high-risk patients who had an elevated BNP ($P = .009$), whereas there was no beneficial effect in low-risk patients who had a normal BNP value.[17]

The safety of ranolazine was confirmed in this large clinical trial. There was no difference in mortality between patients treated with ranolazine versus placebo, nor sudden death. The incidence of symptomatic documented arrhythmias throughout the duration of the study was also similar in the two treatment groups ($P = .84$). Discontinuation of treatment because of an adverse event occurred in 28% in the ranolazine group to 22% in the placebo group ($P < .001$). Discontinuation because of an adverse event was reported significantly more frequently among patients receiving ranolazine compared with patients receiving placebo (8.8% versus 4.7%, $P < .001$). The most frequent adverse events, occurring in more than 4% of patients, were dizziness (13% versus 7%), nausea (9% versus 6%), and constipation (9% versus 3%). Syncope occurred in 3.3% of the patients receiving ranolazine and 2.3% of the patients receiving placebo ($P = .01$). Most of these were believed to be vasovagal syncope. Only two cases of torsades de pointes were noted in the study, one in each treatment group.

Electrophysiologic Effects of Ranolazine and Efficacy as an Antiarrhythmic Agent

Ranolazine exerts several effects on cardiac ion currents at concentrations within the therapeutic

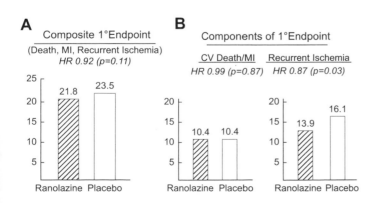

A

Composite 1°Endpoint
(Death, MI, Recurrent Ischemia)
HR 0.92 (p=0.11)

21.8   23.5

Ranolazine Placebo

B

Components of 1°Endpoint

CV Death/MI   Recurrent Ischemia
HR 0.99 (p=0.87)   HR 0.87 (p=0.03)

10.4   10.4   13.9   16.1

Ranolazine Placebo   Ranolazine Placebo

Fig. 9. Effect of ranolazine in patients who have a non–ST elevation ACS: the MERLIN trial. (*From* Morrow DA, Scirica BM, Karwatowska-Prokopczuk E, et al. Effects of ranolazine on recurrent cardiovascular events in patients with non–ST elevation ACS: the MERLIN-TIMI 36 randomized trial. *Data from JAMA* 2007;297:1779.)

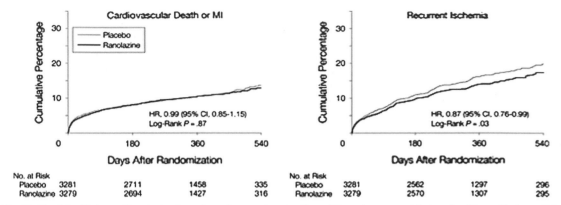

Fig. 10. Kaplain-Meier estimated rates of cardiovascular death or MI and recurrent ischemia. (*From* Morrow DA, Scirica BM, Karwatowska-Prokopczuk E, et al. Effects of ranolazine on recurrent cardiovascular events in patients with non–ST elevation ACS: the MERLIN-TIMI 36 randomized trial. JAMA 2007;297:17780; with permission.)

range of 2 to 6 μmol/L, which include inhibition of I_{Kr}, late I_{Na}, and late $I_{Ca,L}$ (**Fig. 11**).[6] Although inhibition of I_{Kr} by ranolazine prolongs the action potential duration, inhibition of the late I_{Na} and the late I_{Ca} shorten the action potential duration such that the net effect on the action potential duration, or QTc, is usually modest (ie, in the range of 5–10 milliseconds). In experimental animals and tissue preparations ranolazine actually shortens or normalizes the action potential duration that is prolonged from ischemia or exposure to arrhythmogenic compounds, such as d-sotalol (**Fig. 12**A, B).[6]

It is now well appreciated that development of drug-induced torsades de pointes requires not only prolongation of the action potential and the QTc interval, but also the presence of early afterdepolarizations and increased dispersion of repolarization across the myocardium. Although ranolazine exerts a minimal effect of prolonging

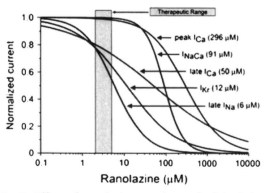

Fig. 11. Effect of ranolazine on electrophysiologic ion currents across the myocyte cell membrane. (*From* Antzelevitch C, Belardinelli L, Zygmunt AC, et al. Electrophysiological effects of ranolazine, a novel antianginal agent with antiarrhythmic properties. Circulation 2004;110:906; with permission.)

the QT interval, it exerts several other protective effects: (i) ranolazine reduces the incidence of early afterdepolarizations (see **Fig. 12**A), and (ii) ranolazine does not exacerbate the transmural dispersion of repolarization, which is associated with ischemia and exposure to arrhythmogenic drugs.[6] In the experimental animal ranolazine does not cause torsades de pointes,[6] and, as noted earlier in the experience in the MERLIN trial, there was only one case of torsades in the patients who had a non–ST elevation ACS, and this was the same incidence as in the placebo group.[16]

Although ranolazine has not been studied as a primary antiarrhythmic agent, it has been efficacious as an antiarrhythmic agent in the large-scale studies that have included continuous ECG monitoring.[16] In the MERLIN trial 97% of the 6560 patients who had ACS had a continuous ECG that was interpretable for analysis. Treatment with ranolazine was associated with a significant reduction in ventricular arrhythmias, including ventricular tachycardia greater than or equal to 3, 4, or 8 beats at a rate of 100 beats per minute (bpm) or greater ($P < .001$), but had no effect on sustained ventricular tachycardia greater than 30 seconds (**Table 2** and **Fig. 13**). Ranolazine also reduced the incidence of supraventricular arrhythmias 120 bpm or greater lasting 4 beats or more ($P < .001$), and was associated with a trend toward reducing the incidence of new-onset atrial fibrillation ($P = .08$) (see **Table 2**). Among several high-risk subgroups, including patients who had prior heart failure, reduced left ventricular function, prolonged QTc interval at baseline, and high TIMI Risk Score (5–7), ranolazine consistently reduced the incidence of ventricular tachycardias lasting 8 beats or more, although there was no difference in sudden cardiac death.[16] Ranolazine also reduced the incidence of bradycardia less than

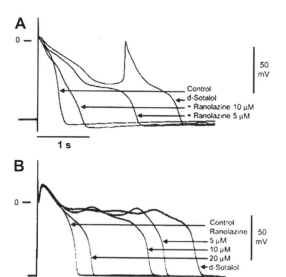

Fig. 12. Effect of ranolazine to normalize the action potential duration and suppress early afterdepolarizations in M cells (*A*) and Purkinje fiber preparations (*B*). (*From* Antzelevitch C, Belardinelli L, Zygmunt AC, et al. Electrophysiological effects of ranolazine, a novel antianginal agent with antiarrhythmic properties. Circulation 2004;110:909; with permission.)

45 bpm for at least 4 beats. It is not clear whether the antiarrhythmic effects observed with ranolazine were attributable to prevention of ischemia-associated arrhythmias by preventing the ischemia itself, or from a more primary antiarrhythmic effect related to its effect on membrane ion channels.

New studies are being considered to investigate the more primary use of ranolazine as an antiarrhythmic agent for atrial or ventricular arrhythmias.

Future Applications

Diastolic heart failure

Evidence in experimental animals suggests that ranolazine may provide a unique role in the management of patients who have heart failure, particularly diastolic heart failure associated with ischemic cardiomyopathy and left ventricular hypertrophy. Abnormal late I_{Na}, and subsequent sodium ion and calcium ion overload, is a common characteristic of myocardial dysfunction associated with myocardial ischemia, left ventricular hypertrophy, and various conditions associated with oxidative stress.[4] Ranolazine is uniquely able to treat the abnormal late I_{Na}, and it can thereby prevent the sodium overload and the consequent calcium overload and the abnormal left ventricular diastolic function that ensues. For example, in isometrically contracting ventricular muscle strips from end-stage failing human hearts, ranolazine (10 μmol/L) significantly reduced the frequency-dependent increase in diastolic dysfunction by approximately 30% without significantly affecting sarcoplasmic reticulum Ca^{++} loading.[18] To investigate the mechanism of this observed amelioration of diastolic dysfunction in the human heart, isolated ventricular rabbit myocytes were exposed to ATX-II, a toxin that mimics the effects of abnormal opening of the late I_{Na}, and ranolazine prevented the increases in late I_{Na} and intracellular sodium and diastolic calcium ions caused by ATX-II.[18] In isolated ejecting/working

Table 2
Effect of ranolazine on tachyarrhythmias detected after non–ST segment elevation myocardial infarction

	Ranolazine n (%)	Placebo n (%)	RR (95% CI)	P value
Ventricular arrhythmias				
VT ≥ 3 beats ≥ 100 bpm	1646 (52.1)	1933 (60.6)	0.86 (0.82–0.90)	<0.001
VT ≥ 4 beats ≥ 100 bpm	662 (20.9)	941 (29.5)	0.71 (0.6–0.78)	<0.001
VT ≥ 8 beats (lasting <30 s)	166 (5.3)	265 (8.3)	0.63 (0.52–0.76)	<0.001
Polymorphic VT ≥ 8 beats	38 (1.2)	46 (1.4)	0.83 (0.54–1.28)	0.40
Sustained VT (≥30 s)	14 (0.44)	14 (0.44)	1.01 (0.48–2.13)	0.98
Monomorphic	4 (0.13)	7 (0.22)	0.59 (0.17–2.06)	0.37
Polymorphic	10 (0.32)	7 (0.22)	1.41 (0.52–3.78)	0.46
Supraventricular arrhythmias				
New-onset atrial fibrillation	55 (1.7)	75 (2.4)	0.74 (0.52–1.05)	0.08
Other SVT ≥ 120 bpm lasting at least 4 beats	1413 (44.7)	1752 (55.0)	0.81 (0.77–0.85)	<0.001

Abbreviations: bpm, beats per minute; SVT, supraventricular tachycardia; VT, ventricular tachycardia.

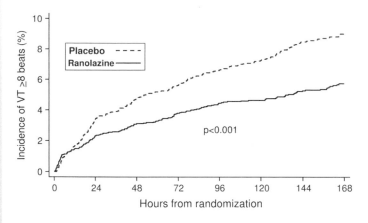

Fig. 13. Kaplan-Meier estimated rates of the first occurrence of an episode of ventricular tachycardia lasting at least 8 beats. The incidence of ventricular tachycardia was significantly lower in patients treated with ranolazine versus placebo at 24 hours after randomization (2.3% versus 3.4%; relative risk [RR], 0.67; 95% CI, 0.50–0.90; P = .008) and 48 hours (3.1% versus 4.7%; RR, 0.65; 95% CI, 0.51–0.84; P < .001). (*From* Scirica BM, Morrow DA, Hod H, et al. Effect of ranolazine, an antianginal agent with novel electrophysiological properties, on the incidence of arrhythmias in patients with non ST-segment elevation ACS: results from the Metabolic Efficiency With Ranolazine for Less Ischemia in Non ST-Elevation Acute Coronary Syndrome Thrombolysis in Myocardial Infarction 36 (MERLIN-TIMI 36) randomized controlled trial. Circulation 2007;116:1650; with permission.)

rat hearts ranolazine prevents the left ventricular systolic and diastolic dysfunction associated with exposure to ischemia (**Fig. 14**).[4] Similarly, isolated rat hearts exposed to hydrogen peroxide, the primary reactive oxygen species associated with detrimental oxidative stress, develop immediate diastolic dysfunction, which can be ameliorated by treatment with ranolazine.[19]

In intact animal models of heart failure ranolazine improves myocardial function. Sabbah and colleagues created chronic heart failure in dogs by intracoronary microembolizations (mean left ventricular ejection fraction 27%) and then administered ranolazine intravenously with a bolus and infusion (1.0 mg/kg/h).[20] Ranolazine significantly increased the ejection fraction (27% to 36%,

P = .0001), the peak left ventricle +dP/dt (1712 to 1900 mm Hg/s, P = .001), and stroke volume (20 to 26 mL, P = .0001) without affecting heart rate or systemic pressure. Using this same model, these investigators subsequently demonstrated that both ranolazine and dobutamine infusions increased left ventricular ejection fraction, stroke volume, cardiac output, and peak +dP/dt, without affecting heart rate or systolic pressure, but that the improvement from ranolazine, in comparison to dobutamine, was related to an increase in left ventricular mechanical efficiency and not to an increase in coronary blood flow or myocardial O_2 consumption.[21] Indices of diastolic dysfunction were not assessed in these studies. In contrast to these studies, Aaker and colleagues created

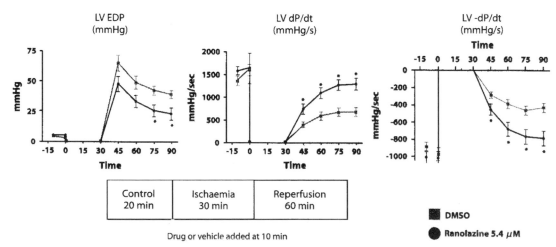

Fig. 14. Ranolazine prevents left ventricular systolic and diastolic dysfunction caused by ischemia in rabbit isolated Langendorff perfused hearts. (*From* Belardinelli L, Antzelevitch C, Fraser H. Inhibition of late (sustained/persistent) sodium current: a potential drug target to reduce intracellular sodium-dependent calcium overload and its detrimental effects on cardiomyocyte function. European Heart Journal 2004;6:16; with permission.)

chronic heart failure in rats by surgically inducing an MI, and then administered ranolazine 50 mg/kg twice a day.[22] They observed that ranolazine did not increase the endurance capacity in these animals, but the doses used in this study were almost 10 times the usual dose in humans.

Preliminary studies in humans suggest that ranolazine may be of clinical usefulness in the management of patients who have diastolic dysfunction associated with ischemic cardiomyopathy. Hayashida and colleagues[23] administered intravenous ranolazine 200 or 500 µg/kg to 15 patients who had previous transmural MI in whom regional left ventricular segments were classified as either normal, ischemia, or infarcted. Administration of ranolazine significantly increased the regional peak filling rate and the regional wall lengthening during the isovolumic relaxation period in the ischemic segments ($P < .05$), indicating an improvement of regional diastolic function, without significant effect on the infarcted segments. Early preliminary experience suggested that ranolazine immediate-release formulation improved the peak filling rate as assessed by echo Doppler analysis of the left ventricular filling dynamics.[24] Similarly, intravenous administration of ranolazine to 15 patients who had ischemic cardiomyopathy led to a significant downward shift of the pressure–volume relationship during diastole accompanied by a reduction in mean diastolic wall stress and increase in end-diastolic volume.[25] A recent preliminary study investigating the proof-of-concept of the effects of ranolazine in patients who had a documented genetic defect in the late sodium channel, the hereditary long QT syndrome LQT3-deltaKPQ, found that intravenous ranolazine shortened the prolonged QTc and significantly improved the associated diastolic dysfunction, as assessed by the left ventricular isovolumic relaxation time and the mitral E-wave velocity.[26]

Further studies in humans investigating the role of ranolazine in treating diastolic dysfunction are ongoing and the results are awaited with great interest.

SUMMARY

Ranolazine is a new compound that has been approved by the FDA for use in patients who have chronic stable angina refractory to conventional antianginal medications. Its mechanism of action does not depend on lowering determinants of myocardial O_2 demand, which is the mechanism used by conventional anti-ischemic medications, but instead it prevents the pathologic persistent opening of the late I_{Na} current, which occurs when the myocardium is exposed to ischemia, heart failure, and oxidative stress. Ranolazine thereby prevents the intracellular sodium and subsequent calcium overload that occurs in these disorders, and the associated myocardial metabolic, electrophysiologic, and mechanical dysfunction. Ranolazine consequently improves diastolic and systolic left ventricular function and preserves myocardial perfusion.

Ranolazine is effective as monotherapy for patients who have stable angina and also effective as part of a combination regimen. In non–ST elevation ACS it reduces recurrent ischemia and ventricular and atrial arrhythmias, but has no effect on mortality or development of MI.

In animal models of heart failure and in preliminary studies in humans, ranolazine improves diastolic and systolic dysfunction.

More studies are needed to evaluate the role of ranolazine as primary therapy for myocardial diastolic and systolic dysfunction and ventricular and atrial arrhythmias.

REFERENCES

1. Gibbons RJ, Abrams J, Chatterjee K, et al. ACC/AHA 2002 guideline update for the management of patients with chronic stable angina—summary article: a report of the American College of Cardiology/American Heart Association Task Force on practice guidelines (Committee on the Management of Patients With Chronic Stable Angina). J Am Coll Cardiol 2003;41:159–68.
2. McCormack JG, Barr RL, Wolff AA, et al. Ranolazine stimulates glucose oxidation in normoxic, ischemic, and reperfused ischemic rat hearts. Circulation 1996;93:135–42.
3. MacInnes A, Fairman DA, Binding P, et al. The antianginal agent trimetazidine does not exert its functional benefit via inhibition of mitochondrial long-chain 3-ketoacyl coenzyme A thiolase. Circ Res 2003;93:e26–32.
4. Belardinelli L, Antzelevitch C, Fraser H. Inhibition of late (sustained/persistent) sodium current: a potential drug target to reduce intracellular sodium-dependent calcium overload and its detrimental effects on cardiomyocyte function. Eur Heart J 2004;6:13–7.
5. Undrovinas AI, Belardinelli L, Undrovinas NA, et al. Ranolazine improves abnormal repolarization and contraction in left ventricular myocytes of dogs with heart failure by inhibiting late sodium current. J Cardiovasc Electrophysiol 2006;17(Suppl 1):S169–77.
6. Antzelevitch C, Belardinelli L, Zygmunt AC, et al. Electrophysiological effects of ranolazine, a novel

antianginal agent with antiarrhythmic properties. Circulation 2004;110:904–10.

7. Belardinelli L, Shryock JC, Fraser H. The mechanism of ranolazine action to reduce ischemia-induced diastolic dysfunction. Eur Heart J 2006;8:A10–3.

8. Song Y, Shryock JC, Wu L, et al. Antagonism by ranolazine of the pro-arrhythmic effects of increasing late INa in guinea pig ventricular myocytes. J Cardiovasc Pharmacol 2004;44:192–9.

9. Chaitman BR. Ranolazine for the treatment of chronic angina and potential use in other cardiovascular conditions. Circulation 2006;113:2462–72.

10. Stone PH, Chaitman BR, Koren A, et al. Effects of ranolazine as monotherapy and combination therapy on rate pressure product at rest and during exercise: results from the MARISA and CARISA trials. Circulation 2006;114(Suppl II):II-715.

11. Rousseau MF, Pouleur H, Cocco G, et al. Comparative efficacy of ranolazine versus atenolol for chronic angina pectoris. Am J Cardiol 2005;95:311–6.

12. Chaitman BR, Skettino SL, Parker JO, et al. Antiischemic effects and long-term survival during ranolazine monotherapy in patients with chronic severe angina. J Am Coll Cardiol 2004;43:1375–82.

13. Chaitman BR, Pepine CJ, Parker JO, et al. Effects of ranolazine with atenolol, amlodipine, or diltiazem on exercise tolerance and angina frequency in patients with severe chronic angina: a randomized controlled trial. JAMA 2004;291:309–16.

14. Stone PH, Gratsiansky NA, Blokhin A, et al. Antianginal efficacy of ranolazine when added to treatment with amlodipine: the ERICA (Efficacy of Ranolazine in Chronic Angina) trial. J Am Coll Cardiol 2006;48: 566–75.

15. Morrow DA, Scirica BM, Karwatowska-Prokopczuk E, et al. Effects of ranolazine on recurrent cardiovascular events in patients with non-ST-elevation acute coronary syndromes: the MERLIN-TIMI 36 randomized trial. JAMA 2007;297:1775–83.

16. Scirica BM, Morrow DA, Hod H, et al. Effect of ranolazine, an antianginal agent with novel electrophysiological properties, on the incidence of arrhythmias in patients with non ST-segment elevation acute coronary syndrome: results from the Metabolic Efficiency With Ranolazine for Less Ischemia in Non ST-Elevation Acute Coronary Syndrome Thrombolysis in Myocardial Infarction 36 (MERLIN-TIMI 36)

randomized controlled trial. Circulation 2007;116: 1647–52.

17. Morrow DA, Scirica BM, Sabatine MS, et al. B-type natriuretic peptide and the effect of ranolazine in patients with non-ST elevation acute coronary syndromes in the MERLIN-TIMI 36 Trial. Circulation 2007;116(Suppl II):II-382.

18. Sossalla S, Wagner S, Rasenack EC, et al. Ranolazine improves diastolic dysfunction in isolated myocardium from failing human hearts—role of late sodium current and intracellular ion accumulation. J Mol Cell Cardiol 2008;45:32–43.

19. Matsumura H, Hara A, Hashizume H, et al. Protective effects of ranolazine, a novel anti-ischemic drug, on the hydrogen peroxide-induced derangements in isolated, perfused rat heart: comparison with dichloroacetate. Jpn J Pharmacol 1998;77: 31–9.

20. Sabbah HN, Chandler MP, Mishima T, et al. Ranolazine, a partial fatty acid oxidation (pFOX) inhibitor, improves left ventricular function in dogs with chronic heart failure. J Card Fail 2002;8:416–22.

21. Chandler MP, Stanley WC, Morita H, et al. Short-term treatment with ranolazine improves mechanical efficiency in dogs with chronic heart failure. Circ Res 2002;91:278–80.

22. Aaker A, McCormack JG, Hirai T, et al. Effects of ranolazine on the exercise capacity of rats with chronic heart failure induced by myocardial infarction. J Cardiovasc Pharmacol 1996;28:353–62.

23. Hayashida W, van Eyll C, Rousseau MF, et al. Effects of ranolazine on left ventricular regional diastolic function in patients with ischemic heart disease. Cardiovasc Drugs Ther 1994;8:741–7.

24. Rousseau MF, Cocco G, Bouvy T, et al. Effects of a novel metabolic modulator, ranolazine, on exercise tolernace and left ventricular filling dynamics in patients with angina pectoris. Circulation 1992; 86(Suppl I):I-714.

25. Rousseau MF, Van Eyll C, Van Mechelen HV, et al. Novel metabolic modulator ranolazine selectively improves diastolic function in heart failure. Circulation 1992;86(Suppl I):I-375.

26. Moss A, Zareba WZ, Schwarz KQ, et al. Ranolazine shortens repolarization and improves myocardial relaxation in patients with type-3 long QT syndrome. J Am Coll Cardiol 2008;51(Suppl A):A15.

Anticoagulants in Coronary Artery Disease

L. Veronica Lee, MD

KEYWORDS
- Anticoagulant • Acute coronary syndrome
- Acute myocardial infarction • Unstable angina • Therapy

Acute coronary syndromes, such as unstable angina (UA) and myocardial infarction (MI), are the result of plaque rupture and the formation of thrombus that occludes the coronary artery. The mechanism of thrombus formation has been a primary target of cardiovascular acute and preventive therapy for half a century. Thrombus formation is the result of the activation of thrombin, and activation and aggregation of platelets. Thrombin has a central role in thrombus formation because it can directly activate platelets, convert fibrinogen to fibrin, and activate factor XIIIa, which crosslinks fibrin forming a stable clot. Medical therapy for acute coronary syndromes has therefore been directed at inhibition of these two targets, thrombin and platelets, through combined therapy. Previously these agents have been referred to as antithrombotics, but because they have multiple affects beyond thrombin the term anticoagulation has been recommended by the current guidelines. The anticoagulants discussed are ones that have been used in clinical trials and are approved or anticipated for use in coronary artery disease.

Anticoagulants can be divided into unfractionated and low molecular weight heparin (LMWH) (enoxaparin, dalteparin, tinzaparin), direct thrombin inhibitors (argatroban, bivalirudin, inogatran, and lepirudin), heparinoids or synthetic heparins (danaparoid, fondaparinux), and the oral anticoagulant warfarin.

UNFRACTIONATED HEPARIN

Unfractionated heparin (UFH) is made primarily from porcine bowel or bovine lung and is composed of many different molecular weight glycosaminoglycans (5,000–30,000 d) with variable antithrombin activity. UFH indirectly inhibits thrombin by binding and causing a conformational change in antithrombin (also known as antithrombin III) increasing its activity against thrombin (factor IIa) 1000-fold and inactivating factor Xa and to a smaller degree factors IXa, XIa, and XIIa. UFH stabilizes and reduces further clot formation, but does not dissolve the thrombus nor does it have action against clot-bound active thrombin. The anticoagulant effect of UFH must be monitored using activated partial thromboplastin time (aPTT) to reach a prespecified target range by using a weight-adjusted nomogram that has been standardized for the health care center providing heparin therapy.[1–3] Body weight, age, sex, smoking, and diabetes are known to be factors that alter the degree of anticoagulation achieved with a specific dose of UFH.[1–5] UFH at high doses is primarily metabolized by the kidneys and should be adjusted if there is a reduction in creatinine clearance.[3]

UNFRACTIONATED HEPARIN IN ST SEGMENT ELEVATION MYOCARDIAL INFARCTION WITH FIBRINOLYTICS

Most of the trial data that support the use of UFH in ST segment elevation myocardial infarction (STEMI) is based on trials that did not use aspirin (ASA). These earlier trials supported the use of UFH and oral anticoagulants for reducing ultimate infarct size, reinfarction, and embolization, but this is not relevant to our current standard of care.[6–8] ASA is now routinely used, although there has

Division of Cardiology, Yale University School of Medicine, 789 Howard Avenue, FMP3, New Haven, CT 06437, USA

E-mail address: lveronica.lee@yale.edu

Cardiol Clin 26 (2008) 615–628
doi:10.1016/j.ccl.2008.07.002

not been a randomized controlled trial to directly evaluate the use of ASA with and without heparin in patients who had or did not have reperfusion therapy. When fibrinolytics are used a procoagulable state is created and coadministration or early administration of anticoagulants, such as heparin, is recommended with fibrin-specific fibrinolytics (eg, alteplase) because recurrent thrombosis has been demonstrated in their absence.[9] When fibrin-specific fibrinolytics are used, a procoagulable state is created that demonstrates a marked increase in fibrinopeptide A as a result of thrombin binding to soluble fibrin degradation products. Non–fibrin-specific fibrinolytics (streptokinase, anistreplase) do not demonstrate a benefit in the reduction of mortality or reinfarction with adjuvant treatment with UFH and are associated with an increased risk for hemorrhage.[10–14]

Fibrin-specific fibrinolytic trials have had variable results in part because of the difficulty in achieving adequate anticoagulation early with UFH without either under- or overshooting the desired target range established to achieve inhibition of the procoagulable state without increasing the risk for hemorrhage. The current American College of Cardiology/American Heart Association (ACC/AHA) guidelines recommend the use of heparin with fibrin-specific fibrinolytics and select patients treated with non–fibrin-specific fibrinolytics who are at an increased risk for systemic embolization (atrial fibrillation, history of embolization, left ventricular thrombus, anterior or extensive MI).[15] UFH is to be administered as a 60 U/kg intravenous bolus (IVB) (≤4000 U) followed by an intravenous infusion (IVF) of UFH at 12 U/kg/h (≤1000 U/h). A target aPTT has been established as 50 to 70 seconds because other studies with more aggressive anticoagulation and a higher upper end target of anticoagulation resulted in increased hemorrhagic complications.[16–20] The length of treatment with UFH after MI has not been established. If a patient is at risk for embolization (atrial fibrillation, history of embolization, left ventricular thrombus, anterior or extensive MI, or heart failure) prolonged administration should be considered.[21]

UNFRACTIONATED HEPARIN IN ST SEGMENT ELEVATION MYOCARDIAL INFARCTION WITH PRIMARY PERCUTANEOUS INTERVENTION

Primary percutaneous intervention (PCI) routinely uses UFH to prevent thrombosis and acute vessel closure. A target activating clotting time (ACT) of 250 to 350 seconds is used. If glycoprotein receptor inhibitors are used the target range is reduced to 200 to 250 seconds.[22–24] Preprocedure and postprocedure heparin administration does not improve efficacy of PCI and is associated with an increased risk for hemorrhage and vascular complications.[25]

UNFRACTIONATED HEPARIN AND EARLY CONSERVATIVE THERAPY FOR UNSTABLE ANGINA / NON–ST SEGMENT ELEVATION MYOCARDIAL INFARCTION

Early studies in patients who had UA and non–ST segment elevation myocardial infarction (UA/NSTEMI) with UFH and ASA demonstrated a 54% reduction compared with placebo in the composite endpoint of reinfarction or death during the first week of therapy and the addition of UFH to ASA versus ASA alone yielded a relative risk (RR) of 33% at follow-up during weeks 2 to 12.[26,27] The benefit to therapy is of short duration and there is evidence of a prothrombotic state once UFH is discontinued leading to the observed heparin rebound that has also been seen with other anticoagulants.[19,28–32] The now recommended weight-adjusted regimen is an initial 60 U/kg IVB (maximum 4000 U) followed by 12 U/kg/h IVF (maximum 1000 U/h) with an appropriate aPTT target range and nomograms for adjusting dose determined by local laboratory protocol that corresponds to anti-factor Xa concentration of 0.3 to 0.7 U/mL.[5] Dosing should be monitored every 6 hours until two measures are within the prespecified target range, then once daily with platelet count and hemoglobin measurement unless there is a clinical change that warrants additional testing of aPTT and blood counts (hypotension, recurrent ischemia, or suspected hemorrhage). Duration of UFH therapy for UA/NSTEMI has not been clearly defined.

UNFRACTIONATED HEPARIN AND EARLY INVASIVE THERAPY FOR ACUTE CORONARY SYNDROME

Unfractionated heparin has been used in PCI as the gold standard until more recent randomized clinical trials have been performed against newer agents. Results of these trials are discussed later under the particular agents. UFH remains the preferred choice if a patient is going to require emergent coronary artery bypass graft (CABG) (<24 h).

HEPARIN-INDUCED THROMBOCYTOPENIA

One of the obstacles to heparin therapy is heparin-induced thrombocytopenia (HIT), an immune-mediated reduction in platelets that occurs in 2.5% to 3.0% of patients who have prior exposure to heparin or exposure for approximately 4 days with a platelet count decline of 50% or greater.[33]

It is caused by antibodies that are formed against the unit formed by platelet factor 4 bound to heparin. HIT has been connected to both arterial and venous thrombosis. Delayed HIT has been seen with a median onset of 14 days after heparin has been stopped.[34] HIT is often underdiagnosed and it is recommended that daily platelet counts be made while on UFH; this is not needed for LMWH or the heparinoid fondaparinux.[35] In the case of a suspected or known history of HIT, anticoagulation should be changed to bivalirudin in patients who have STEMI. Patients who have a history of HIT have been able to have limited use of heparin during cardiopulmonary bypass with success after absence of HIT antibodies has been confirmed.[36–38]

LOW MOLECULAR WEIGHT HEPARINS

LMWHs come from depolymerized UFH and because of their similar smaller weights have a more reproducible antithrombin activity. Approximately 25% to 50% of a LMWH is long enough ($\geq$18 polysaccharides) to have both factor Xa and thrombin activity. LMWH has a greater effect on factor Xa than thrombin and cannot be measured using aPTT, although monitoring of Xa activity is possible. LMWH delivers a more uniform and predictable level of anticoagulation and has a lower association with HIT. LMWHs, because of their longer half-life, lack of reliance on aPTT measurement, and more reliable anticoagulant effect, can be given subcutaneously with less frequent dosing than UFH to achieve a similar benefit. Protamine is more effective in reversing the anticoagulant effects of UFH than LMWH. The prolonged anticoagulant effect with LMWH has been of importance clinically when anticoagulation is changed for an invasive procedure or in anticipation of surgery, as discussed later.

LOW MOLECULAR WEIGHT HEPARIN AND ST SEGMENT ELEVATION MYOCARDIAL INFARCTION AND FIBRINOLYTICS

Trials suggest that there is a benefit when using LMWH as compared with UFH with nonspecific fibrinolytics (eg, streptokinase) with improved clinical outcomes.[39] Benefit has also been found when used in STEMI patients treated with fibrin-specific fibrinolytics and LMWH versus UFH.[40–45] A large meta-analysis of more than 27,000 patients receiving enoxaparin used a combined primary efficacy and safety endpoint of mortality and reinfarction within 30 days of initial STEMI and found a reduction in the enoxaparin-treated group as compared with the UFH group (11.1% versus 12.9%, odds ratio [OR] 0.84, 95% CI 0.73–0.9).[46] Major hemorrhage occurred more frequently in the enoxaparin group as compared with UFH treated patients (2.6% versus 1.8%), which translates into a decrease in 21 deaths or reinfarctions for an increase of four nonfatal major hemorrhages. Increased hemorrhage risk was found in patients 75 years or older and with reduced renal function.

LOW MOLECULAR WEIGHT HEPARIN AND EARLY CONSERVATIVE THERAPY FOR UNSTABLE ANGINA/NON–ST SEGMENT ELEVATION MYOCARDIAL INFARCTION

There are eight major randomized trials that have explored the effect of LMWH as an alternative therapy of UFH in UA/NESTMI patients. Most data from trials comparing UFH and LMWH are with enoxaparin. Trials with dalteparin and nadroparin did not demonstrate improved efficacy for death and reinfarction.[28,47,48] Enoxaparin was found to decrease mortality and nonfatal MI event rates in five of six trials, when analyzed together demonstrating an OR of 0.91 (95% CI 0.83–0.99).[49–54] Hemorrhage rates are in general more prominent in LMWH as compared with UFH heparin, but these are primarily minor and related to the injection site.[40,41] Because none of these studies directly compared the different LMWHs the presence or absence of a class effect cannot be determined in these dissimilar trials that allowed open-label use of anticoagulants before randomization, and different doses, study designs, and populations. The exception is the Enoxaparin Versus Tinzaparin (EVET) (n = 436) trial that compared enoxaparin and tinzaparin in patients who had UA/NSTEMI with LMWH administered for 7 days. There was a decreased rate of the composite endpoint of death, nonfatal MI, or recurrent angina present at 7 days that persisted to the 6-month endpoint in the enoxaparin group as compared with tinzaparin (6 month 22.5% versus 44.0%, $p<.001$) without a difference in hemorrhage.[55,56] Other studies that did not directly compare LMWH to UFH but used placebo are not discussed here.[57]

LOW MOLECULAR WEIGHT HEPARIN AND EARLY INVASIVE THERAPY FOR ACUTE CORONARY SYNDROME

LMWH during PCI cannot be monitored by ACT and in earlier trials UFH was used during PCI for a target ACT greater than 350 seconds with LMWH being stopped before CABG successfully.[50,58,59] The Superior Yield of the New Strategy of Enoxaparin, Revascularization and Glycoprotein IIb/IIIa Inhibitors (SYNERGY) trial (n = 9978) studied high-risk UA/NSTEMI patients during PCI randomized to receive either enoxaparin or UFH.[54] Although there was no significant difference in efficacy, there was a significant increase in TIMI-defined major hemorrhage (9.1% versus 7.6%, p = .008) that post hoc seemed related to the use of UFH in enoxaparin patients at PCI.[60] It is therefore suggested that anticoagulant therapy not be changed if possible during PCI until this can be evaluated further.[26] The guidelines suggest that if substitution is necessary that LMWH be stopped approximately 8 hours before PCI and UFH use and that LMWH be discontinued 24 hours before CABG when possible to minimize hemorrhage.

DIRECT THROMBIN INHIBITORS

Direct thrombin inhibitors directly bind to thrombin and inactivate at least one of its active sites. Unlike heparin they do not require a cofactor to work, can inactivate clot-bound thrombin, are less affected by circulating inhibitors than heparin (eg, platelet factor 4), and inhibit thrombin activation of platelets. They also interact less with circulating plasma proteins. Hirudin was the first to be developed as a recombinant protein derived from the one produced from the salivary gland of the medicinal leech (Hirudo medicinalis). Hirudin blocks thrombin's action by binding to the substrate (fibrinogen binding) and catalytic sites. Hirulog, now known as bivalirudin, is a peptide analog that binds thrombin at the same two sites as hirudin.[61] Argatroban is an arginine derivative that competitively binds the catalytic site of thrombin. It is approved for use in patients who have heparin-induced thrombocytopenia, but is not recommended for use in ACS in the current guidelines.[62,63] The dose of argatroban is given as a continuous infusion of 2 μg/kg/m and then adjusted according to aPTT or ACT. It is hepatically metabolized. Oral direct thrombin inhibitors have not been successful to date in cardiac patients; ximelagatran, the last tested, was associated with an increase in MI and severe liver damage.

DIRECT THROMBIN INHIBITORS AND ST SEGMENT ELEVATION MYOCARDIAL INFARCTION

Small clinical trials HIT, TIMI-5, and TIMI-6 suggested that direct thrombin inhibition in STEMI receiving either fibrin-specific or nonspecific fibrinolytics suggested a benefit as compared with treatment with UFH.[64,65] After an increased rate of intracranial hemorrhage in both treatment arms

in GUSTO-IIA and TIMI-9a caused the trials to be halted, further evaluation of hirudin was performed at a lower dose in GUSTO-IIb (also included UA/NSTEMI and PCI), TIMI-9B, and HIT-4.[31,66] There were no significant differences found in the primary efficacy endpoints or hemorrhage in these trials.

Hirulog (bivalirudin) in the HERO pilot trial of STEMI patients receiving fibrinolytics therapy with streptokinase and ASA demonstrated an increase in TIMI grade 3 flow without an increase in hemorrhage with bivalirudin.[67] HERO-2, which compared bivalirudin with UFH in STEMI treated with streptokinase, demonstrated a significant reduction in reinfarction at 96 hours (1.6% bivalirudin versus 2.3% UFH) and a trend toward increased major hemorrhage (0.7% versus 0.5%, p = .07) and intracranial hemorrhage (0.6 % versus 0.4 % p = .09). The ACC/AHA guidelines (2004) have recommended that bivalirudin be considered as a reasonable therapy in patients treated with streptokinase and with a history of HIT to heparin therapy.[15] Dosing of bivalirudin is to include an initial IVB of 0.25 mg/kg followed by a continuous IVF of 0.5 mg/kg/h for 12 hours and then dose reduction to 0.25 mg/kg/h for 36 hours. The dose of bivalirudin should be adjusted in renal insufficiency and if during the first 12 hours an aPTT is greater than 75 seconds.

PCI was evaluated in the HORIZON study (n = 3600) in STEMI patients randomized to treatment with UFH and GP IIb/IIIa inhibitors or bivalirudin and "provisional" GP IIb/IIIa inhibitors.[68,69] Bivalirudin was given in an IVB of 0.75 mg/kg followed by a continuous IVF of 1.75 mg/kg/h until post-PCI. There was no significant difference in the primary efficacy endpoint of death, reinfarction, ischemic target vessel revascularization, or stroke (5.4% versus 5.5%). Non-CABG major hemorrhage was less in the bivalirudin group, however (4.9% versus 8.3%).

There are limited data with argatroban from the MINT trial (n= 125) in which STEMI patients treated with alteplase were randomized to receive either argatroban or UFH.[70] There was improved attainment of TIMI 3 flow especially in patients presenting late (>3 hours) and a reduction in major hemorrhage in the argatroban group compared with UFH. Clinical efficacy could not be assessed in this preliminary study.

DIRECT THROMBIN INHIBITORS AND EARLY CONSERVATIVE STRATEGY NON–ST SEGMENT ELEVATION MYOCARDIAL INFARCTION AND UNSTABLE ANGINA

GUSTO IIB evaluated 8011 patients who had suspected NSTEMI treated with ASA and then randomly assigned to either intravenous hirudin (0.1 mg/kg IVB and 0.1 mg/kg/h IVF for 3 to 5 days) or UFH.[17] At 30 days the primary efficacy endpoint of death, nonfatal MI, or reinfarction was reduced in the hirudin group 9.1% versus 8.3% in the UFH group, respectively (OR 0.90, $p = .22$). The Organization to Assess Strategies for Ischemic Syndromes (OASIS-2) trial (n = 10,141) used the middle dose found in their pilot to again assess the benefit of hirudin (0.4 mg/kg IVB and 0.15 mg/kg/h IVF) versus UFH (5000 IU IVB plus 15 U/kg/h IVF) administered for 72 hours in patients who had UA/NSTEMI.[71] The composite efficacy endpoint of death or new infarction was decreased in the hirudin group (3.6 %) versus the UFH group (4.2%) at 7 days (RR 0.84, $p = .06$), but more transfusions were required in the hirudin group (1.2% versus 0.7% with heparin, $p = .014$). At present bivalirudin is not recommended for UA/NSTEMI treated conservatively.

DIRECT THROMBIN INHIBITORS AND EARLY INVASIVE STRATEGY NON–ST SEGMENT ELEVATION MYOCARDIAL INFARCTION AND UNSTABLE ANGINA

A subset of patients in the GUSTO IIB trial (n = 1410) were treated with PCI and were found with hirudin to have a benefit in death and reinfarction rates versus UFH with a small increase in hemorrhage.[72] RE-PLACE 2 found bivalirudin (0.75 mg/kg IVB followed by 1.75 mg/kg/h IVF) to be non-inferior at one year compared with UFH (65 U/kg IVB) in patients undergoing elective or urgent PCI treated with provisional GP IIb/IIIa inhibition.[73–75] The Acuity trial compared in a 2 × 2 open-label randomized factorial design the use of UFH versus enoxaparin with and without GP IIb/IIIa inhibition with and without upstream bivalrudin.[76] PCI was done using an early invasive approach with a mean time to PCI of 4 hours. Non-inferiority was demonstrated in the heparin versus bivalirudin groups receiving GP IIb/IIIa inhibitors for the 30 day composite endpoints of ischemia or major bleeding. Non-inferiority in the composite endpoints was also found in the group receiving bivalirudin alone compared with the group receiving heparin and GP IIb/IIIa inhibitors with less hemorrhage (3.0% versus 5.7%, $p<.001$, RR 0.53, 95% CI 0.43–0.65) and statistically significant superiority in clinical outcome at 30 days (10.1% versus 11.7%, respectively, $p = 0.015$, RR 0.86, 95% CI 0.77–0.97). Thienopyridine before PCI demonstrated a 7.0% composite endpoint reduction in the bivalirudin alone group (9.1% without thienopyridine) versus 7.3% in the heparin plus GP IIb/IIIa inhibition (7.1% without thienopyridine). Bivalirudin is approved for UA/NSTEMI in patients

who have a planned early invasive strategy, including PCI. It is recommended that in patients who have delayed PCI or early ischemia who are using bivalirudin or heparin, a thienopyridine or GP IIb/IIIa inhibitor should be given before PCI to achieve the most benefit.[26] Unlike the heparins there are few data and there is no specific protocol for controlling the increase in hemorrhage associated with changing therapy at the time of PCI.

HEPARINOIDS

Fondaparinux, which is a synthetic heparin pentapeptide, has direct action on antithrombin that specifically inhibits factor Xa. In the setting of hemorrhage protamine can be used to reverse UFH and LMWH, but not fondaparinux, which requires transfusion of fresh frozen plasma to restore coagulation factors. Danaparoid is a combination of heparin, chondroitin, and dermatan sulfates and as a result can be used in patients who have HIT with less than 10% cross-reactivity.[77] The synthetic heparin fondaparinux was used in OASIS-6 (n = 12,000) in two different groups. In one group UFH was not indicated (majority had streptokinase fibrinolysis) and patients were randomized to receive fondaparinux (2.5 mg/d for 8 days) or placebo, and in the other group heparin was indicated (primary PCI, fibrin-specific fibrinolysis, or no reperfusion) and patients were randomized to receive UFH (24–48 hours) or fondaparinux (2.5 mg/d for 8 days).[78] Both groups compared with no heparin or UFH demonstrated a significant reduction in death and nonfatal reinfarctions at 30 days (9.7% versus 11.2%, hazards ratio 0.86, 95% CI 0.77–0.96). Both endpoint reductions of mortality and nonfatal reinfarctions were independently significant at 30 days. Analysis of the separate groups did not find a significant difference in patients who required heparin therapy because of a trend toward worse clinical outcomes in patients who had primary PCI (increase in catheter thrombosis, abrupt closure, dissection, and lack of flow). In the group of patients who did not require heparin the benefit seen may have been the result of the prolonged anticoagulation. Based on current data use in primary PCI is contraindicated and use with fibrinolysis requires further evaluation.

OASIS 5 was designed to evaluate the use of enoxaparin (1.0 mg/kg subcutaneously twice a day, with renal dosing for creatinine clearance less than 30 mL/min) versus fondaparinux (2.5 mg subcutaneously every day) for a mean of 6 days in ACS patients (n = 20,078) undergoing PCI.[79] Initially PCI was performed with UFH (65 U/kg with GP IIb/IIIa inhibitor, 100 U/kg without) in the enoxaparin arm if more than 6 hours from last dose because there was a lack of data and the FDA had not approved enoxaparin for PCI. OASIS 5 was revised after there was found to be more catheter-related thrombus in the fondaparinux arm during PCI to include UFH IVB at the operator's discretion. Non-inferiority was demonstrated at 9 and 30 days for the composite endpoint of death, MI, or refractory ischemia. There was a significant decrease in mortality at 30 days (295 fondaparinux versus 352 enoxaparin, $p = .02$) and at 180 days, and in the combined endpoint of reinfarctions, stroke, and death at 180 days ($p = .007$). Major hemorrhage was significantly lower in fondaparinux group (2.2%) versus enoxaparin (4.1%, $p<.001$), although this may have to do with the crossover to UFH in the enoxaparin group, which was associated with increased hemorrhage in SYNERGY. Fondaparinux has been recommended in the treatment of UA/NSTEMI with the use of UFH 50 to 60 U/kg intravenously during PCI, although further evaluation is warranted because UFH use was not prespecified and controlled in OASIS 5.[26] UFH is still preferred in patients who may require CABG within 24 hours.

WARFARIN: LONG-TERM ANTICOAGULATION AND ORAL ANTICOAGULANTS

Although there have been attempts to find a substitute for warfarin as an oral anticoagulant, warfarin remains the only approved option for cardiac use. Warfarin is composed of S and R enantiomers and when strongly bound to protein, chiefly albumin, is inactive. If warfarin is displaced from the proteins that bind it activity is increased. The S form, more physiologically active, is metabolized in the liver by the CYP2C9 enzyme system, which is inducible by medications. Warfarin inhibits the vitamin K–dependent coagulation factors II, VII, IX, and X, and inhibitor proteins C and S increasing factors VIII and V activity. The effect of warfarin does not reach full potency until 36 to 72 hours after the first dose is given and factor II levels are reduced. Typically a higher dose of warfarin is given the first 2 days of therapy (2–5 mg at bedtime).[80–82] Higher doses have been found to lead to a hypercoagulable state from initial effects on protein C and a falsely elevated international normalized ratio (INR) through isolated effects on the extrinsic pathway and factor VII without complete inhibition of intrinsic pathways. As a result heparin therapy is typically recommended to overlap for 4 to 5 days when initiating therapy to prevent protein C–related effects and allow for complete inhibition of the intrinsic pathway. A black box warning has been added to labeling by the FDA because of the association of warfarin and hemorrhage and death. Risk factors for hemorrhage include increasing age, female, hypertension, diabetes, liver or renal disease, alcoholism, malignancy, anemia, diarrhea, heart failure, fever, prior hemorrhage (eg, intracranial, active gastrointestinal), bleeding disorder (platelet or coagulation disorder, concomitant medications affecting platelets or coagulation factors), prior stroke, genetic variations in hepatic enzyme pathway, prior hemorrhage on therapeutic warfarin, noncompliance, abnormal INR or difficult-to-regulate INR. If the INR is less than 5.0 but above the desired target range then the risk for hemorrhage is lower and withholding a dose and decreasing the subsequent dose should be sufficient to attain a therapeutic INR in target range with close monitoring.[83] If the INR is between 5.0 and 9.0, however, then there is a 1% risk for hemorrhage within the next 30 days that remains even after the anticoagulation has been corrected.[84] If there is no active bleeding and the INR is between 5.0 and 9.0, holding the dose with or without oral vitamin K is recommended.[85] INR greater than 9.0 without bleeding should have warfarin therapy stopped temporarily and oral vitamin K administered. If there is active bleeding on warfarin therapy warfarin should be stopped, and intravenous vitamin K and fresh frozen plasma administered.[86–91] If the hemorrhage is more emergent prothrombin complex or recombinant human factor VIIa can be administered.

Warfarin requires careful monitoring so that the predetermined target INR is reached and not exceeded. Any changes in a patient's diet or over-the-counter or prescription medications that affect vitamin K levels require increased vigilance for side effects, alterations in INR, and appropriate adjustment of warfarin dosing. A meta-analysis demonstrated in more than 50,000 patients that INR is outside of the target range 64% of the time with self-monitoring achieving the best rates at 72%.[92]

Currently warfarin is not indicated for patients who have a diagnosis of ACS, unless there is a secondary indication. Secondary indications include left ventricular thrombus, left ventricular aneurysm, atrial fibrillation, mechanical valve replacement, and so forth. There are numerous trials that have been performed in STEMI patients comparing ASA to the addition of warfarin to ASA with different INR target ranges from high to low intensity (<1.5–4.8). Of the trials that demonstrated benefit to warfarin therapy after STEMI (WARIS II, APRICOT-2, ASPECT-2) there was often difficulty maintaining target range INR, high discontinuation rates, and increased bleeding.[93–96] Patients were also not treated with newer antiplatelet agents, which limits the applicability of data from these

Table 1
Summary of 2007 anticoagulant for therapy of ST segment elevation myocardial infarction, American College of Cardiology/American Heart Association guideline update

Reperfusion/PCI/Supportive	Dosing	Evidence
Reperfusion with fibrinolytic	IV anticoagulant ≥48 h (max 8 d)	Class I, Level C
IV anticoagulation ≥48 h	Avoid UFH, reduce HIT	Class I, Level A
UFH dosing for maximum 48 h	60 U IVB per kg (maximum 4000 U) followed by IV infusion of 12 U/kg/h (maximum 1000 U/h) adjust to aPTT of 1.5–2.0 times control (approximately 50–70 s)	Class I, Level C
Enoxaparin (Cr<2.5 mg/dL men, <2.0 women)	<75 y old IVB 30 mg and SC 1.0 mg/kg q 12 h start 15 min after IVB	Class I, Level A
Duration of hospitalization or for maximum 8 days	≥75 y old No IVB, SC 0.75 mg/kg q 12 h CrCl<30 mL/min SC 1.0 mg/kg q 24 h	
Fondaparinux (Cr<3.0 mg/dL) Duration of hospitalization or for maximum 8 days	First dose 2.5 mg IV then 2.5 mg SC once daily	Class I, Level B
Post-PCI	Dosing to adjust if GPIIb/IIIa receptor inhibitor given for UFH and enoxaparin	Class I, Level C
PCI with prior UFH	Bolus with UFH to support procedure Bolus with bivalirudin to support procedure	Class I, Level C Class I, Level C
PCI with prior enoxaparin	Within 8 h: no additional enoxaparin Within 8–12 h: 0.3 mg/kg enoxaparin IV	Class I, Level B
PCI with prior fondaparinux	Anti-IIa anticoagulant adjusting if GPIIb/IIIa receptor inhibitor given	Class I, Level C
Fondaparinux in PCI	Not to be used alone as anticoagulant because of increase in catheter thrombosis	Class III, Level C
Supportive therapy for STEMI (no reperfusion)	IV or SC UFH or SC LMWH for ≥48 h or ambulatory	Class IIa, Level C
LMWH Fondaparinux	For more than 48 h and up to 8 d to reduce HIT as dosed above for patients treated with fibrinolytics	Class IIa, Level C Class IIa, Level B

Data from Antman EM, Hand M, Armstrong PW, et al. 2007 focused update of the ACC/AHA 2004 guidelines for the management of patients with ST-elevation myocardial infarction. J Am Coll Cardiol 2008;51:172–209.

trials to current standard of care, such as for patients receiving stents and clopidogrel.

Although there is a possible theoretic advantage to long-term anticoagulation with warfarin or subcutaneous LMWH after discontinuation of intravenous anticoagulation (eg, prothrombotic state noted post–intravenous anticoagulant therapy and exposed prothrombotic material at healing site of infarct-related artery) data have not supported long-term use.[97,98] In the setting of UA there are limited trial data; however, two study groups have suggested benefit in reduction of ischemic events with a small increased risk for hemorrhagic complications in some patient groups (ATACS, OASIS, OASIS 2) from warfarin after UA.[99–101] Currently our approach to patients who have UA/NSTEMI has changed to include an early invasive strategy with stent placement and the use of newer antiplatelet agents, such as clopidogrel. Clopidogrel is frequently used in patients who are allergic to ASA who in the past might have been recommended to receive warfarin. As a result warfarin should only be used in the setting of a secondary indication, and when adding antiplatelet therapy post-stent with ASA and clopidogrel assessment of hemorrhagic risk and careful

Table 2
Intravenous anticoagulants for unstable angina/non–ST segment elevation myocardial infarction from American College of Cardiology/American Heart Association guidelines

Drug	Initial Medical Treatment	Received Initial Treatment	Did not Receive Initial Treatment	After PCI
Bivalirudin	0.1 mg/kg bolus, 0.25 mg/kg/h infusion	0.5 mg/kg bolus, increase infusion to 1.75 mg/kg/h	0.75 mg/kg bolus, 1.75 mg/kg/h infusion	No additional treatment or continue infusion for up to 4 h
Dalteparin	120 IU/kg SC every 12 h (maximum 10,000 IU twice daily)	IV GP IIb/IIIa planned: target ACT 200 s using UFH. No IV GP IIb/IIIa planned: target ACT 250–300 s for HemoTec; 300–350 s for Hemochron using UFH	IV GP IIb/IIIa planned: 60–70 U/kg of UFH. No IV GP IIb/IIIa planned: 100–140 U/kg of UFH	No additional treatment
Enoxaparin	LD of 30 mg IV bolus may be given. 1 mg/kg SC every 12 h; extend dosing interval to 1 mg/kg every 24 h if estimated creatinine clearance less than 30 mL per min	Last SC dose less than 8 h: no additional therapy. Last SC dose greater than 8 h: 0.3 mg/kg IV bolus	0.5–0.75 mg/kg IV bolus	No additional treatment
Fondaparinux	2.5 mg SC once daily. Avoid for creatinine clearance less than 30 mL/min	50–60 U/kg IV bolus of UFH is recommended by the OASIS 5 investigators	50–60 U/kg IV bolus of UFH is recommended by the OASIS 5 investigators	No additional treatment
Unfractionated heparin	LD of 60 U/kg (max 4000 U) as IV bolus. IV infusion of 12 U/kg/h (max 1000 U/h) to maintain aPTT at 1.5 to 2.0 times control (approximately 50–70 s)	IV GP IIb/IIIa planned: target ACT 200 s. No IV GP IIb/IIIa planned: target ACT 250–300 s for HemoTec; 300–350 s for Hemochron	IV GP IIb/IIIa planned: 60–70 U/kg. No IV GP IIb/IIIa planned: 100–140 U/ kg	No additional treatment

Data from Antman EM, Hand M, Armstrong PW, et al. 2007 focused update of the ACC/AHA 2004 guidelines for the management of patients with ST-elevation myocardial infarction. J Am Coll Cardiol 2008;51:172–209.

Table 3
Summary of anticoagulant therapy unstable angina/non–ST segment elevation myocardial infarction from American College of Cardiology/American Heart Association guidelines

Evidence	Therapy	Evidence
Early invasive/conservative	Anticoagulant in addition to antiplatelet therapy without delay at presentation	Class I, Level A
Early invasive choice of anticoagulant	Enoxaparin UFH Bivalirudin Fondaparinux	Class I, Level A Class I, Level A Class I, Level B Class I, Level B
Conservative therapy choice of anticoagulant	Enoxaparin UFH Fondaparinux	Class I, Level A Class I, Level A Class I, Level B
Conservative therapy at increased risk for hemorrhage	Fondaparinux	Class I, Level B
Conservative without CABG in 24 h	Enoxaparin or fondaparinux preferred over UFH	Class IIa, Level B
Conservative therapy duration of anticoagulation	UFH for 48 h or enoxaparin or fondaparinux for hospitalization or up to 8 days	Class I, Level A
Anticipated CABG		
UFH	Continue UFH preoperatively	Class I, Level B
Enoxaparin	Discontinue 12–24 h before CABG and change to UFH	Class I, Level B
Fondaparinux	Discontinue 24 h before CABG and change to UFH	Class I, Level B
Bivalirudin	Discontinue 3 h before CABG and change to UFH	Class I, Level B
Post–uncomplicated PCI	Discontinue anticoagulant therapy	Class I, Level B
Post-PCI: medical management	No significant obstructive coronary artery disease at discretion of clinician	Class I, Level C
UFH	Continue for at least 48 h or until discharge	Class I, Level A
Enoxaparin	Continue duration of hospitalization or maximum of 8 days	Class I, Level A
Fondaparinux	Continue duration of hospitalization or maximum of 8 days	Class I, Level B
Bivalirudin	Discontinue or reduce dose to 0.25 mg/kg/h for a maximum of 72 h	Class I, Level B
Conservative therapy with no additional angiography or stress testing	UFH for 48 h or fondaparinux or enoxaparin continue duration of hospitalization or maximum of 8 days	Class I, Level A

Data from Antman EM, Hand M, Armstrong PW, et al. 2007 focused update of the ACC/AHA 2004 guidelines for the management of patients with ST-elevation myocardial infarction. J Am Coll Cardiol 2008;51:172–209.

monitoring are recommended until further studies can assess combination therapy.

SUMMARY

Anticoagulant therapy has evolved greatly in the past allowing for more options than before, and a better understanding of the risk and benefit of using these medications has been achieved through elaborate clinical trials. We have achieved better control of UFH through weight-adjusted nomograms and found other agents that achieve a longer, more predictable level of anticoagulation. Newer agents also have been able to directly affect clot-bound thrombin. We are now in need of further investigation into the interaction of antiplatelet and anticoagulant agents with our newer invasive therapies to improve efficacy and safety.

In addition, further investigation into procedures for crossover therapy that is still necessary at times, especially when CABG is required, and methods to further reduce hemorrhage perioperatively in the presence of the newer antiplatelet agents are needed.

Present clinical guideline recommendations are summarized in **Table 1** for STEMI and in **Tables 2** and **3** for UA/NSTEMI. Long-term anticoagulation with an oral agent is not recommended at present unless there is a compelling secondary reason, such as left ventricular thrombus, left ventricular aneurysm, atrial fibrillation, mechanical valve replacement, and so forth. Careful monitoring for bleeding and dose reduction after an assessment of hemorrhagic risk should be performed. Future oral anticoagulants that have more predictable anticoagulation have yet to be found, although the oral once a day rivaroxaban (Xarelto) has just recently had promising data released when used in symptomatic venous thromboembolic disease.

REFERENCES

1. Hassan WM, Flaker GC, Feutz C, et al. Improved anticoagulation with a weight-adjusted heparin nomogram in patients with acute coronary syndromes: a randomized trial. J Thromb Thrombolysis 1995;2:245–9.

2. Becker RC, Ball SP, Eisenberg P, et al. A randomized, multicenter trial of weight-adjusted intravenous heparin dose titration and point-of-care coagulation monitoring in hospitalized patients with active thromboembolic disease: Antithrombotic Therapy Consortium Investigators. Am Heart J 1999;137:59–71.

3. Hochman JS, Wali AU, Gavrila D, et al. A new regimen for heparin use in acute coronary syndromes. Am Heart J 1999;138:313–8.

4. Hirsh J, Warkentin TE, Raschke R, et al. Heparin and low-molecular-weight heparin: mechanisms of action, pharmacokinetics, dosing considerations, monitoring, efficacy, and safety. Chest 1998;114: 489S–510S.

5. Hirsh J, Raschke R. Heparin and low-molecular-weight heparin: the seventh ACCP conference on antithrombotic and thrombolytic therapy. Chest 2004;126:188S–203S.

6. Assessment of short-anticoagulant administration after cardiac infarction. Report of the working party on anticoagulant therapy in coronary thrombosis to the medical research council. Br Med J 1969;1:335–42.

7. Drapkin A, Merskey C. Anticoagulant therapy after acute myocardial infarction. Relation of therapeutic benefit to patient's age, sex, and severity of infarction. JAMA 1972;222:541–8.

8. Anticoagulants in acute myocardial infarction. Results of a cooperative clinical trial. JAMA 1973; 225:724–9.

9. Eisenberg PR. Role of heparin in coronary thrombolysis. Chest 1992;101:131S–9S.

10. The GUSTO Angiographic Investigators. The effects of tissue plasminogen activator, streptokinase, or both on coronary-artery patency, ventricular function, and survival after acute myocardial infarction. N Engl J Med 1993;329:1615–22.

11. O'Connor CM, Meese R, Carney R, et al. A randomized trial of intravenous heparin in conjunction with anistreplase (anisoylated plasminogen streptokinase activator complex) in acute myocardial infarction: The Duke University Clinical Cardiology Study (DUCCS) 1. J Am Coll Cardiol 1994;23:1–8.

12. Gruppo Italiano per lo Studio della Sopravvivenza nell'Infarto Miocardico. GISSI-2: a factorial randomised trial of alteplase versus streptokinase and heparin versus no heparin among 12,490 patients with acute myocardial infarction. Lancet 1990;336: 65–71.

13. The International Study Group. In-hospital mortality and clinical course of 20,891 patients with suspected acute myocardial infarction randomised between alteplase and streptokinase with or without heparin. Lancet 1990;336:71–5.

14. ISIS-3 (Third International Study of Infarct Survival) Collaborative Group. ISIS-3: a randomised comparison of streptokinase vs tissue plasminogen activator vs anistreplase and of aspirin plus heparin vs aspirin alone among 41,299 cases of suspected acute myocardial infarction. Lancet 1992;339: 753–70.

15. Antman EM, Hand M, Armstrong PW, et al. 2007 focused update of the ACC/AHA 2004 guidelines for the management of patients with ST-elevation myocardial infarction: a report of the American College of Cardiology/American Heart Association Task Force on practice guidelines (Writing Group to review new evidence and update the acc/aha 2004 guidelines for the management of patients with st-elevation myocardial infarction). J Am Coll Cardiol 2008;51:XXX. Available at: www. acc.org/qualityandscience/clinical/statements.htm Accessed March 15, 2008.

16. The GUSTO investigators. An international randomized trial comparing four thrombolytic strategies for acute myocardial infarction. N Engl J Med 1993; 329:673–82.

17. The Global Use of Strategies to Open Occluded Coronary Arteries (GUSTO) IIa Investigators. Randomized trial of intravenous heparin versus recombinant hirudin for acute coronary syndromes. Circulation 1994;90:1631–7.

18. Antman EM, For the TIMI 9A Investigators. Hirudin in acute myocardial infarction. Safety report from

the thrombolysis and thrombin inhibition in myocardial infarction (TIMI) 9A trial. Circulation 1994;90: 1624–30:

19. Granger CB, Hirsch J, Califf RM, et al. Activated partial thromboplastin time and outcome after thrombolytic therapy for acute myocardial infarction: results from the GUSTO-I trial. Circulation 1996;93:870–8.

20. Nallamothu BK, Bates ER, Hochman JS, et al. Prognostic implication of activated partial thromboplastin time after reteplase or half-dose reteplase plus abciximab: results from the GUSTO-V trial. Eur Heart J 2005;26:1506–12.

21. Vaitkus PT, Barnathan ES. Embolic potential, prevention and management of mural thrombus complicating anterior myocardial infarction: a meta-analysis. J Am Coll Cardiol 1993;22:1004–9.

22. Tolleson TR, O'Shea JC, Bittl JA, et al. Relationship between heparin anticoagulation and clinical outcomes in coronary stent intervention: observations from the ESPRIT trial. J Am Coll Cardiol 2003;41: 386–93.

23. The EPILOG Investigators. Platelet glycoprotein IIb/IIIa receptor blockade and low-dose heparin during percutaneous coronary revascularization. N Engl J Med 1997;336:1689–96.

24. Brener SJ, Moliterno DJ, Lincoff AM, et al. Relationship between activated clotting time and ischemic or hemorrhagic complications: analysis of 4 recent randomized clinical trials of percutaneous coronary intervention. Circulation 2004;110:994–8.

25. Liem A, Zijlstra F, Ottervanger JP, et al. High dose heparin as pretreatment for primary angioplasty in acute myocardial infarction: the Heparin in Early Patency (HEAP) randomized trial. J Am Coll Cardiol 2000;35:600–4.

26. Anderson JL, Adams CD, Antman EM, et al. ACC/AHA guidelines for the management of patients with unstable angina/non-ST-elevation myocardial infarction: a report of the American College of Cardiology and American Heart Association Task Force on practice guidelines. J Am Coll Cardiol 2007;50:e1–157.

27. Oler A, Whooley MA, Oler J, et al. Adding heparin to aspirin reduces the incidence of myocardial infarction and death in patients with unstable angina. A meta-analysis. JAMA 1996;276:811–5.

28. Fragmin during Instability in Coronary Artery Disease (FRISC) Study Group. Low-molecular-weight heparin during instability in coronary artery disease. Lancet 1996;347:561–8.

29. Theroux P, Waters D, Lam J, et al. Reactivation of unstable angina after the discontinuation of heparin. N Engl J Med 1992;327:141–5.

30. Serruys PW, Herrman JP, Simon R, et al. A comparison of hirudin with heparin in the prevention of restenosis after coronary angioplasty. Helvetica Investigators. N Engl J Med 1995;333:757–63.

31. The Global Use of Strategies to Open Occluded Coronary Arteries (GUSTO) IIb Investigators. A comparison of recombinant hirudin with heparin for the treatment of acute coronary syndromes. N Engl J Med 1996;335:775–82.

32. Granger CB, Miller JM, Bovill EG, et al. Rebound increase in thrombin generation and activity after cessation of intravenous heparin in patients with acute coronary syndromes. Circulation 1995;91: 1929–35.

33. Martel N, Lee J, Wells PS. Risk for heparin-induced thrombocytopenia with unfractionated and low-molecular-weight heparin thromboprophylaxis: a meta-analysis. Blood 2005;106:2710–5.

34. Rice L, Attisha WK, Drexler A, et al. Delayed-onset heparin-induced thrombocytopenia. Ann Intern Med 2002;136:210–5.

35. Antman EM, Anbe DT, Armstrong PW, et al. ACC/AHA guidelines for the management of patients with ST-elevation myocardial infarction. Available at: www. acc.org/qualityandscience/clinical/statements.htm. Accessed May 20, 2008.

36. Warkentin TE. Heparin-induced thrombocytopenia: a clinicopathologic syndrome. Thromb Haemost 1999;82:439–47.

37. Potzsch B, Klovekorn WP, Madlener K. Use of heparin during cardiopulmonary bypass in patients with a history of heparin-induced thrombocytopenia. N Engl J Med 2000;343:515 [letter].

38. Follis F, Schmidt CA. Cardiopulmonary bypass in patients with heparin-induced thrombocytopenia and thrombosis. Ann Thorac Surg 2000;70: 2173–81.

39. Eikelboom JW, Quinlan DJ, Mehta SR, et al. Unfractionated and low-molecular-weight heparin as adjuncts to thrombolysis in aspirin-treated patients with ST-elevation acute myocardial infarction: a meta-analysis of the randomized trials. Circulation 2005;112.3855–67.

40. Ross AM, Molhoek P, Lundergan C, et al. Randomized comparison of enoxaparin, a low-molecular-weight heparin, with unfractionated heparin adjunctive to recombinant tissue plasminogen activator thrombolysis and aspirin: second trial of heparin and aspirin reperfusion therapy (Hart II). Circulation 2001;104:648–52.

41. Wallentin L, Goldsten D, Armstrong PW, et al. Efficacy and safety of tenecteplase in combination with enoxaparin, abciximab, or unfractionated heparin: the ASSENT-3 randomised trial in acute myocardial infarction. Lancet 2001;358:605–13.

42. Van de Werf F. ASSENT-3: implications for future trial design and clinical practice. Eur Heart J 2002;23:911–2.

43. Antman EM, Louwerenburg HW, Baars HF, et al. Enoxaparin as adjunctive antithrombin therapy for ST-elevation myocardial infarction: results of the ENTIRE-Thrombolysis in Myocardial Infarction (TIMI) 23 trial. Circulation 2002;105:1642–9.

44. Wallentin L, Goldstein P, Armstrong PW, et al. Efficacy and safety of tenecteplase in combination with the low-molecular-weight heparin enoxaparin or unfractionated heparin in the prehospital setting: the Assessment of the Safety and Efficacy of a New Thrombolytic Regimen (ASSENT)-3 PLUS randomized trial in acute myocardial infarction. Circulation 2003;108:135–42.

45. Antman EM, Morrow DA, McCabe CH, et al. Enoxaparin versus unfractionated heparin with fibrinolysis for ST-elevation myocardial infarction. N Engl J Med 2006;354:1477–88.

46. Murphy SA, Gibson CM, Morrow DA, et al. Efficacy and safety of the low-molecular weight heparin enoxaparin compared with unfractionated heparin across the acute coronary syndrome spectrum: a meta-analysis. Eur Heart J 2007;28:2077–86.

47. Klein W, Buchwald A, Hillis SE, et al. Comparison of low molecular-weight heparin with unfractionated heparin acutely and with placebo for 6 weeks in the management of unstable coronary artery disease. Fragmin in unstable coronary artery disease study (FRIC). [published erratum appears in Circulation 1998;97:413]. Circulation 1997;96:61–8.

48. The F.R.A.I.S. Study Group. Comparison of two treatment durations (6 days and 14 days) of a low molecular weight heparin with a 6-day treatment of unfractionated heparin in the initial management of unstable angina or non-Q wave myocardial infarction: FRAX.I.S. (FRAxiparine in Ischaemic Syndrome). Eur Heart J 1999;20:1553–62.

49. Cohen M, Demers C, Gurfinkel EP, et al. A comparison of low-molecular-weight heparin with unfractionated heparin for unstable coronary artery disease. Efficacy and safety of subcutaneous enoxaparin in non-Q-wave coronary events study group. N Engl J Med 1997;337:447–52.

50. Antman EM, McCabe CH, Gurfinkel EP, et al. Enoxaparin prevents death and cardiac ischemic events in unstable angina/non-Q wave myocardial infarction: results of the Thrombolysis In Myocardial Infarction (TIMI) 11B trial. Circulation 1999;100: 1593–601.

51. Cohen M, Theroux P, Borzak S, et al. Randomized double-blind safety study of enoxaparin versus unfractionated heparin in patients with non-ST-segment elevation acute coronary syndromes treated with tirofiban and aspirin: the ACUTE II study. The antithrombotic combination using tirofiban and enoxaparin. Am Heart J 2002;144:470–7.

52. Goodman SG, Fitchett D, Armstrong PW, et al. Randomized evaluation of the safety and efficacy of enoxaparin versus unfractionated heparin in high-risk patients with non-ST-segment elevation acute coronary syndromes receiving the glycoprotein IIb/IIIa inhibitor eptifibatide. Circulation 2003;107: 238–44.

53. Blazing MA, de Lemos JA, White HD, et al. Safety and efficacy of enoxaparin vs unfractionated heparin in patients with non-ST segment elevation acute coronary syndromes who receive tirofiban and aspirin: a randomized controlled trial. JAMA 2004; 292:55–64.

54. Ferguson JJ, Califf RM, Antman EM, et al. Enoxaparin vs unfractionated heparin in high-risk patients with non-ST-segment elevation acute coronary syndromes managed with an intended early invasive strategy: primary results of the SYNERGY randomized trial. JAMA 2004;292:45–54.

55. Michalis LK, Katsouras CS, Papamichael N, et al. Enoxaparin versus tinzaparin in non-ST-segment elevation acute coronary syndromes: the EVET trial. Am Heart J 2003;146:304–10.

56. Antman EM. Low molecular weight heparins for acute coronary syndrome: tackling the issues head-on. Am Heart J 2003;146:191–3.

57. Yusuf S, Mehta SR, Xie C, et al. CREATE Trial Group Investigators. Effects of reviparin, a low-molecular-weight heparin, on mortality, reinfarction, and strokes in patients with acute myocardial infarction presenting with ST-segment elevation. JAMA 2005; 293(4):427–35.

58. Fox KA. Low molecular weight heparin (enoxaparin) in the management of unstable angina: the ESSENCE study. Efficacy and safety of subcutaneous enoxaparin in non-Q wave coronary events. Heart 1999;82(Suppl 1):I12–4.

59. Collet JP, Montalescot G, Lison L, et al. Percutaneous coronary intervention after subcutaneous enoxaparin pretreatment in patients with unstable angina pectoris. Circulation 2001;103:658–63.

60. Mahaffey KW, Ferguson JJ. Exploring the role of enoxaparin in the management of high-risk patients with non-ST-elevation acute coronary syndromes: the SYNERGY trial. Am Heart J 2005;149:S81–90.

61. Bittl JA, Strony J, Brinker JA, et al. Treatment with bivalirudin (Hirulog) as compared with heparin during coronary angioplasty for unstable or postinfarction angina. N Engl J Med 1995;333:764–9.

62. Argatroban package insert. Available at: us.gsk.com/products/assets/us_argatroban.pdf. Accessed August 10, 2006.

63. The Direct Thrombin Inhibitor Trialists' Collaborative Group. Direct thrombin inhibitors in acute coronary syndromes: principal results of a meta-analysis based on individual patients' data. Lancet 2002; 359:294–302.

64. Cannon CP, McCabe CH, Henry TD, et al. A pilot trial of recombinant desulfatohirudin compared

with heparin in conjunction with tissue-type plasminogen activator and aspirin for acute myocardial infarction: results of the Thrombolysis In Myocardial Infarction (TIMI) 5 trial. J Am Coll Cardiol 1994;23: 993–1003.

65. Lee LV, For the TIMI 6 Investigators. Initial experience with hirudin and streptokinase in acute myocardial infarction: results of the Thrombolysis In Myocardial Infarction (TIMI) 6 trial. Am J Cardiol 1995;75:7–13.

66. Antman EM. Hirudin in acute myocardial infarction. Thrombolysis and Thrombin Inhibition in Myocardial Infarction (TIMI) 9B Trial. Circulation 1996;94: 911–21.

67. White HD, Aylward PE, Frey MJ, et al. on behalf of the Hirulog Early Reperfusion/Occlusion (HERO) Trial Investigators. Randomized, double-blind comparison of hirulog versus heparin in patients receiving streptokinase and aspirin for acute myocardial infarction (HERO) Hirulog Early Reperfusion/Occlusion (HERO) Trial Investigators. Circulation 1997;96:2155–61.

68. HORIZONS AMI. A prospective, randomized comparison of bivalirudin vs. heparin plus glycoprotein IIb/IIIa inhibitors during primary angioplasty in acute myocardial infarction—30 day results. Presented at the 2007 Transcatheter Cardiovascular Therapeutics. Available at: http://www.tct2007. com/. Accessed March 15, 2008.

69. Stone GW, Witzenbichler B, Guagliumi G, et al. HORIZONS-AMI Trial Investigators. Bivalirudin during primary PCI in acute myocardial infarction. N Engl J Med 2008;358(21):2218–30.

70. Jang IK, Brown DF, Giugliano RP, et al. A multicenter, randomized study of argatroban versus heparin as adjunct to tissue plasminogen activator (TPA) in acute myocardial infarction: myocardial infarction with novastan and TPA (MINT) study. J Am Coll Cardiol 1999;33:1879–85.

71. Organisation to Assess Strategies for Ischemic Syndromes (OASIS-2) Investigators. Effects of recombinant hirudin (lepirudin) compared with heparin on death, myocardial infarction, refractory angina, and revascularisation procedures in patients with acute myocardial ischaemia without ST elevation: a randomised trial. Lancet 1999;353: 429–38.

72. Roe MT, Granger CB, Puma JA, et al. Comparison of benefits and complications of hirudin versus heparin for patients with acute coronary syndromes undergoing early percutaneous coronary intervention. Am J Cardiol 2001;88:1403–6.

73. Lincoff AM, Bittl JA, Harrington RA, et al. Bivalirudin and provisional glycoprotein IIb/IIIa blockade compared with heparin and planned glycoprotein IIb/IIIa blockade during percutaneous coronary intervention: REPLACE-2 randomized trial. JAMA 2003;289:853–63.

74. Antman EM. Should bivalirudin replace heparin during percutaneous coronary interventions? JAMA 2003;289:903–5.

75. Lincoff AM, Kleiman NS, Kereiakes DJ, et al. Long-term efficacy of bivalirudin and provisional glycoprotein IIb/IIIa blockade vs heparin and planned glycoprotein IIb/IIIa blockade during percutaneous coronary revascularization: REPLACE-2 randomized trial. JAMA 2004;292:696–703.

76. Stone GW, McLaurin BT, Cox DA, et al. Bivalirudin for patients with acute coronary syndromes. N Engl J Med 2006;355:2203–16.

77. Chuang YJ, Swanson R, et al. Heparin enhances the specificity of antithrombin for thrombin and factor Xa independent of the reactive center loop sequence. Evidence for an exosite determinant of factor Xa specificity in heparin-activated antithrombin. J Biol Chem 2001;276(18):14961–71.

78. Yusuf S, Mehta SR, Chrolavicius S, et al. Effects of fondaparinux on mortality and reinfarction in patients with acute ST-segment elevation myocardial infarction: the OASIS-6 randomized trial. JAMA 2006;295:1519–30.

79. Yusuf S, Mehta SR, Chrolavicius S, et al. Comparison of fondaparinux and enoxaparin in acute coronary syndromes. N Engl J Med 2006;354:1464–76.

80. Gage BF, Fihn SD, White RH. Management and dosing of warfarin therapy. Am J Med 2000;109: 481–8.

81. Harrison L, Johnston M, Massicotte MP, et al. Comparison of 5 mg and 10 mg loading doses in initiation of warfarin therapy. Ann Intern Med 1997;126: 133–6.

82. Crowther MA, Ginsberg JB, Kearon C, et al. A randomized trial comparing 5-mg and 10-mg warfarin loading doses. Arch Intern Med 1999;159:46–8.

83. Banet GA, Waterman AD, Milligan PE, et al. Warfarin dose reduction vs watchful waiting for mild elevations in the international normalized ratio. Chest 2003;123:499–503.

84. Garcia DA, Regan S, Crowther M, et al. The risk of hemorrhage among patients with warfarin-associated coagulopathy. J Am Coll Cardiol 2006;47: 804–8.

85. Kucher N, Connolly S, Beckman JA, et al. International normalized ratio increase before warfarin-associated hemorrhage: brief and subtle. Arch Intern Med 2004;164:2176–9.

86. Schulman S. Care of patients receiving long-term anticoagulant therapy. N Engl J Med 2003;349:675–83.

87. O'Shaughnessy DF, Atterbury C, Bolton Maggs P, et al. Guidelines for the use of fresh-frozen plasma, cryoprecipitate and cryosupernatant. Br J Haematol 2004;126:11–28.

88. Evans G, Luddington R, Baglin T. Beriplex P/N reverses severe warfarin-induced overanticoagulation immediately and completely in patients presenting with major bleeding. Br J Haematol 2001; 115:998–1001.

89. Preston FE, Laidlaw ST, Sampson B, et al. Rapid reversal of oral anticoagulation with warfarin by a prothrombin complex concentrate (Beriplex): efficacy and safety in 42 patients. Br J Haematol 2002; 116:619–24.

90. Deveras RA, Kessler CM. Reversal of warfarin-induced excessive anticoagulation with recombinant human factor VIIa concentrate. Ann Intern Med 2002;137:884–8.

91. Lin J, Hanigan WC, Tarantino M, et al. The use of recombinant activated factor VII to reverse warfarin-induced anticoagulation in patients with hemorrhages in the central nervous system: preliminary findings. J Neurosurg 2003;98:737–40.

92. van Walraven C, Jennings A, Oake N, et al. Effect of study setting on anticoagulation control: a systematic review and meta regression. Chest 2006; 129:1155–66.

93. Rothberg MB, Celestin C, Fiore LD, et al. Warfarin plus aspirin after myocardial infarction or the acute coronary syndrome: meta-analysis with estimates of risk and benefit. Ann Intern Med 2005;143: 241–50.

94. Hurlen M, Abdelnoor M, Smith P, et al. Warfarin, aspirin, or both after myocardial infarction. N Engl J Med 2002;347:969–74.

95. van Es RF, Jonker JJ, Verheugt FW, et al. Aspirin and Coumadin after acute coronary syndromes (the ASPECT-2 study): a randomised controlled trial. Lancet 2002;360:109–13.

96. Brouwer MA, van den Bergh PJ, Aengevaeren WR, et al. Aspirin plus coumarin versus aspirin alone in the prevention of reocclusion after fibrinolysis for acute myocardial infarction: results of the Antithrombotics in the Prevention of Reocclusion In Coronary Thrombolysis (APRICOT)-2 trial. Circulation 2002;106:659–65.

97. Eikelboom JW, Anand SS, Malmberg K, et al. Unfractionated heparin and low-molecular-weight heparin in acute coronary syndrome without ST elevation: a meta-analysis. Lancet 2000;355: 1936–42.

98. Long-term low-molecular-mass heparin in unstable coronary-artery disease: FRISC II prospective randomised multicentre study. Fragmin and Fast Revascularisation During Instability In Coronary Artery Disease Investigators. Lancet 1999;354: 701–7.

99. Cohen M, Adams PC, Parry G, et al. Antithrombitic Therpy in Acute Coronary Syndromes Research Group. Combination antithrombotic therapy in unstable rest angina and non-Q-wave infarction in nonprior aspirin users. Primary end points analysis from the ATACS trial. Circulation 1994;89:81–8.

100. Anand SS, Yusuf S, Pogue J, et al. Long-term oral anticoagulant therapy in patients with unstable angina or suspected non-Q-wave myocardial infarction: organization to assess strategies for ischaemic syndromes (OASIS) pilot study results. Circulation 1998;98:1064–70.

101. Effects of long-term, moderate-intensity oral anticoagulation in addition to aspirin in unstable angina. The Organization to Assess Strategies for Ischemic Syndromes (OASIS) investigators. J Am Coll Cardiol 2001;37:475–84.

Intensity of Antiplatelet Therapy in Patients with Acute Coronary Syndromes and Percutaneous Coronary Intervention: the Promise of Prasugrel?

Stephen D. Wiviott, MD[a,b],*

KEYWORDS
- Platelet • Antiplatelet therapy • Acute coronary syndrome
- Percutaneous coronary intervention

Platelet activation and aggregation are key contributors to the pathophysiology of acute coronary syndromes (ACS) and to ischemic complications of percutaneous coronary intervention (PCI), including spontaneous and periprocedural myocardial infarction (MI) and stent thrombosis. Platelets adhere to the site of vascular injury (whether spontaneous with ACS or iatrogenic with PCI). This initial adherence is followed by activation, which includes shape change and secretion of various procoagulant, proinflammatory, and vasoconstrictive secondary messengers, including ADP, thromboxane A2, and serotonin. Among the effects of these messengers is further activation of platelets, resulting in a feedback loop and explosive amplification of activation. ADP in particular interacts with puranergic receptors (P2Y1 and P2Y12) to amplify and sustain this activation.[1] In addition to shape change and secretion, platelet activation leads to the exposure of glycoprotein IIb/IIIa integrin receptors, which allows for crosslinking of platelets and fibrinogen to form platelet aggregates. Local vasoconstriction and inflammation, combined with the accumulation and embolization of platelet aggregates, result in thrombosis, ischemia, and infarction.

With this pathophysiology, it is not surprising that antiplatelet agents play a key role in the prevention of ischemic complications of ACS and PCI.[2–6] Three key classes of antiplatelet agents play major roles in the management of patients with these conditions: aspirin, intravenous glycoprotein IIb/IIIa integrin receptor antagonists, and thienopyridine antiplatelet agents. Aspirin inhibits the cyclooxygenase enzyme, a key mediator of arachadonic acid metabolism, resulting in a decrease in the production of proinflammatory and procoagulant mediators, including thromboxane A2, and has been demonstrated to reduce ischemic events in the setting of ST-elevation and non–ST-elevation ACS.[7,8] The glycoprotein IIb/IIIa integrin receptor antagonists block platelet aggregation by interfering with the formation of platelet fibrinogen crosslinks and have also been demonstrated to improve clinical outcomes of selected patients with ACS, especially those at high risk of recurrent ischemic events and those being managed with an invasive (coronary angiography directed) strategy of care.[9,10]

The thienopyridine class of antiplatelet agents has three members: ticlopidine, clopidogrel, and the subject of this review, prasugrel. All three

a Cardiovascular Division, Brigham and Women's Hospital, 75 Francis Street, Boston, MA 02115, USA
b Harvard Medical School, Boston, MA, USA
* Cardiovascular Division, Brigham and Women's Hospital, 75 Francis Street, Boston, MA 02115.
E-mail address: swiviott@partners.org

Cardiol Clin 26 (2008) 629–637
doi:10.1016/j.ccl.2008.07.003

drugs are prodrugs, orally inactive, and require metabolism to an active metabolite. The active metabolite of the thienopyridine binds irreversibly to the P2Y12 receptor, blocking the binding of ADP, and thereby inhibiting platelet activation and aggregation.[11] Ticlopidine, the first-generation thienopyridine was initially developed and tested in patients with previous transient ischemic attack or stroke.[12,13] The major utility of ticlopidine, however, was as a component of dual antiplatelet therapy in combination with aspirin for patients with PCI and intracoronary stents.[14–17] The utility of this agent was shown in a series of trials comparing dual antiplatelet therapy to aspirin plus an oral anticoagulant.[14,15] The utility of ticlopidine, however, was limited by the need to take the drug twice daily, and by issues with tolerability, including gastrointestinal distress and, most importantly, rare but severe hematological side effects, such as bone marrow aplasia,[18] which required frequent monitoring. As such, the clinical use of ticlopidine is largely historical. However, the results of studies of ticlopidine in cardiovascular disease set the stage for the use of the second-generation thienopyridine, clopidogrel, in cardiovascular disease, including ACS and PCI.

Clopidogrel plus aspirin dual antiplatelet therapy has become the standard of care for the support of patients undergoing PCI with stenting regardless of the indication for PCI.[19] In the Clopidogrel Aspirin Stent International Cooperative Study (CLASSICS)[20] comparing ticlopidine plus aspirin to clopidogrel (with or without a loading dose) plus aspirin in patients with stenting, clopidogrel was found to have a significantly better safety/tolerability profile, but no difference between the two agents was observed in recurrent ischemic events.

The Clopidogrel in Unstable Angina to Prevent Recurrent Events (CURE) trial compared clopidogrel plus aspirin with aspirin alone in patients with non–ST-elevation ACS[21] and observed an improvement ischemic outcomes and an increase in minor bleeding events. Of the patients enrolled in the CURE trial who underwent PCI, reported as the PCI-CURE,[22] analysis demonstrated 30% relative reduction in the key composite end point of cardiovascular death, MI, and urgent revascularization.[22] On the basis of these and other studies, the American College of Cardiology/American Heart Association (ACC/AHA) guidelines recommend dual antiplatelet therapy with aspirin and clopidogrel in patients with ACS for up to 1 year regardless of treatment strategy (medical, PCI, or surgery).[5]

Patients with ST-segment elevation MI (STEMI) were not included in the CURE trial but also have strong clinical trial evidence for the use of dual antiplatelet therapy, including aspirin and clopidogrel. In the Clopidogrel as Adjunctive Reperfusion Therapy—Thrombolysis in Myocardial Infarction 28 (CLARITY-TIMI 28) trial, subjects with STEMI receiving fibrinolytic therapy were randomized to dual antiplatelet therapy with aspirin or to aspirin alone. The composite end point of death, MI, or an occluded infarct-related artery was reduced by 36%, which was highly statistically significant, without an observed increase in major bleeding or a difference in intracranial hemorrhage.[23] The results of CLARITY-TIMI 28 were complemented by the report of the Clopidogrel and Metoprolol in Myocardial Infarction Trial—Second Chinese Cardiac Study (COMMIT-CCS 2),[24] a large simple trial with more than 45,000 subjects enrolled within 24 hours of MI and allocated to clopidogrel daily plus aspirin or aspirin alone until hospital discharge. Clopidogrel resulted in a 0.9% absolute reduction in death, which was statistically significant.[24] These studies together have resulted in the recommendation by national guidelines committees for the use of clopidogrel in patients with STEMI treated medically with or without fibrinolytic therapy.[3]

PHARMACOLOGIC LIMITATIONS OF CLOPIDOGREL

Despite the profound successes of clopidogrel alone and in combination with aspirin for patients with ACS and those undergoing PCI, there are pharmacologic limitations of this agent.[25] The antiplatelet effects of clopidogrel have a delayed onset and substantial variability among patients. With a growing number of studies using a variety of measures linking poor antiplatelet response to clopidogrel and in turn to adverse clinical outcomes, particularly coronary ischemia and stent thrombosis,[26–29] an interest has emerged in the development of antiplatelet therapy that is more intensive than that offered with clopidogrel.

One such agent, prasugrel, a third-generation thienopyridine, is the focus of this review.

PHARMACOLOGY AND EARLY PHASE CLINICAL STUDIES OF PRASUGREL

Like ticlopidine and clopidogrel, prasugrel is a prodrug that requires activation (**Fig. 1**) to form an active metabolite with platelet inhibitory properties.[30] Prasugrel is metabolized in a two-step process, including initial activation by plasma esterases followed by a single cytochrome P-450 (CYP)–dependent step.[31] In contrast, clopidogrel is largely inactivated by plasma esterases before a two-step CYP-dependent activation.[31] These

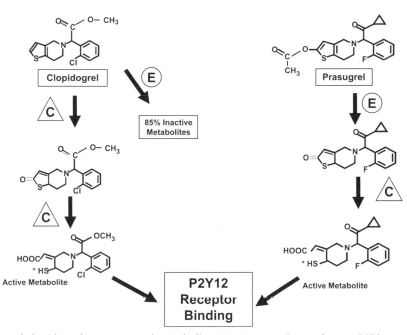

Fig. 1. Prasugrel and clopidogrel structure and metabolism. E, esterases; C, cytochrome-P450.

metabolic disparities appear to underlie the key pharmacodynamic differences: quicker onset, greater potency, and greater consistency of antiplatelet activity with prasugrel compared with clopidogrel.

In healthy subjects, prasugrel has been demonstrated to be approximately 10-fold more potent (on a milligram basis) than clopidogrel as measured by ADP-induced platelet aggregation (IPA). Ten milligrams of prasugrel achieved higher levels of platelet inhibition than 75 mg of clopidogrel, both alone and in combination with aspirin.[31] A key early-phase study of prasugrel included a crossover design of healthy subjects receiving both prasugrel 60 mg and clopidogrel 300 mg in random order and separated by a washout period.[32] As early as 30 minutes, and throughout the follow-up period, higher levels of IPA were observed with prasugrel, with maximum IPA of 79%, compared with 35% with clopidogrel. In addition to higher overall levels, there was less variability in response to prasugrel and, in contrast to clopidogrel, no patients with an IPA less than 20% (a level of inhibition that cannot reliably be differentiated from placebo). As would have been predicted by the metabolic differences, substantially greater concentrations of the active metabolite of prasugrel were observed compared with the active metabolite of clopidogrel.[32]

In results similar to those for healthy subjects, prasugrel was demonstrated to achieve higher levels of IPA in patients with stable coronary artery disease.[33] In this study, 101 subjects with

coronary artery disease were randomized to standard-dose clopidogrel (300-mg loading dose followed by 75 mg daily) or one of four dose regimens of prasugrel (40-mg loading dose followed by 5 mg daily; 40-mg loading dose followed by 7.5 mg daily; 60-mg loading dose followed by 10 mg daily; or 60-mg loading dose followed by15 mg daily). Greater levels of IPA and fewer predefined poor responders (<20% IPA) were observed in patients receiving either 40- or 60-mg loading doses. In the maintenance phase, both 10-mg and 15-mg doses of prasugrel achieved higher IPA and had fewer poor responders than did clopidogrel. Though no significant differences were observed for bleeding events, bruising and bleeding tended to be higher in the prasugrel 15-mg treatment arm.[33]

The Prasugrel in Comparison to Clopidogrel for Inhibition of Platelet Activation and Aggregation—Thrombolysis in Myocardial Infarction 44 (PRINCIPLE-TIMI 44) trial extended the pharmacodynamic comparison of prasugrel and clopidogrel in two important ways.[34] First, the study compared prasugrel (60-mg loading dose followed by 10 mg daily) to higher loading- and maintenance-dose clopidogrel (600-mg loading dose followed by 150 mg daily) and, second, this comparison was performed in patients with coronary artery disease undergoing cardiac catheterization with PCI if coronary anatomy was suitable. Two hundred one subjects were enrolled and randomized to receive either 60 mg of prasugrel or 600 mg of clopidogrel pretreatment before cardiac catheterization in the loading-dose phase of the study. Patients who received PCI entered the maintenance-dose phase, which was a two-period crossover study of 10 mg of prasugrel versus 150 mg of clopidogrel daily, with the initial treatment corresponding to the loading-dose assignment. The primary end point of the loading-dose phase, IPA at 6 hours, was higher in the prasugrel arm 75% versus 32% (P < .0001). The greater antiplatelet effects were apparent at 30 minutes and persisted through 24 hours. In addition, the effects were consistent across a broad range of platelet-function measures. At 6 hours, 27% of clopidogrel-treated patients and none of the prasugrel-treated patients had IPA less than 20%, a predefined measure of poor response. Though the absolute differences were less, a highly significant difference in IPA was also observed in the maintenance phase with mean IPA of 61% with prasugrel compared with 46% with clopidogrel (P < .0001).[34]

CLINICAL EVALUATION

Early-phase evaluations of prasugrel established the pharmacologic differences between prasugrel and clopidogrel outlined above: that prasugrel resulted in more rapid, more consistent, and more complete inhibition of ADP-mediated platelet aggregation. Though several studies had suggested that IPA was related to clinical outcomes,[35,36] no one had shown that the pharmacologic advantages of prasugrel translated to improved clinical outcomes. The Joint Utilization of Medications to Block Platelets Optimally—Thrombolysis in Myocardial Infarction 26 (JUMBO-TIMI 26) trial was a randomized, dose-ranging safety study of prasugrel compared with clopidogrel in 904 patients with coronary artery disease undergoing planned elective or urgent PCI.[37] Patients were randomized to standard-dose clopidogrel or three loading- and maintenance-

dose regimens of prasugrel (40-mg loading dose followed by 7.5 mg daily; 60-mg loading dose followed by 10 mg daily; 60-mg loading dose followed by 15 mg daily). The primary end point of the study was the combination of thrombolysis in myocardial infarction (TIMI) major or minor bleeding. All treatment arms had low rates of bleeding. However, the composite end point tended to be higher in prasugrel-treated patients (1.7% versus 1.2%, hazard ratio 1.42 [0.40–5.08]), and no difference was observed in major bleeding.[37] Though not powered for clinical events, major adverse clinical events tended to be lower with prasugrel (7.2% versus 9.4%, P = .31) driven primarily by a trend toward less MI (5.7% versus 7.9%, P = .23). Though no clear trend was seen among the doses of prasugrel studied for major or minor bleeding, less severe bleeding episodes tended to be more frequent with the highest dose of prasugrel, which aided in the choice of doses (prasugrel 60-mg loading dose and 10-mg maintenance dose) for the Trial to Assess Improvement in Therapeutic Outcomes by Optimizing Platelet Inhibition with Prasugrel—Thrombolysis in Myocardial Infarction 38 (TRITON-TIMI 38).[38]

The TRITON-TIMI 38 trial was, therefore, designed with two key aims: to evaluate a novel drug and to test a scientific concept. The trial was thus designed to answer two questions: (1) Is prasugrel (60-mg loading dose followed by 10 mg daily) safe and effective for the reduction of major ischemic events in patients with ACS undergoing PCI compared with standard-dose clopidogrel (300-mg loading dose followed by 75 mg daily)? and (2) Does a thienopyridine dose regimen (in this case prasugrel 60-mg loading dose followed by 10 mg daily), which is known to achieve higher and more consistent levels of platelet aggregation than standard-dose clopidogrel, reduce ischemic events? TRITON-TIMI 38 (**Fig. 2**) was designed to be a trial of patients undergoing PCI. Therefore, the inclusion criteria were designed so

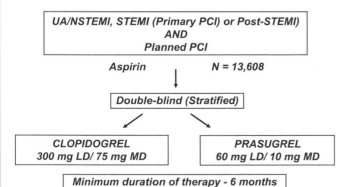

Fig. 2. Design of TRITON-TIMI 38. LD, loading dose; MD, maintenance dose; UA/STEMI, unstable angina–non-STEMI. (*Adapted from* Wiviott SD, Antman EM, Gibson CM, et al. Evaluation of prasugrel compared with clopidogrel in patients with acute coronary syndromes: design and rationale for the TRial to assess Improvement in Therapeutic Outcomes by optimizing platelet InhibitioN with prasugrel Thrombolysis In Myocardial Infarction 38 [TRITON-TIMI 38]. Am Heart J 2006;152(4):627–35; with permission.)

that all patients would undergo PCI. So, 13,608 patients were enrolled with one of the following: (1) moderate- to high-risk unstable angina–non-STEMI with coronary anatomy known to be suitable for PCI, (2) planned primary PCI for STEMI (regardless of known coronary anatomy), or (3) following medical therapy for STEMI with coronary anatomy known suitable for PCI. Key exclusion criteria were high risk for bleeding and prior thienopyridine use within the previous 5 days. Unlike many previous studies of anticoagulants, there were no exclusions for advanced age or renal dysfunction. Patients were treated with study medications for a minimum of 6 months and a maximum of 15 months. The primary end point of the trial was the composite of cardiovascular death, nonfatal MI, and nonfatal stroke.

In TRITON-TIMI 38, randomization to prasugrel resulted in a highly significant reduction in ischemic events with prasugrel as measured by the primary end point (9.9% versus 12.1%, hazard ratio 0.81 [0.73–0.90], P = .0004) (**Fig. 3**).[39] This included similar reductions in events likely related to the loading dose (within 3 days: 4.7% versus 5.6%, hazard ratio 0.82, P = .01) and the maintenance dose (after 3 days: 5.6% versus 6.9%, hazard ratio 0.80, P = .003).[40] The reduction in the primary end point was primarily driven by a substantial reduction in fatal or nonfatal MI (7.4% versus 9.7%, hazard ratio 0.76, P < .001). However, stroke was neutral and cardiovascular death (2.1% versus 2.4%, hazard ratio 0.89, P = .31) tended to favor prasugrel. These reductions in ischemic events were similar to those noted in the CURE study comparing clopidogrel to placebo.[21]

Perhaps the most striking finding in the TRITON-TIMI 38 study was the efficacy of prasugrel in the reduction of stent thrombosis (ST).[39,41] Stent thrombosis events were serious with nearly 90% of patients experiencing death or MI associated with the stent thrombosis event. Stent thrombosis was reduced overall by more than 50% with prasugrel (1.1% versus 24%, hazard ratio 0.48, P < .0001). The reduction in stent thrombosis was robust with respect to stent thrombosis definition, stent type (bare metal or drug-eluting stents), timing, and across several key clinical characteristics.[41]

As with previous studies of antiplatelet agents, more potent inhibition of platelet aggregation with prasugrel resulted in more bleeding than with standard-dose clopidogrel. The key safety end point of non–coronary artery bypass graft–related TIMI major bleeding was increased with prasugrel (2.4% versus 1.8%, hazard ratio 1.32; P − .03).[39] This increase in bleeding was consistent across several definitions of bleeding, including major plus minor (5.0% versus 3.8%, hazard ratio 1.31, P = .002), and included significant increases in rare but serious events, including life-threatening bleeding (1.4% versus 0.9%, P = .01) and fatal bleeding (0.4% versus 0.1%, P = .002).[39]

To weigh the benefits of improved ischemic outcomes against the risks of higher rates of bleeding, a net clinical outcome (net clinical benefit) was calculated using the prespecified definition of all-cause death, nonfatal MI, nonfatal stroke, and nonfatal TIMI major bleed. This calculation favored prasugrel overall (12.2% versus 13.9%, hazard ratio 0.87, P = .004),[39] a finding that was robust to multiple net benefit end points, including

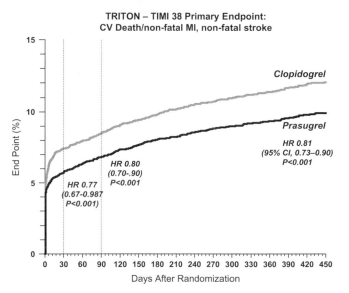

Fig. 3. Primary Results of TRITON-TIMI 38. CV, cardiovascular; HR, hazard ratio. (*Data from* Wiviott SD, Braunwald E, McCabe CH, et al. Prasugrel versus clopidogrel in patients with acute coronary syndromes. N Engl J Med 2007;357(20):2001–5.

the addition of less severe bleeding.[42] In a post hoc effort to identify patients for whom the net benefit did not favor prasugrel, we identified two subgroups with a neutral benefit (the reduction of ischemic events was balanced by the increase in major bleeding): the elderly ($\geq$75 years) and those with low body weight (<60 kg). We also identified a single major subgroup where the net outcome was worse with prasugrel: patients with a history of prior stroke or transient ischemic attack.[39] Patients without these features had a greater relative net benefit of prasugrel compared with clopidogrel (10.2% versus 12.5%, hazard ratio 0.80, $P < .001$, P interaction = 0.006) than those who had at least one of these (20.2% versus 19.0%, hazard ratio 1.07, $P = .43$).[39]

LESSONS LEARNED

The study of prasugrel compared with clopidogrel outlined above has significant implications both for the management of patients with ACS and those undergoing PCI, and for the understanding of the role of the platelet activation and aggregation in the clinical outcomes of these patients. In TRITON-TIMI 38, despite an active comparison with standard-dose clopidogrel, an extremely effective medication, prasugrel demonstrated superiority in the reduction of ischemic events, including MI and stent thrombosis. In addition to the benefits seen, an increase in hemorrhagic complications, including severe bleeding was observed with prasugrel. For the significant majority of patients enrolled, without specific features (prior stroke or transient ischemic attack, advanced age, or low body weight) the balance of safety and efficacy favored prasugrel treatment.[39]

In addition to offering implications for prasugrel specifically, TRITON-TIMI 38 served as a "proof of concept" study. This trial is the first adequately powered clinical trial to show that an agent (or a dose of an agent) that achieves higher and more consistent levels of IPA than standard-dose clopidogrel results in improved ischemic outcomes. These results serve as support for the growing body of literature that relates laboratory measures of platelet function, and the variability of response, to clopidogrel and to clinical outcomes.[43] Some have criticized TRITON-TIMI 38 for the use of a 300-mg loading dose of clopidogrel, stating that 600 mg is the standard of care.[44] In fact, before TRITON-TIMI 38, the frequent use of higher-dose clopidogrel was based on pharmacodynamic studies and small clinical trials with few end points.[45] Until the definitive trial of clopidogrel dosing (Clopidogrel Optimal Loading Dose Usage to Reduce Recurrent Events—Optimal Antiplatelet

Strategy for Interventions 7 [CURRENT-Oasis 7]) is reported, the TRITON-TIMI trial stands as the single greatest support for the use of higher-dose clopidogrel in clinical practice. Though 600 mg of clopidogrel has substantially less antiplatelet effect than the prasugrel dose in TRITON-TIMI 38,[34] 600 mg of clopidogrel has greater antiplatelet effect than 300 mg and therefore may have a portion of the benefits observed with prasugrel. Had TRITON-TIMI 38 not shown a reduction in ischemic events, it would have been difficult to expect a less potent thienopyridine dose regimen to improve outcomes compared with standard dosing. In addition, these data support the continued development of potent antiplatelet agents for the reduction of cardiovascular events.

REMAINING QUESTIONS

While the evaluation of prasugrel to date has answered several important questions about the safety and efficacy of the drug and has provided support for the importance of intensive platelet inhibition in ACS and PCI, it has also raised several more questions for both the clinician and the platelet biologist. First, which aspect of the pharmacologic profile of prasugrel is most important for the improvement in outcomes: the speed of onset, the level of inhibition on a population basis, or the consistency of inhibition? Is the same aspect of the profile responsible for the excess bleeding? In each case (both for safety and efficacy), can we use clinical features or laboratory measures (biomarkers, genetics, platelet function testing) to better identify the patients who are most likely to benefit with the least harm from intensive antiplatelet therapy to better target therapy on an individual basis? Will prasugrel result in improved outcomes with adequate safety in patients with ACS treated medically (this question is being evaluated in the ongoing Targeted Platelet Inhibition to Clarify the Optimal Strategy to Medically Manage Acute Coronary Syndromes [TRILOGY] study)?

Studies will address additional question that the prasugrel experience has raised. Can the results of TRITON-TIMI 38 be replicated with the lesser difference in antiplatelet effect obtained by the use of higher-dose clopidogrel? This will be addressed by CURRENT-Oasis 7. Will blocking the P2Y12 receptor with nonthienopyridine antiplatelet agents with different pharmacologic profiles, such as cangrelor or AZD6140,[25] have similar effects to prasugrel? Cangrelor is being evaluated in the ongoing Clinical Trial Comparing Cangrelor to Clopidogrel in Subjects Who Require Percutaneous Coronary Intervention (CHAMPION PCI). AZD6140 is being studied in the Platelet Inhibition and Patient

Outcomes (PLATO) study. Will antiplatelet agents that target other platelet receptors, such as the PAR-1 receptor, improve clinical outcomes. The ongoing Thrombin Receptor Antagonist in Secondary Prevention of Atherothrombotic Ischemic Events—Thrombolysis in Myocardial Infarction (TRA 2P–TIMI 50) and Trial to Assess the Effects of SCH530348 in Preventing Heart Attack and Stroke in Patients with Acute Coronary Syndromes (TRACER) will address this question. Other questions remain: What is the role of platelet function testing in the future of patient management? Will there come a time that antiplatelet therapy will be tailored not only to patient risk, but also to respond to a single agent or a series of agents?

SUMMARY

Platelet activation and aggregation play key roles in the management of ischemic complications of ACS and PCI. Dual antiplatelet therapy with aspirin and the thienopyridine clopidogrel has become the standard of care for prevention of such complications. Prasugrel, a novel thienopyridine antiplatelet agent, has been demonstrated to have favorable pharmacologic properties including rapid onset and potent and consistent inhibition of platelet aggregation. When compared directly against clopidogrel in the TRITON-TIMI 38 trial, prasugrel resulted in significant reductions in ischemic events including MI and stent thrombosis, but with more bleeding. Prasugrel shows promise for improvements in patient care, for better understanding of platelet biology, and for more helpful evaluations of antiplatelet therapy.

REFERENCES

1. Storey F. The P2Y12 receptor as a therapeutic target in cardiovascular disease. Platelets 2001;12(4): 197–209.
2. Antman EM, Anbe DT, Armstrong PW, et al. ACC/AHA guidelines for the management of patients with ST-elevation myocardial infarction: a report of the American College of Cardiology/American Heart Association Task Force on Practice Guidelines (Committee to Revise the 1999 Guidelines for the Management of Patients with Acute Myocardial Infarction). Circulation 2004;110(9):e82–292.
3. Antman EM, Hand M, Armstrong PW, et al. 2007 Focused Update of the ACC/AHA 2004 Guidelines for the Management of Patients With ST-Elevation Myocardial Infarction: a report of the American College of Cardiology/American Heart Association Task Force on Practice Guidelines: developed in collaboration with the Canadian Cardiovascular Society endorsed by the American Academy of Family Physicians: 2007 Writing Group to Review New Evidence and Update the ACC/AHA 2004 Guidelines for the Management of Patients With ST-Elevation Myocardial Infarction, Writing on Behalf of the 2004 Writing Committee. Circulation 2008;117(2):296–329.
4. Smith SC Jr, Feldman TE, Hirshfeld JW Jr, et al. ACC/AHA/SCAI 2005 guideline update for percutaneous coronary intervention: a report of the American College of Cardiology/American Heart Association Task Force on Practice Guidelines (ACC/AHA/SCAI Writing Committee to Update 2001 Guidelines for Percutaneous Coronary Intervention). Circulation 2006;113(7):e166–286.
5. Braunwald E, Antman EM, Beasley JW, et al. ACC/AHA guideline update for the management of patients with unstable angina and non-ST-segment elevation myocardial infarction–2002: summary article: a report of the American College of Cardiology/American Heart Association Task Force on Practice Guidelines (Committee on the Management of Patients With Unstable Angina). Circulation 2002; 106(14):1893–900.
6. Silber S, Albertsson P, Aviles FF, et al. Guidelines for percutaneous coronary interventions. The Task Force for Percutaneous Coronary Interventions of the European Society of Cardiology. Eur Heart J 2005;26(8):804–47.
7. Catella-Lawson F, Reilly MP, Kapoor SC, et al. Cyclooxygenase inhibitors and the antiplatelet effects of aspirin. N Engl J Med 2001;345(25):1809–17.
8. Clarke RJ, Mayo G, Price P, et al. Suppression of thromboxane A2 but not of systemic prostacyclin by controlled-release aspirin. N Engl J Med 1991; 325(16):1137–41.
9. Lincoff AM, Califf RM, Moliterno DJ, et al. Complementary clinical benefits of coronary-artery stenting and blockade of platelet glycoprotein IIb/IIIa receptors. Evaluation of Platelet IIb/IIIa Inhibition in Stenting Investigators. N Engl J Med 1999;341(5):319–27.
10. Montalescot G, Barragan P, Wittenberg O, et al. Platelet glycoprotein IIb/IIIa inhibition with coronary stenting for acute myocardial infarction. N Engl J Med 2001;344(25):1895–903.
11. Herbert JM, Savi P. P2Y12, a new platelet ADP receptor, target of clopidogrel. Semin Vasc Med 2003;3(2):113–22.
12. Hass WK, Easton JD, Adams HP Jr, et al. A randomized trial comparing ticlopidine hydrochloride with aspirin for the prevention of stroke in high-risk patients. Ticlopidine Aspirin Stroke Study Group. N Engl J Med 1989;321(8):501–7.
13. Gent M, Blakely JA, Easton JD, et al. The Canadian American Ticlopidine Study (CATS) in thromboembolic stroke. Lancet 1989;1(8649):1215–20.
14. Bertrand ME, Legrand V, Boland J, et al. Randomized multicenter comparison of conventional anticoagulation versus antiplatelet therapy in unplanned

and elective coronary stenting. The full anticoagulation versus aspirin and ticlopidine (Fantastic) study. Circulation 1998;98(16):1597–603.

15. Leon MB, Baim DS, Popma JJ, et al. A clinical trial comparing three antithrombotic-drug regimens after coronary-artery stenting. Stent Anticoagulation Restenosis Study Investigators. N Engl J Med 1998;339(23):1665–71.

16. Schomig A, Neumann FJ, Kastrati A, et al. A randomized comparison of antiplatelet and anticoagulant therapy after the placement of coronary-artery stents. N Engl J Med 1996;334(17):1084–9.

17. Urban P, Macaya C, Rupprecht HJ, et al. Randomized evaluation of anticoagulation versus antiplatelet therapy after coronary stent implantation in high-risk patients: the multicenter aspirin and ticlopidine trial after intracoronary stenting (MATTIS). Circulation 1998;98(20):2126–32.

18. Elias M, Reichman N, Flatau E. Bone marrow aplasia associated with ticlopidine therapy. Am J Hematol 1993;44(4):289–90.

19. Smith SC Jr, Feldman TE, Hirshfeld JW Jr, et al. ACC/AHA/SCAI 2005 guideline update for percutaneous coronary intervention-summary article: a report of the American College of Cardiology/American Heart Association Task Force on Practice Guidelines (ACC/AHA/SCAI Writing Committee to Update the 2001 Guidelines for Percutaneous Coronary Intervention). Catheter Cardiovasc Interv 2006; 37(1):87–112.

20. Bertrand ME, Rupprecht HJ, Urban P, et al. Double-blind study of the safety of clopidogrel with and without a loading dose in combination with aspirin compared with ticlopidine in combination with aspirin after coronary stenting: the clopidogrel aspirin stent international cooperative study (CLASSICS). Circulation 2000;102(6):624–9.

21. Yusuf S, Zhao F, Mehta SR, et al. Effects of clopidogrel in addition to aspirin in patients with acute coronary syndromes without ST-segment elevation. N Engl J Med 2001;345(7):494–502.

22. Mehta SR, Yusuf S, Peters RJ, et al. Effects of pretreatment with clopidogrel and aspirin followed by long-term therapy in patients undergoing percutaneous coronary intervention: the PCI-CURE study. Lancet 2001;358(9281):527–33.

23. Sabatine MS, Cannon CP, Gibson CM, et al. Addition of clopidogrel to aspirin and fibrinolytic therapy for myocardial infarction with ST-segment elevation. N Engl J Med 2005;352(12):1179–89.

24. Chen ZM, Jiang LX, Chen YP, et al. Addition of clopidogrel to aspirin in 45,852 patients with acute myocardial infarction: randomised placebo-controlled trial. Lancet 2005;366(9497):1607–21.

25. O'Donoghue M, Wiviott SD. Clopidogrel response variability and future therapies: clopidogrel: Does one size fit all? Circulation 2006;114(22):e600–6.

26. Buonamici P, Marcucci R, Migliorini A, et al. Impact of platelet reactivity after clopidogrel administration on drug-eluting stent thrombosis. J Am Coll Cardiol 2007;49(24):2312–7.

27. Gurbel PA, Bliden KP, Samara W, et al. Clopidogrel effect on platelet reactivity in patients with stent thrombosis: results of the CREST Study. J Am Coll Cardiol 2005;46(10):1827–32.

28. Hochholzer W, Trenk D, Bestehorn HP, et al. Impact of the degree of peri-interventional platelet inhibition after loading with clopidogrel on early clinical outcome of elective coronary stent placement. J Am Coll Cardiol 2006;48(9):1742–50.

29. Wenaweser P, Dorffler-Melly J, Imboden K, et al. Stent thrombosis is associated with an impaired response to antiplatelet therapy. J Am Coll Cardiol 2005;45(11):1748–52.

30. Sugidachi A, Asai F, Yoneda K, et al. Antiplatelet action of R-99224, an active metabolite of a novel thienopyridine-type G(i)-linked P2T antagonist, CS-747. Br J Pharmacol 2001;132(1):47–54.

31. Jakubowski JA, Winters KJ, Naganuma H, et al. Prasugrel: a novel thienopyridine antiplatelet agent. A review of preclinical and clinical studies and the mechanistic basis for its distinct antiplatelet profile. Cardiovasc Drug Rev 2007;25(4): 357–74.

32. Brandt JT, Payne CD, Wiviott SD, et al. A comparison of prasugrel and clopidogrel loading doses on platelet function: magnitude of platelet inhibition is related to active metabolite formation. Am Heart J 2007;153(1):e9–e16.

33. Jernberg T, Payne CD, Winters KJ, et al. Prasugrel achieves greater inhibition of platelet aggregation and a lower rate of non-responders compared with clopidogrel in aspirin-treated patients with stable coronary artery disease. Eur Heart J 2006;27(10): 1166–73.

34. Wiviott SD, Trenk D, Frelinger AL, et al. Prasugrel compared with high loading- and maintenance-dose clopidogrel in patients with planned percutaneous coronary intervention: the Prasugrel in Comparison to Clopidogrel for Inhibition of Platelet Activation and Aggregation—Thrombolysis in Myocardial Infarction 44 trial. Circulation 2007;116(25): 2923–32.

35. Gurbel PA, Bliden KP, Zaman KA, et al. Clopidogrel loading with eptifibatide to arrest the reactivity of platelets: results of the Clopidogrel Loading With Eptifibatide to Arrest the Reactivity of Platelets (CLEAR Platelets) study. Circulation 2005;111(9): 1153–9.

36. Matetzky S, Shenkman B, Guetta V, et al. Clopidogrel resistance is associated with increased risk of recurrent atherothrombotic events in patients with acute myocardial infarction. Circulation 2004; 109(25):3171–5.

37. Wiviott SD, Antman EM, Winters KJ, et al. Randomized comparison of prasugrel (CS-747, LY640315), a novel thienopyridine P2Y12 antagonist, with clopidogrel in percutaneous coronary intervention: results of the Joint Utilization of Medications to Block Platelets Optimally (JUMBO)-TIMI 26 trial. Circulation 2005;111(25):3366–73.

38. Wiviott SD, Antman EM, Gibson CM, et al. Evaluation of prasugrel compared with clopidogrel in patients with acute coronary syndromes: design and rationale for the TRial to assess Improvement in Therapeutic Outcomes by optimizing platelet Inhibition with prasugrel Thrombolysis In Myocardial Infarction 38 (TRITON-TIMI 38). Am Heart J 2006;152(4): 627–35.

39. Wiviott SD, Braunwald E, McCabe CH, et al. Prasugrel versus clopidogrel in patients with acute coronary syndromes. N Engl J Med 2007;357(20):2001–15.

40. Antman EM, Wiviott SD, Murphy SA, et al. Early and late benefits of prasugrel in patients with acute coronary syndromes undergoing percutaneous coronary intervention: a TRITON-TIMI 38 (TRial to Assess Improvement in Therapeutic Outcomes by Optimizing Platelet InhibitioN with Prasugrel-Thrombolysis In Myocardial Infarction) analysis. J Am Coll Cardiol 2008;51(21):2028–33.

41. Wiviott SD, Braunwald E, McCabe CH, et al. Intensive oral antiplatelet therapy for reduction of ischaemic events including stent thrombosis in patients with acute coronary syndromes treated with percutaneous coronary intervention and stenting in the TRITON-TIMI 38 trial: a subanalysis of a randomised trial. Lancet 2008;371(9621):1353–63.

42. Wiviott SD, Braunwald E, Murphy SA, et al. A perspective on the efficacy and safety of intensive antiplatelet therapy in the trial to assess improvement in therapeutic outcomes by optimizing platelet inhibition with prasugrel-thrombolysis in myocardial infarction 38. Am J Cardiol 2008;101(9):1367–70.

43. Wiviott SD. Clopidogrel response variability, resistance, or both? Am J Cardiol 2006;98(10A): 18N–24N.

44. Pasceri V, Patti G, Di Sciascio G. Prasugrel versus clopidogrel. N Engl J Med 2008;358(12):1298–9 [author reply 1299–301].

45. Patti G, Colonna G, Pasceri V, et al. Randomized trial of high loading dose of clopidogrel for reduction of periprocedural myocardial infarction in patients undergoing coronary intervention: results from the ARMYDA-2 (Antiplatelet therapy for Reduction of MYocardial Damage during Angioplasty) study. Circulation 2005;111(16):2099–106.

Dipeptidyl Peptidase-4 as a New Target of Action for Type 2 Diabetes Mellitus: A Systematic Review

Javaid H. Wani, MD, PhD[a], Jennifer John-Kalarickal, MD[b],
Vivian A. Fonseca, MD[a],*

KEYWORDS

- Dipeptidyl peptidase-4 inhibitor • DPP-4 inhibitors
- Sitagliptin • Vildagliptin • Diabetes type 2
- Glycohemoglobin A1c • Incretins

Diabetes mellitus type 2 is a consequence of decreased glucose uptake by cells either because of lack of insulin or defective insulin action or both, leading to hyperglycemia. The underlying mechanisms of reduced insulin secretion include the loss of β-cell function and mass, and apoptotic β-cell death in the pancreas.[1,2] Insulin resistance, usually associated with obesity, is an impaired biological response to insulin, either endogenous or exogenous, leading to unregulated hepatic production of glucose and decreased insulin-stimulated peripheral insulin uptake and utilization.[3] Chronic hyperglycemia leads to microvascular and macrovascular damage, causing multiple diseases including retinopathy, neuropathy, nephropathy, gastroparesis, coronary artery disease, and stroke. These diseases are responsible for a significant increase in morbidity and mortality in the general population, particularly in people who have other comorbid conditions. There is a direct relationship between the level of glycemic control and the risk of these complications. Therefore, glycemic control is important for managing diabetes.

In addition to insulin, glucagon plays a role in the pathophysiology of diabetes. In starvation, glucagon, which is produced by the α-cells of the pancreas, helps to maintain glucose levels by stimulating hepatic glycogenolysis or gluconeogenesis. Normally, meals stimulate insulin for glucose uptake and suppress glucagon secretion to decrease endogenous production of glucose. In diabetes, this regulation is disturbed, resulting in a diminished and delayed insulin response to a meal. Furthermore, glucagon is not suppressed appropriately and even may be elevated, resulting in postprandial hyperglycemia. Disturbance in the regulation of insulin and glucagon, coupled with insulin resistance, leads to alterations in the metabolism of carbohydrates, proteins, and fats.

Treatment of diabetes is intended to control blood glucose and minimize the secondary complications of hyperglycemia.[1] Treatment modalities for type 2 diabetes include lifestyle modifications (eg, weight reduction, exercise, or dietary changes), oral medications, and subcutaneous medications, including insulin. Oral medications include biguanides, sulfonylurea and nonsulphonylurea secretagogues, thiazolidinediones, and α-glucosidase inhibitors. The management of type 2 diabetes continues to be a challenge, as less than half of United States adults who have diabetes achieve HgA1c of less

a Tulane University Health Sciences Center, 1430 Tulane Avenue, SL-53, New Orleans, LA 70112-2632, USA
b Medical Center of Louisiana, Tulane University Health Sciences Center, 1430 Tulane Avenue, SL-53, New Orleans, LA 70112-2632, USA
* Corresponding author.
E-mail address: vfonseca@tulane.edu (V.A. Fonseca).

Cardiol Clin 26 (2008) 639–648
doi:10.1016/j.ccl.2008.06.008
0733-8651/08/$ – see front matter. Published by Elsevier Inc.

than 7%. Progressive decline in β-cell function contributes to poor diabetes control.

In recent years, new classes of oral and subcutaneous medications have been introduced including incretin mimetic exenatide. The new oral diabetes medications are the inhibitors of the enzyme dipeptidyl peptidase isozyme 4 (DPP-4), and the subcutaneous medications include the incretin-based therapy (pramlintide and exenatide). In the United States, one DPP-4 inhibitor, namely sitagliptin (MK-04310), has been approved by the US Food and Drug Administration (FDA) for managing type 2 diabetes mellitus as monotherapy and combination therapy with other oral agents. Other DPP-4 inhibitors, namely vildagliptin (LAF237) and saxagliptin (BMS-477118) are available in other countries.

This article provides an overview of the effectiveness of DPP-4 inhibitors in glycemic control in type 2 diabetes mellitus. To have a comprehensive understanding of DPP-4 inhibitors, one must understand the role of incretins.

THE INCRETIN SYSTEM

It was observed that oral administration of glucose caused 50% to 70% higher insulin secretion as compared with an equivalent dose of intravenous glucose. This augmentation in response, called incretin effect, is caused by the gut-derived hormones, gastric inhibitory peptide (GIP) and glucagon-like peptide-1 (GLP-1).[4,5] These hormones, called incretins, are stimulated by oral feeding and are secreted by the K-cells and L-cells of the intestinal mucosa, respectively. GLP-1 is more potent than GIP in stimulating insulin secretion. GLP-1 and GIP control glucose metabolism by their effects on the pancreas, gastrointestinal (GI) tract, and central nervous system (CNS). In the pancreas, GLP-1 causes a glucose-dependent increase in insulin and inhibits glucagon secretion. In the GI tract, it inhibits gastric emptying and increases gastric acid production, and in the central nervous system, it inhibits food intake and promotes postprandial satiety and weight loss.[6,7]

Glucose-Dependent Insulinotropic Peptide

This incretin is produced by neuroendocrine K-cells, which exist in duodenum and jejunum. It is released in response to fats and, to a lesser extent, carbohydrate. It causes glucose-dependent release of insulin by binding to the highly specific GIP receptors on pancreatic β-cells. In diabetic patients, the levels of GIP are found to be normal, but the incretin response is decreased. The cause of this resistance is not known, but various

mechanisms have been suggested, including a defect in the GIP receptor, rapid desensitization, and decreased expression of the receptor.[8-11]

Glucagon-Like Peptide-1

GLP-1 and GLP-2 are intestinal peptide hormones derived from proglucagon, and they bear significant amino acid homology with glucagon (thus the name). GLP-1 is the most potent of all the incretins. Its level begins to rise immediately after food ingestion. Although the mechanism of release is not known, a neural stimulus and close contact of nutrients with L-cells have been proposed as the mechanisms. GLP-1 interacts with its receptors in the pancreas, resulting in release of insulin. GLP-1 also decreases glucagon from the α-cells of the pancreas and promotes satiety in the CNS. GLP-1 has been found to stimulate growth and increase survival of β-cells and also to stimulate the proliferation and differentiation of new β-cells. The degradation product of GLP-1, GLP-1(9-36)-amide, from DPP-4 enzymatic activity, does not possess glucose-lowering activity.[12]

In diabetic patients, the postprandial release of GLP-1 is impaired, and the later (60 to 120 minutes postprandial) response is reduced also, which results in a late- phase hypoinsulinemia. The glucagon-reducing action also is impaired in diabetes mellitus, causing glycogenolysis, which results in postprandial hyperglycemia.

DIPEPTIDYL PEPTIDASE-4 AS A THERAPEUTIC TARGET

Once in circulation, incretins have a very short half-life, because they are degraded rapidly by DPP-4, also known as CD 26. The enzyme DPP-4 is extremely diverse in terms of its distribution and function. It is located in the kidneys, intestines, liver, placenta, uterus, prostate, skin, capillary endothelium, plasma, and body fluids. It cleaves incretins and many other proteins that have proline or alanine in the second position by cleaving two N-terminal amino acids.[13] These two amino acids are important for the biological activity of the incretins GIP and GLP-1, which are rendered inactive by the proteolytic activity of DPP-4. DPP-4 is present in gut mucosa adjacent to L-cells, and 50% of GLP-1 is degraded even before it is released from gut mucosa. Both GIP and GLP-1 are inactivated in circulation, and the degradation products are cleared renally. In addition to DPP-4, another enzyme neutral endopeptidase 24.11 (NEP 24.11) cleaves GLP-1; however, its physiologic significance is unknown.

In addition to incretins, DPP-4 cleaves various neuropeptides. These include pituitary adenylate cyclase activation polypeptide (PACAP), vasoactive intestinal polypeptide (VIP), gastrin-releasing peptide (GRP), neuropeptide Y (NPY), growth hormone-releasing hormone (GHRH), GLP-2, and peptide YY. Furthermore, DPP-4 has been found to play a role in the cellular uptake of HIV-1, malignant transformation, and tumor invasion. Additionally, it may be a tumor marker for certain malignancies.[14,15] The clinical significance of these roles of the DPP family of enzymes and DPP-4 in particular is unknown.

Inhibition of DPP-4 enzyme results in prolonging the physiologic effect of endogenously produced incretins. The DPP-4 inhibitors are α-amino acid derivatives that can be modified to increase their affinity, potency, selectivity, oral bioavailability, and duration of action. DPP-4 inhibition caused a sixfold increase in GLP-1 given exogenously by infusion, but a similar response was not observed in endogenous GLP-1 secretion.[16] In most animal studies, DPP-4 inhibition was associated with mild increase in GLP-1 level, and it is uncertain if this modest increase in GLP-1 alone could be responsible for insulinotropic and antihyperglycemic effect of DPP-4 inhibitors. Increasing the half-life of other substrates, other than GIP and GLP-1, also may contribute to the therapeutic potential of DPP-4 inhibitors. The major mechanism by which DPP-4 inhibitors exert their antidiabetic effect is by inhibition of glucagon secretion. In addition, DPP-4 inhibition improves β-cell function. Although the insulin level is not increased, the threshold of glucose level to secrete insulin is lowered by DPP-4 inhibitors, thereby increasing the insulinogenic index. This improvement in β-cell function has been demonstrated by multiple indices, including improvement in the homeostasis model assessment (HOMA) β-cell, fasting proinsulin:insulin ratios, and 3-hour postmeal insulin: glucose area-under-the- curve (AUC) ratios.[17]

A comparison between use of DPP-4 inhibitors and GLP-1 mimetics indicates that an increase in GLP-1 is not the sole mechanism of action of DPP-4 inhibitors. Various DPP-4 inhibitors are either in preclinical or clinical use. These include sitagliptin, vildagliptin, and saxagliptin. The data on the efficacy of DPP-4 inhibitors suggest that not only are they effective as antihyperglycemic agents in the treatment of diabetes, but they also have disease-modifying abilities by attenuating or reversing the loss of β-cell mass and function. Treatment of streptozotocin-treated animal models with DPP-4 inhibitors resulted in restoration of β-cell function.[18] DPP-4 inhibitor use also resulted in dose-dependent increases in the number of β-cells in islets and increased glucose-stimulated insulin secretion in isolated islets. There are various other DPP-4 inhibitors that are at various stages of clinical trials.

DATA SOURCES AND SEARCHES

The authors conducted a search of MEDLINE (1966 to April 2008) and the Cochran Central Register of Controlled trials (first quarter of 2008) for English language randomized–controlled trials of DPP-4 inhibitor therapy in adults who had type 2 diabetes. They used the following search terms: diabetes, blood glucose, hemoglobin A1c, glycohemoglobin, GLP-1, dipeptidyl peptidase, DPP, LAF237, MK-0431, sitagliptin, vildagliptin, saxagliptin, human, and clinical trial. The authors also searched the clinical trials Web site (www.clinical trials.gov) and the references from the previously mentioned searches. Here the focus is on sitagliptin and vildagliptin as these are the most commonly used DPP-4 inhibitors.

EFFICACY OF DIPEPTIDYL PEPTIDASE-4 INHIBITORS
Sitagliptin

Sitagliptin causes an effective dose-dependent inhibition of DPP-4 enzyme, resulting in an increase in incretin levels without causing hypoglycemia. It is highly selective for the DPP-4 enzyme, well-tolerated at high doses (up to 600 mg daily) with no GI adverse effects.[19,20] A single dose of sitagliptin (50 to 200 mg) caused greater than 80% reduction in DPP-4 activity, producing two- to threefold increase in GLP-1 and GIP levels, increasing insulin and C-peptide levels, reducing plasma glucagon levels, and reducing hyperglycemia after oral glucose tolerance test (OGTT).[19,21]

Sitagliptin does not inhibit CYP enzymes in vitro,[22] and its half-life is 8 to 14 hours, achieving a steady-state concentration in 3 days.[19,20,23] The renal clearance is independent of the dose, and over 80% of the dose is excreted in urine unchanged. The pharmacokinetic and pharmacodynamic profile on multiple doses of sitagliptin in healthy, normoglycemic male subjects was similar to the daily doses, indicating once daily is a suitable dosing schedule.[20] Food intake does not affect the pharmacokinetics of sitagliptin, indicating that the medication can be taken with or without food.[24]

In animal studies done on a high fat diet (HFD) streptozotocin (STZ)-induced diabetic mice, it has been demonstrated that chronic treatment with des-fluoro-sitagaliptin, an analog of sitagliptin, not only improved postprandial and fasting hyperglycemia and HgA1c, but also caused a dose-dependent increase in insulin-producing β-cells in islets, resulting in normalization of β-cell mass and β-cell to α-cell ratio.[18]

The efficacy of sitagliptin in controlling hyperglycemia has been demonstrated in several studies (**Table 1**).[21,25–28] Patients who had diabetes for less than 3 years had greater benefit than those who had longer duration of disease. Also, the patients with higher HgA1c (greater than 9%) had a greater decrease in HgA1c than those who had lower (less than 8%) HgA1c. In addition, fasting blood sugar, postmeal glucose, proinsulin:insulin ratio, and β-cell function also improved. Patients on sitagliptin experienced higher incidence of nasopharyngitis, back pain, osteoarthritis, and pain in extremities compared with the placebo groups. Apart from very small increases in white blood cells (WBCs) and absolute neutrophil counts (ANCs), there were no meaningful changes in routine laboratory tests. Various trials have looked at the effect of sitagliptin on lipid parameters; however, the results have been inconsistent. It is likely the lipid profile is unchanged.

Sitagliptin is approved as initial monotherapy, as well as combination therapy, and also is marketed as a combination product with metformin. Metformin has been demonstrated to increase GLP-1 levels;[29] therefore a combination of metformin with a DPP-4 inhibitor is theoretically appealing. Initial therapy with sitagliptin (50 mg twice daily and 100 mg daily) and metformin (500 mg and 1000 mg twice daily) as monotherapy and combination therapy in 1,091 patients who had type 2 diabetes (ages 18 to 78 years) over a 24-week period showed that the two medications were effective individually in improving β-cell function, insulin resistance, and glycemic control. Additionally, metformin exhibited additive effect in the combination therapy.[17,30–33] Metformin treatment resulted in a small but significant weight reduction, while sitagliptin was weight neutral.

Sitagliptin has been studied in type 2 diabetic patients who were controlled poorly on glimepiride alone or glimepiride and metformin combination.

Table 1
Efficacy studies

Drug	Add on to	Decrease in A1c	Study
Sitagliptin	Monotherapy	0.38% to 0.77%	Scott et al (2007)[28]
Sitagliptin	Monotherapy	0.48% to 0.6%	Raz et al (2006)[26]
Sitagliptin	Monotherapy	0.79% to 0.94%	Aschner et al (2006)[27]
Sitagliptin	Monotherapy	0.4% to 0.6%	Hanefeld et al (2005)[25]
Sitagliptin	Monotherapy	1.05%	Nonaka et al (2008)[61]
Sitagliptin	Metformin	0.77%	Goldstein et al (2007)[30]
Sitagliptin	Metformin	1.00%	Raz et al (2008)[17]
Sitagliptin	Metformin	0.67%	Nauck et al (2007)[35]
Sitagliptin	Metformin	0.65%	Charbonnel et al (2006)[33]
Sitagliptin	Pioglitazone	0.70%	Rosenstock et al (2006)[36]
Sitagliptin	Glimepiride	0.74%	Hermansen et al (2007)[34]
Sitagliptin	Glimepiride + Metformin	0.89%	Hermansen et al (2007)[34]
Vildagliptin	Monotherapy	0.53% to 0.56%	Ristic et al (2005)[42]
Vildagliptin	Monotherapy	0.6% to 1.2%	Pratley et al (2006)[44]
Vildagliptin	Monotherapy	0.5% to 0.9%	Pi-Sunyer et al (2007)[45]
Vildagliptin	Monotherapy	0.7% to 0.9%	Dejager et al (2007)[46]
Vildagliptin	Monotherapy	0.30%	Mari et al (2008)[51]
Vildagliptin	Monotherapy	1.0% to 1.2%	Pratley et al (2007)[53]
Vildagliptin	Monotherapy	0.15%	Rosenstock et al (2008)[52]
Vildagliptin	Metformin	0.70%	Ahren et al (2004)[56]
Vildagliptin	Metformin	0.7% to 1.1	Bosi et al (2007)[57]
Vildagliptin	Pioglitazone	0.8% to 1.0%	Garber et al (2007)[57]
Vildagliptin	Pioglitazone	1.7% to 1.9%	Rosenstock et al (2007)[59]
Vildagliptin	Insulin	0.60%	Fonseca et al (2007)[60]

In this 24-week study of 441 patients 18 to 75 years of age, sitagliptin 100 mg daily improved glycemic control and β-cell function in both groups.[34] Sitagliptin caused a small increase in hypoglycemia and weight gain, possibly because of the sulfonylurea. Similar results were obtained when sitagliptin was compared with another sulfonylurea glipizide in a 52-week study involving 1,172 type 2 diabetic patients who were controlled inadequately on metformin alone.[35] At the end of the study, proinsulin:insulin ratio, which is a function of β-cell dysfunction was higher in glipizide treated diabetic patients compared with sitagliptin-treated patients. This deterioration in β-cell function is most likely because of chronic β-cell stimulation by glipizide.

The efficacy of sitagliptin added to on going pioglitazone therapy was studied in a 24-week study of 175 patients who had type 2 diabetes.[36] The addition of sitagliptin 100 mg daily to pioglitazone (30 or 40 mg daily) therapy resulted in a drop of HgA1c from 7.82% to 7.17%, a reduction of 0.70%. In the combination therapy group alone, 45.4% of patients achieved HgA1c of less than 7.0%, compared with only 23.0% in the pioglitazone treatment group. Fasting serum proinsulin and the proinsulin:insulin ratio also were reduced by the addition of sitagliptin. Sitagliptin and rosiglitazone have not been studied in combination therapy, but in a two-period crossover study of 5 days on 18 adult healthy patients, where sitagliptin was not found to change the pharmacokinetics of rosiglitazone.[37]

Incretins have been reported to have some relationship, not yet fully understood, with hypertension. Although GLP-1 and GLP-1 receptor agonists have been reported to increase blood pressure and heart rate in animal models, continuous intravenous administration of GLP-1 resulted in a mild decrease in blood pressure in patients who had type 2 diabetes.[38–40] Because sitagliptin increases GLP-1, its effect on hypertension was studied by Mistry and colleagues,[41] who found no significant effect on blood pressure.

Vildagliptin

Vildagliptin is a selective DPP-4 inhibitor that enhances islet cell function by increasing α- and β-cell responsiveness to glucose, resulting in meal-stimulated increase in biologically active GLP-1. Additionally, it improves glucose tolerance. Vildagliptin was studied in 279 patients who had type 2 diabetes over 12 weeks, in which vildagliptin was used from 25 to 100 mg daily doses; 50 mg and 100 mg daily doses resulted in a reduction in HgA1c by 0.56% and 0.53%, respectively.[42] The number of patients who achieved HgA1c less than 7% was higher among patients who received doses of 100 mg daily, 50 mg daily, or 25 mg twice daily, compared with 25 mg daily or placebo groups. As seen with sitagliptin, patients who had higher HgA1c and those who had body mass index (BMI) of greater than 30 kg/m² had increased reduction in HgA1c. In this study, an improvement in β-cell function was observed. Other studies have demonstrated similar effects of vildagliptin increasing β-cell mass.[43–47] Vildagliptin treatment resulted in a decrease in glucagon levels, with no effect on insulin levels over the study period. Baseline GLP-1 levels were increased with increased GLP-1 response to breakfast, with a reduced glucose and glucagon response. Balas and colleagues also found a sustained elevation in the incretins for a period beyond the duration of DPP-4 inhibition.[47]

The potential effect of vildagliptin on pancreatic mass was studied, which showed that 2 to 3 months of treatment results in a dose-dependent increase in pancreatic β-cell mass and improved islet function in high-fat fed streptozotocin-injected diabetic mice.[18] Studies done on animals have shown that GLP-1 may increase β-cell mass by reducing apoptosis and also by helping endocrine precursor cells to differentiate into β-cells, stimulating replication of β-cells, and forming new islets. A long-duration study was conducted by Ahren and colleagues,[48] however, in which 55 type 2 diabetic patients on metformin were randomized to receive either vildagliptin or placebo. The patients had an average age of 56 ± 1.5 years with BMI of 29.6 ± 0.5 kg/m² and HgA1c of 7.7 ± 0.1%. At baseline and after 52 weeks of treatment, proinsulin related to insulin secretion was measured with C-peptide in the fasting and postprandial (4 hours after meal) states to assess β-cell function. It was observed that the dynamic proinsulin to C-peptide ratio (DynP/C) relative to glucose was reduced significantly with vildagliptin compared with placebo, both in the fasting state ($p = 0.023$) and postprandially ($p = 0.004$). This indicates that vildagliptin treatment improves β-cell function as evident by a more efficient β-cell insulin processing capacity.

Because GLP-1 is an inhibitor of gastric emptying, a study was conducted to see the effect of vildagliptin, which increases GLP-1, on gastric emptying.[49,50] It was concluded that although DPP-4 inhibition results in doubling of the postprandial concentration of GLP-1, it is does not alter the gastric emptying.

To evaluate the effect of vildagliptin on patients with mild hyperglycemia, 306 patients with HgA1c of 6.2 to 7.5% were studied over 2 weeks using vildagliptin at 50 mg daily dose.[51] Vildagliptin showed statistically significant increase in fasting insulin, glucose sensitivity, and rate sensitivity, but the total insulin secretion excursion during meals were unchanged. These changes caused reduction in glucose and an improvement in HgA1c by $-0.3 \pm 0.1\%$ ($p = <0.001$). Vildagliptin also has been studied in a 12-week, double blind and randomized study on 179 patients with impaired glucose tolerance (IGT) with average HgA1c 5.9%.[52] This unique study on pre-diabetic patients showed that vildagliptin 50 mg twice daily decreased HgA1c by 0.15% and glucagon by 3.3 pmol/L/h, and increased insulin by 37 pmol/L/h, GLP-1 by 8.8 pmol/L/h, and GIP by 51.3 pmol/L/h. Postprandial hyperglycemia was decreased. The decrease in HgA1c occurred despite normal baseline HgA1c, and contrary to previous studies on patients who had type 2 diabetes, there was no change in FPG. It is evident that vildagliptin is effective in improving glycemic control and the β-cell function in patients who have mild hyperglycemia, as in patients who have severe hyperglycemia.

A study was conducted to evaluate the efficacy and risks of vildagliptin as monotherapy in elderly patients.[53] Vildagliptin as monotherapy in 100 mg daily doses (50 mg twice daily or 100 mg once a day) were studied over 24 weeks in younger (less than 65 years; n = 1,231) and older ($\geq$65 years; n = 338) patients and the data from five double-blind, randomized, placebo-controlled trials were pooled. The study also included active groups who were treated with either metformin (1,000 mg twice daily) or one of the TZDs (pioglitazone 30 mg daily or rosiglitazone 8 mg daily). The baseline HgA1c in older patients was $8.3 \pm 0.1\%$, which dropped by $1.2 \pm 0.1\%$ whereas the baseline HgA1c in younger patients was $8.7 \pm 0.0\%$, which dropped by $1.0 \pm 0.0\%$. Vildagliptin did not increase the adverse side effects in 62% of the older patient population with mild renal impairment and hypoglycemia was rare (0.8%). These results showed that vildagliptin is effective and tolerated well in elderly patients.

Vildagliptin (50 mg twice daily) was compared with metformin (1000 mg twice daily) on 780 type 2 drug-naïve patients with baseline HgA1c between 7.5% and 11.0%.[54] In this 52-week double-blind, randomized, multicenter, parallel group study HgA1c was measured over the study period. At the end of the study, both vildagliptin and metformin reduced HgA1c by $1.0\% \pm 0.1\%$ ($p = <0.001$) and $1.4\% \pm 0.1\%$ ($p \leq 0.001$), respectively. The number of patients who experienced adverse effects was almost similar in the vildagliptin (70.1%) and metformin (75.4%) groups. However, metformin was associated with three- to fourfold greater incidence of diarrhea, nausea and abdominal pain. The incidence of hypoglycemia was equally low with both drugs.

Vildagliptin (50 mg twice daily) also has been compared with rosiglitazone (8 mg once a day) as monotherapy in a 24-week study on 786 patients who had type 2 diabetes.[55] In this double-blind, randomized study, monotherapy with vildagliptin and rosiglitazone decreased HgA1c to a similar extent during the 24-week period. At the end of the study, vildagliptin caused a reduction in HgA1c by $1.1 \pm 0.1\%$ ($p = <0.001$), whereas rosiglitazone decreased HgA1c by $1.3 \pm 0.1\%$ ($p = <0.001$). FPG decreased more with rosiglitazone (-2.3 mmol/L) compared with vildagliptin (-1.3 mmol/L). Rosiglitazone, but not vildagliptin, caused an increase in body weight ($+1.6 \pm 0.3$ kg; $p \leq 0.001$). Incidence of edema was greater with rosiglitazone (4.1%) compared with vildagliptin (2.1%), but the incidence of other adverse effects was similar between the two drugs.

Vildagliptin has been shown to be efficacious in treating type 2 diabetes as an add-on therapy with metformin.[56,57] Vildagliptin in 50 and 100 mg daily doses was evaluated for its antihyperglycemic effect on 544 type 2 diabetic patients who were controlled inadequately (HgA1c 7.5% to 11.0%) on metformin ($\geq$1500 mg daily) therapy.[57] At the end of 24-week study period, the between-treatment difference (vildagliptin – placebo) was $-0.7\% \pm 0.1\%$ ($p < 0.001$) and $-1.1\% \pm 0.1\%$ ($p < 0.001$) with 50 and 100 mg daily doses of vildagliptin, respectively. The between-treatment difference in FPG was -1.8 ± 0.3 mmol/L ($P = 0.003$) and -1.7 ± 0.3 mmol/L ($p < 0.001$) in patients receiving 50 or 100 mg vildagliptin daily, respectively. Two doses of vildagliptin and placebo had similar incidence of adverse effect; however, GI adverse effects were higher in the placebo group than groups receiving either of the two doses. This study shows that vildagliptin at both doses is effective in improving glycemic control in patients who are not optimally controlled with metformin monotherapy. Hypoglycemia was rare and weight gain was insignificant. Similar results were observed in another study by Ahren and colleagues.[56]

Vildagliptin also has been demonstrated to be effective in improving glycemic control when added to the on-going treatment with pioglitazone.[58] In this 24-week multicenter, double-blind, randomized, parallel group study, vildagliptin at 50 and 100 mg daily doses was compared with placebo as an add-on therapy to maximum-dose pioglitazone (45 mg daily) treatment in 463 type 2 diabetic patients who were controlled inadequately with prior TZD monotherapy. Vildagliptin showed a dose-dependent decrease in HgA1c; 50 and 100 mg daily doses reduced HgA1c by 0.8% ± 0.1% (p = 0.001 versus placebo) and 1.0% ± 0.1% (p < 0.001 versus placebo), respectively. With a similar aim as in the previous study but a different study design, vildagliptin was compared with pioglitazone as monotherapy, and the two drugs were tested as a combination therapy.[59] In this 24-week randomized, double-blind, multicenter study 607 type 2 diabetic patients had baseline HgA1c of approximately 8.7%. Pioglitazone (30 mg daily), vildagliptin:pioglitazone (50/15 mg daily) combination, vildagliptin:pioglitazone (100/30 mg daily) combination, and vildagliptin (100 mg daily) showed an adjusted mean change in HgA1c of −1.4% ± 0.1%, −1.7% ± 0.1%, −1.9 ± 0.1%, and −1.1% ± 0.1% from baseline, respectively. These results indicate that both combinations were more potent in reducing HgA1c compared with pioglitazone alone (p = 0.039 and p < 0.001, respectively). In the high-dose combination therapy, 65% patients achieved HgA1c of 7%, with a tolerability profile similar to pioglitazone 30 mg daily monotherapy. Furthermore, the low-dose combination (50/15 mg daily) had better efficacy and tolerability benefit over pioglitazone 30 mg daily monotherapy. The adverse events ranged from 45.8% in the low-dose combination group to 51.6% in the pioglitazone monotherapy group. Pioglitazone monotherapy was associated with dose-dependent peripheral edema (up to 9.3%). Hypoglycemic events were minimal. These results indicate that vildagliptin/pioglitazone combination may be a more effective initial oral pharmacotherapy than either drug alone for managing type 2 diabetes.

Often type 2 diabetes remains uncontrolled on both oral medications and insulin. Vildagliptin was studied as an add-on therapy to insulin in a 24-week multicenter, double-blind, randomized, placebo-controlled, parallel-group study on 296 type 2 diabetic patients who were controlled inadequately (HgA1c =7.5% to 11%) on insulin.[60] While on insulin therapy, 144 patients received vildagliptin (50 mg twice daily), and 152 patients received placebo. Patients had a baseline HgA1c of 8.4% ± 0.1%. The adjusted mean change in HgA1c from baseline (AMΔ) was −0.5% ± 0.1% for vildagliptin group and −0.2% ± 0.1% for the placebo group, with a significant difference between the interventions (p = 0.01). In patients older than 65 years, the AMΔ HgA1c was −0.7% ± 0.1% in the vildagliptin group versus −0.1% ± 0.1% in the placebo group (p ≤ 0.001). Vildagliptin treatment and placebo were associated with equal number of adverse events (81.3% and 82.9%, respectively). Hypoglycemic events with vildagliptin, however, were less common (p < 0.001) and less severe (p < 0.05) compared with the placebo group. This study demonstrated that vildagliptin improves glycemic control in patients who are not at goal with insulin. Furthermore, the drug is associated with fewer incidents of hypoglycemia.

SUMMARY

Type 2 diabetes mellitus is a major risk factor for coronary artery disease (CAD) and is considered as a CAD-equivalent. The optimal control of diabetes is often daunting, requiring multiple medications. New medications also are needed when the adverse effects (eg, fluid retention, heart failure, hypoglycemia, weight gain) of the currently available medications limit their use. DPP-4 inhibitors such as sitagliptin and vildagliptin are effective in controlling diabetes as monotherapy and combination therapy, including their use with insulin.

ACKNOWLEDGEMENTS

Dr. Fonseca is supported in part by the American Diabetes Association, National Institutes of Health (ACCORD and TINSAL T2D trials) and the Earl Madison Ellis fund and the Tullis-Tulane Alumni Chair in Diabetes supporting diabetes research at Tulane University Health Sciences Center. Dr. Fonseca and Tulane University have Research Support Grants and honoraria for consulting and lectures from Glaxo Smith Kline, Novo- Nordisk, Takeda, Astra -Zeneca, Pfizer, Sanofi- Aventis, Eli Lilly, Daiichi- Sankyo and Novartis.

Dr. John-Kalarickal is supported in part by the American Diabetes Association and National Institutes of Health (ACCORD trial). Dr. John-Kalarickal and Tulane University have Research Support Grants from Glaxo Smith Kline, Novo- Nordisk, Takeda, Astra -Zeneca, Pfizer, Sanofi-Aventis, Eli Lilly, Daiichi- Sankyo and Novartis.

REFERENCES

1. Turner RC, Holman RR. The UK prospective diabetes study. UK Prospective Diabetes Study Group. Ann Med 1996;28(5):439–44.
2. Butler AE, Janson J, Bonner-Weir S, et al. Beta-cell deficit and increased beta-cell apoptosis in humans with type 2 diabetes. Diabetes 2003;52(1):102–10.
3. DeFronzo RA, Bonadonna RC, Ferrannini E. Pathogenesis of NIDDM. A balanced overview. Diabetes Care 1992;15(3):318–68.

4. Creutzfeldt W. The [pre-] history of the incretin concept. Regul Pept 2005;128(2):87–91.

5. Perley MJ, Kipnis DM. Plasma insulin responses to oral and intravenous glucose: studies in normal and diabetic subjects. J Clin Invest 1967;46(12): 1954–62.

6. Verdich C, Flint A, Gutzwiller JP, et al. A meta-analysis of the effect of glucagon-like peptide-1 (7-36) amide on ad libitum energy intake in humans. J Clin Endocrinol Metab 2001;86(9):4382–9.

7. Willms B, Werner J, Holst JJ, et al. Gastric emptying, glucose responses, and insulin secretion after a liquid test meal: effects of exogenous glucagon-like peptide-1 (GLP-1)-(7-36) amide in type 2 (noninsulin-dependent) diabetic patients. J Clin Endocrinol Metab 1996;81(1):327–32.

8. Nauck M, Stockmann F, Ebert R, et al. Reduced incretin effect in type 2 (noninsulin-dependent) diabetes. Diabetologia 1986;29(1):46–52.

9. Meier JJ, Hucking K, Holst JJ, et al. Reduced insulinotropic effect of gastric inhibitory polypeptide in first-degree relatives of patients with type 2 diabetes. Diabetes 2001;50(11):2497–504.

10. Lynn FC, Pamir N, Ng EH, et al. Defective glucose-dependent insulinotropic polypeptide receptor expression in diabetic fatty Zucker rats. Diabetes 2001;50(5):1004–11.

11. Lynn FC, Thompson SA, Pospisilik JA, et al. A novel pathway for regulation of glucose-dependent insulinotropic polypeptide (GIP) receptor expression in beta-cells. FASEB J 2003;17(1):91–3.

12. Zander M, Madsbad S, Deacon CF, et al. The metabolite generated by dipeptidyl–peptidase 4 metabolism of glucagon-like peptide-1 has no influence on plasma glucose levels in patients with type 2 diabetes. Diabetologia 2006;49(2):369–74.

13. Barnett A. DPP-4 inhibitors and their potential role in the management of type 2 diabetes. Int J Clin Pract 2006;60(11):1454–70.

14. Tanaka T, Umeki K, Yamamoto I, et al. CD26 (dipeptidyl peptidase IV/DPP IV) as a novel molecular marker for differentiated thyroid carcinoma. Int J Cancer 1995;64(5):326–31.

15. Cordero OJ, Ayude D, Nogueira M, et al. Preoperative serum CD26 levels: diagnostic efficiency and predictive value for colorectal cancer. Br J Cancer 2000;83(9):1139–46.

16. Deacon CF, Hughes TE, Holst JJ. Dipeptidyl peptidase IV inhibition potentiates the insulinotropic effect of glucagon-like peptide 1 in the anesthetized pig. Diabetes 1998;47(5):764–9.

17. Raz I, Chen Y, Wu M, et al. Efficacy and safety of sitagliptin added to ongoing metformin therapy in patients with type 2 diabetes. Curr Med Res Opin 2008;24(2):537–50.

18. Mu J, Woods J, Zhou YP, et al. Chronic inhibition of dipeptidyl peptidase-4 with a sitagliptin analog preserves pancreatic beta-cell mass and function in a rodent model of type 2 diabetes. Diabetes 2006;55(6):1695–704.

19. Herman GA, Stevens C, Van Dyck K, et al. Pharmacokinetics and pharmacodynamics of sitagliptin, an inhibitor of dipeptidyl peptidase IV, in healthy subjects: results from two randomized, double-blind, placebo-controlled studies with single oral doses. Clin Pharmacol Ther 2005;78(6): 675–88.

20. Bergman AJ, Stevens C, Zhou Y, et al. Pharmacokinetic and pharmacodynamic properties of multiple oral doses of sitagliptin, a dipeptidyl peptidase-IV inhibitor: a double-blind, randomized, placebo-controlled study in healthy male volunteers. Clin Ther 2006;28(1):55–72.

21. Herman GA, Bergman A, Stevens C, et al. Effect of single oral doses of sitagliptin, a dipeptidyl peptidase-4 inhibitor, on incretin and plasma glucose levels after an oral glucose tolerance test in patients with type 2 diabetes. J Clin Endocrinol Metab 2006; 91(11):4612–9.

22. Herman G, Bergman A, Wagner JA. Sitagliptin, a DPP-4 inhibitor: an overview of the pharmacokinetic (PK) profile and the propensity for drug–drug interactions (DDI). [abstract]. Diabetologia 2006; 49(Suppl 1):481–2.

23. Herman GA, Bergman A, Liu F, et al. Pharmacokinetics and pharmacodynamic effects of the oral DPP-4 inhibitor sitagliptin in middle-aged obese subjects. J Clin Pharmacol 2006;46(8):876–86.

24. Bergman A, Ebel D, Liu F, et al. Absolute bioavailability of sitagliptin, an oral dipeptidyl peptidase-4 inhibitor, in healthy volunteers. Biopharm Drug Dispos 2007;28(6):315–22.

25. Hanefeld M, Herman G, Mickel C, et al. Effect of MK-0431, a dipeptidyl peptidase IV (DPP-4) inhibitor, on glycemic control after 12 weeks in patients with type 2 diabetes. Diabetologia 2005;48(Suppl 1):287–8.

26. Raz I, Hanefeld M, Xu L, et al. Efficacy and safety of the dipeptidyl peptidase-4 inhibitor sitagliptin as monotherapy in patients with type 2 diabetes mellitus. Diabetologia 2006;49(11):2564–71.

27. Aschner P, Kipnes MS, Lunceford JK, et al. Effect of the dipeptidyl peptidase-4 inhibitor sitagliptin as monotherapy on glycemic control in patients with type 2 diabetes. Diabetes Care 2006;29(12):2632–7.

28. Scott R, Wu M, Sanchez M, et al. Efficacy and tolerability of the dipeptidyl peptidase-4 inhibitor sitagliptin as monotherapy over 12 weeks in patients with type 2 diabetes. Int J Clin Pract 2007;61(1):171–80.

29. Mannucci E, Ognibene A, Cremasco F, et al. Effect of metformin on glucagon-like peptide 1 (GLP-1) and leptin levels in obese nondiabetic subjects. Diabetes Care 2001;24(3):489–94.

30. Goldstein BJ, Feinglos MN, Lunceford JK, et al. Effect of initial combination therapy with sitagliptin,

a dipeptidyl peptidase-4 inhibitor, and metformin on glycemic control in patients with type 2 diabetes. Diabetes Care 2007;30(8):1979–87.

31. Herman GA, Bergman A, Yi B, et al. Tolerability and pharmacokinetics of metformin and the dipeptidyl peptidase-4 inhibitor sitagliptin when coadministered in patients with type 2 diabetes. Curr Med Res Opin 2006;22(10):1939–47.

32. Brazg R, Xu L, Dalla Man C, et al. Effect of adding sitagliptin, a dipeptidyl peptidase-4 inhibitor, to metformin on 24-h glycaemic control and beta-cell function in patients with type 2 diabetes. Diabetes Obes Metab 2007;9(2):186 93.

33. Charbonnel B, Karasik A, Liu J, et al. Efficacy and safety of the dipeptidyl peptidase-4 inhibitor sitagliptin added to ongoing metformin therapy in patients with type 2 diabetes inadequately controlled with metformin alone. Diabetes Care 2006; 29(12):2638–43.

34. Hormancon K, Kipnes M, Luo E, et al. Efficacy and safety of the dipeptidyl peptidase-4 inhibitor, sitagliptin, in patients with type 2 diabetes mellitus inadequately controlled on glimepiride alone or on glimepiride and metformin. Diabetes Obes Metab 2007;9(5):733–45.

35. Nauck MA, Meininger G, Sheng D, et al. Efficacy and safety of the dipeptidyl peptidase-4 inhibitor, sitagliptin, compared with the sulfonylurea, glipizide, in patients with type 2 diabetes inadequately controlled on metformin alone: a randomized, double-blind, noninferiority trial. Diabetes Obes Metab 2007;9(2):194–205.

36. Rosenstock J, Brazg R, Andryuk PJ, et al. Efficacy and safety of the dipeptidyl peptidase-4 inhibitor sitagliptin added to ongoing pioglitazone therapy in patients with type 2 diabetes: a 24-week, multicenter, randomized, double-blind, placebo-controlled, parallel-group study. Clin Ther 2006;28(10):1556–68.

37. Mistry GC, Bergman AJ, Luo WL, et al. Multiple-dose administration of sitagliptin, a dipeptidyl peptidase-4 inhibitor, does not alter the single dose pharmacokinetics of rosiglitazone in healthy subjects. J Clin Pharmacol 2007;47(2):159–64.

38. Barragan JM, Rodriguez RE, Blazquez E. Changes in arterial blood pressure and heart rate induced by glucagon-like peptide-1-(7-36) amide in rats. Am J Physiol 1994;266(3 Pt 1):E459–66.

39. Yamamoto H, Lee CE, Marcus JN, et al. Glucagon-like peptide-1 receptor stimulation increases blood pressure and heart rate and activates autonomic regulatory neurons. J Clin Invest 2002;110(1):43–52.

40. Toft-Nielsen MB, Madsbad S, Holst JJ. Continuous subcutaneous infusion of glucagon-like peptide 1 lowers plasma glucose and reduces appetite in type 2 diabetic patients. Diabetes Care 1999;22(7):1137–43.

41. Mistry GC, Maes AL, Lasseter KC, et al. Effect of sitagliptin, a dipeptidyl peptidase-4 inhibitor, on blood pressure in nondiabetic patients with mild-to-moderate hypertension. J Clin Pharmacol 2008; 48(5):592–8.

42. Ristic S, Byiers S, Foley J, et al. Improved glycaemic control with dipeptidyl peptidase-4 inhibition in patients with type 2 diabetes: vildagliptin (LAF237) dose response. Diabetes Obes Metab 2005;7(6):692–8.

43. Ahren B, Landin-Olsson M, Jansson PA, et al. Inhibition of dipeptidyl peptidase-4 reduces glycemia, sustains insulin levels, and reduces glucagon levels in type 2 diabetes. J Clin Endocrinol Metab 2004; 89(5):2078–84.

44. Pratley RE, Jauffret-Kamel S, Galbreath E, et al. Twelve-week monotherapy with the DPP-4 inhibitor vildagliptin improves glycemic control in subjects with type 2 diabetes. Horm Metab Res 2006;38(6):423–8.

45. Pi-Sunyer FX, Schweizer A, Mills D, et al. Efficacy and tolerability of vildagliptin monotherapy in drug-naive patients with type 2 diabetes. Diabetes Res Clin Pract 2007;76(1):132–8.

46. Dejager S, Razac S, Foley JE, et al. Vildagliptin in drug-naive patients with type 2 diabetes: a 24-week, double-blind, randomized, placebo-controlled, multiple-dose study. Horm Metab Res 2007;39(3):218–23.

47. Balas B, Baig MR, Watson C, et al. The dipeptidyl peptidase IV inhibitor vildagliptin suppresses endogenous glucose production and enhances islet function after single-dose administration in type 2 diabetic patients. J Clin Endocrinol Metab 2007; 92(4):1249–55.

48. Ahren B, Pacini G, Tura A, et al. Improved meal-related insulin processing contributes to the enhancement of B-cell function by the DPP-4 inhibitor vildagliptin in patients with type 2 diabetes. Horm Metab Res 2007;39(11):826–9.

49. Meier JJ, Gallwitz B, Salmen S, et al. Normalization of glucose concentrations and deceleration of gastric emptying after solid meals during intravenous glucagon-like peptide 1 in patients with type 2 diabetes. J Clin Endocrinol Metab 2003;88(6):2719–25.

50. Vella A, Bock G, Giesler PD, et al. Effects of dipeptidyl peptidase-4 inhibition on gastrointestinal function, meal appearance, and glucose metabolism in type 2 diabetes. Diabetes 2007;56(5):1475–80.

51. Mari A, Scherbaum WA, Nilsson PM, et al. Characterization of the influence of vildagliptin on model-assessed cell function in patients with type 2 diabetes and mild hyperglycemia. J Clin Endocrinol Metab 2008;93(1):103–9.

52. Rosenstock J, Foley JE, Rendell M, et al. Effects of the dipeptidyl peptidase-IV inhibitor vildagliptin on

incretin hormones, islet function, and postprandial glycemia in subjects with impaired glucose tolerance. Diabetes Care 2008;31(1):30–5.

53. Pratley RE, Rosenstock J, Pi-Sunyer FX, et al. Management of type 2 diabetes in treatment-naive elderly patients: benefits and risks of vildagliptin monotherapy. Diabetes Care 2007;30(12): 3017–22.

54. Schweizer A, Couturier A, Foley JE, et al. Comparison between vildagliptin and metformin to sustain reductions in HbA(1c) over 1 year in drug-naive patients with type 2 diabetes. Diabet Med 2007; 24(9):955–61.

55. Rosenstock J, Baron MA, Dejager S, et al. Comparison of vildagliptin and rosiglitazone monotherapy in patients with type 2 diabetes: a 24-week, double-blind, randomized trial. Diabetes Care 2007; 30(2):217–23.

56. Ahren B, Gomis R, Standl E, et al. Twelve- and 52-week efficacy of the dipeptidyl peptidase IV inhibitor LAF237 in metformin-treated patients with type 2 diabetes. Diabetes Care 2004;27(12):2874–80.

57. Bosi E, Camisasca RP, Collober C, et al. Effects of vildagliptin on glucose control over 24 weeks in patients with type 2 diabetes inadequately controlled with metformin. Diabetes Care 2007;30(4):890–5.

58. Garber AJ, Schweizer A, Baron MA, et al. Vildagliptin in combination with pioglitazone improves glycaemic control in patients with type 2 diabetes failing thiazolidinedione monotherapy: a randomized, placebo-controlled study. Diabetes Obes Metab 2007;9(2):166–74.

59. Rosenstock J, Baron MA, Camisasca RP, et al. Efficacy and tolerability of initial combination therapy with vildagliptin and pioglitazone compared with component monotherapy in patients with type 2 diabetes. Diabetes Obes Metab 2007;9(2):175–85.

60. Fonseca V, Schweizer A, Albrecht D, et al. Addition of vildagliptin to insulin improves glycaemic control in type 2 diabetes. Diabetologia 2007;50(6):1148–55.

61. Nonaka K, Kakikawa T, Sato A, et al. Efficacy and safety of sitagliptin monotherapy in Japanese patients with type 2 diabetes. Diabetes Res Clin Pract 2008;79(2):291–8.

Index

Note: Page numbers of article titles are in **boldface** type.

Cardiol Clin 26 (2008) 649–655
doi:10.1016/S0733-8651(08)00083-0
0733-8651/08/$ – see front matter © 2008 Elsevier Inc. All rights reserved.

cardiology.theclinics.com

Moving?

Make sure your subscription moves with you!

To notify us of your new address, find your **Clinics Account Number** (located on your mailing label above your name), and contact customer service at:

E-mail: elspcs@elsevier.com

800-654-2452 (subscribers in the U.S. & Canada)
1-407-563-6020 (subscribers outside of the U.S. & Canada)

Fax number: 407-363-9661

Elsevier Periodicals Customer Service
6277 Sea Harbor Drive
Orlando, FL 32887-4800

*To ensure uninterrupted delivery of your subscription, please notify us at least 4 weeks in advance of move.

ELSEVIER

United States Postal Service

Statement of Ownership, Management, and Circulation
(All Periodicals Publications Except Requestor Publications)

1. Publication Title	2. Publication Number	3. Filing Date
Cardiology Clinics	0 0 0 - 7 0 1	9/15/08

4. Issue Frequency	5. Number of Issues Published Annually	6. Annual Subscription Price
Feb, May, Aug, Nov	4	$226.00

7. Complete Mailing Address of Known Office of Publication (Not printer) (Street, city, county, state, and ZIP+4)

Elsevier Inc.
360 Park Avenue South
New York, NY 10010-1710

Contact Person
Stephen Bushing

Telephone (Include area code)
215-239-3688

8. Complete Mailing Address of Headquarters or General Business Office of Publisher (Not printer)

Elsevier Inc., 360 Park Avenue South, New York, NY 10010-1710

9. Full Names and Complete Mailing Addresses of Publisher, Editor, and Managing Editor (Do not leave blank)

Publisher (Name and complete mailing address)

John Schrefer , Elsevier, Inc. , 1600 John F. Kennedy Blvd. Suite 1800, Philadelphia, PA 19103-2899

Editor (Name and complete mailing address)

Barbara Cohen-Kligerman, Elsevier, Inc., 1600 John F. Kennedy Blvd. Suite 1800, Philadelphia, PA 19103-2899

Managing Editor (Name and complete mailing address)

Catherine Bewick, Elsevier, Inc., 1600 John F. Kennedy Blvd. Suite 1800, Philadelphia, PA 19103-2899

10. Owner (Do not leave blank. If the publication is owned by a corporation, give the name and address of the corporation immediately followed by the names and addresses of all stockholders owning or holding 1 percent or more of the total amount of stock. If not owned by a corporation, give the names and addresses of the individual owners. If owned by a partnership or other unincorporated firm, give its name and address as well as those of each individual owner. If the publication is published by a nonprofit organization, give its name and address.)

Full Name	Complete Mailing Address
Wholly owned subsidiary of	4520 East-West Eighway
Reed/Elsevier, US holdings	Bethesda, MD 20814

11. Known Bondholders, Mortgagees, and Other Security Holders Owning or Holding 1 Percent or More of Total Amount of Bonds, Mortgages, or Other Securities. If none, check box. ☐ None

Full Name	Complete Mailing Address
N/A	

12. Tax Status (For completion by nonprofit organizations authorized to mail at nonprofit rates) (Check one)
The purpose, function, and nonprofit status of this organization and the exempt status for federal income tax purposes:
☐ Has Not Changed During Preceding 12 Months
☐ Has Changed During Preceding 12 Months (Publisher must submit explanation of change with this statement)

PS Form 3526, September 2006 (Page 1 of 3 (Instructions Page 3)) PSN 7530-01-000-9931 PRIVACY NOTICE: See our Privacy policy in www.usps.com

---

13. Publication Title	14. Issue Date for Circulation Data Below
Cardiology Clinics	August 2008

15. Extent and Nature of Circulation		Average No. Copies Each Issue During Preceding 12 Months	No. Copies of Single Issue Published Nearest to Filing Date
a. Total Number of Copies (Net press run)		2225	2000
b. Paid Circulation (By Mail and Outside the Mail)	(1) Mailed Outside-County Paid Subscriptions Stated on PS Form 3541. (Include paid distribution above nominal rate, advertiser's proof copies, and exchange copies)	944	856
	(2) Mailed In-County Paid Subscriptions Stated on PS Form 3541 (Include paid distribution above nominal rate, advertiser's proof copies, and exchange copies)		
	(3) Paid Distribution Outside the Mails Including Sales Through Dealers and Carriers, Street Vendors, Counter Sales, and Other Paid Distribution Outside USPS®	450	461
	(4) Paid Distribution by Other Classes Mailed Through the USPS (e.g. First-Class Mail®)		
c. Total Paid Distribution (Sum of 15b (1), (2), (3), and (4))	►	1394	1317
d. Free or Nominal Rate Distribution (By Mail and Outside the Mail)	(1) Free or Nominal Rate Outside-County Copies Included on PS Form 3541	73	78
	(2) Free or Nominal Rate In-County Copies Included on PS Form 3541		
	(3) Free or Nominal Rate Copies Mailed at Other Classes Mailed Through the USPS (e.g. First-Class Mail)		
	(4) Free or Nominal Rate Distribution Outside the Mail (Carriers or other means)		
e. Total Free or Nominal Rate Distribution (Sum of 15d (1), (2), (3) and (4)	►	73	78
f. Total Distribution (Sum of 15c and 15e)	►	1467	1395
g. Copies not Distributed (See instructions to publishers #4 (page #3))	►	758	605
h. Total (Sum of 15f and g)	►	2225	2000
i. Percent Paid (15c divided by 15f times 100)		95.02%	94.41%

16. Publication of Statement of Ownership

☑ If the publication is a general publication, publication of this statement is required. Will be printed
in the **November 2008** issue of this publication.   ☐ Publication not required

17. Signature and Title of Editor, Publisher, Business Manager, or Owner

[signature]
Jam Panecer
James Panecci – Executive Director of Subscription Services

Date: September 15, 2008

I certify that all information furnished on this form is true and complete. I understand that anyone who furnishes false or misleading information on this form or who omits material or information requested on the form may be subject to criminal sanctions (including fines and imprisonment) and/or civil sanctions (including civil penalties).

PS Form 3526, September 2006 (Page 2 of 3)